Auditory Neuroscience

Auditory Neuroscience

Making Sense of Sound

Jan Schnupp, Israel Nelken, and Andrew King

The MIT Press
Cambridge, Massachusetts
London, England

First MIT Press paperback edition, 2012

© 2011 Massachusetts Institute of Technology

For information about special quantity discounts, please email special_sales@mitpress.mit.edu

This book was set in Stone Sans and Stone Serif by Toppan Best-set Premedia Limited. Printed and bound in the United States of America.

Library of Congress Cataloging-in-Publication Data

Schnupp, Jan, 1966–
Auditory neuroscience : making sense of sound / Jan Schnupp, Israel Nelken, and Andrew King.
    p. cm.
Includes bibliographical references and index.
ISBN 978-0-262-11318-2 (hardcover : alk. paper)—978-0-262-51802-4 (pb.) 1. Auditory perception. 2. Auditory pathways. 3. Hearing. I. Nelken, Israel, 1961– II. King, Andrew, 1959– III. Title.
QP461.S36   2011
612.8′5—dc22

                                                                    2010011991

10   9   8   7   6   5   4   3

Contents

Preface

What This Book Is About

As I write these lines, a shiver is running down my back. Not that writing usually has that effect on me. But on this occasion, I am allowing myself a little moment of indulgence. As I am writing, I am also listening to one of my favorite pieces of music, the aria "Vorrei spiegarvi, oh dio!" composed by Mozart and masterfully performed by the soprano Kathleen Battle. A digital audio player sits in my pocket. It is smaller than a matchbox and outwardly serene; yet inside the little device is immensely busy, extracting 88,200 numerical values every second from computer files stored in its digital memory, which it converts into electrical currents. The currents, in turn, generate electric fields that incessantly push and tug ever so gently on a pair of delicate membranes in the ear buds of my in-ear headphones. And, voilà, there she is, Kathleen, hypnotizing me with her beautiful voice and dragging me through a brief but intense emotional journey that begins with a timid sadness, grows in intensity to plumb the depths of despair only to resolve into powerful and determined, almost uplifting defiance.

But Kathleen is not alone. She brought a small orchestra with her, prominently featuring a number of string instruments and an oboe. They were all hidden in the immaterial stream of 88,200 numbers a second. Pour these numbers into a pair of ears, and together they make music. Their sounds overlap and weave together, yet my brain easily distinguishes the different instruments from each other and from Kathleen's voice, hears some on the left, others on the right, and effortlessly follows the melodic line each plays. The violins sing, too, but not like Kathleen. Kathleen sings in Italian. My knowledge of Italian is not as good as I would like it to be, and when I first heard this piece of music I spoke no Italian at all, but even on my first hearing it was obvious to me, as it would be to anyone, that this was a song with words, even if I couldn't understand the words. Now I am learning Italian, and each time I hear this song, I understand a little bit more. In other words, each time, this by now so familiar song is engaging new parts of my brain that were previously deaf to some small aspect of it. The title of the song, "Vorrei spiegarvi, oh dio!," by the way, means "I would like to explain to you, oh Lord!" It seems a curiously appropriate title for the purpose at hand.

Every time we listen, not just to music, but to anything at all, our auditory perception is the result of a long chain of diverse and fascinating processes and phenomena that unfold within the sound sources themselves, in the air that surrounds us, in our ears, and, most of all, in our brains. Clearly you are interested in these phenomena, otherwise you would not have picked up this book, and as you learn more about hearing, you will increasingly appreciate that the sense of hearing is truly miraculous. But it is an "everyday miracle," one which, most of the time, despite its rich intricacy and staggering complexity, works so reliably that it is easily amenable to scientific inquiry. In fact, it is usually so reliable and effortless that we come to overlook what a stunning achievement it is for our ears and brains to be able to hear, and we risk taking auditory perception for granted, until it starts to go wrong.

"Vorremo spiegarvi, caro lettore!" we would like to try and explain to you how it all works. Why do instruments and voices make sounds in the first place, and why and in what ways do these sounds differ from one another? How is it possible that our ears can capture these sounds even though the vibrations of sound waves are often almost unimaginably tiny? How can the hundreds of thousands of nerve impulses traveling every second from your ears through your auditory nerves to your brain convey the nature of the incoming sounds? How does your brain conclude from these barrages of nerve impulses that the sounds make up a particular melody? How does it decide which sounds are words, and which are not, and what the words might mean? How does your brain manage to separate the singer's voice from the many other sounds that may be present at the same time, such as those of the accompanying instruments, and decide that one sound comes from the left, the other from the right, or that one sound contains speech, and the other does not? In the pages that follow, we try to answer these questions, insofar as the answers are known.

Thus, in this book we are trying to explain auditory perception in terms of the neural processes that take place in different parts of the auditory system. In doing so, we present selected highlights from a very long and large research project: It started more than 400 years ago and it may not be completed for another 400 years. As you will see, some of the questions we raised above can already be answered very clearly, while for others our answers are still tentative, with many important details unresolved. Neurophysiologists are not yet in a position to give a complete account of how the stream of numbers in the digital audio player is turned into the experience of music. Nevertheless, progress in this area is rapid, and many of the deep questions of auditory perception are being addressed today in terms of the responses of nerve cells and the brain circuits they make up. These are exciting times for auditory neuroscientists, and we hope that at least some of our readers will be inspired by this book to join the auditory neuroscience community and help complete the picture that is currently emerging. We, the authors, are passionate about science: We believe that miracles become more miraculous, not less, if we try to lift the lid to understand their inner workings. Perhaps you will come to share our point of view.

How to Use This Book

People are interested in sound and hearing for many reasons, and they come to the subject from very diverse backgrounds. Because hearing results from the interplay of so many physical, biological, and psychological processes, a student of hearing needs at least a sprinkling of knowledge from many disciplines. A little physical acoustics, at least an intuitive and superficial understanding of certain mathematical ideas, such as Fourier spectra, and a fairly generous helping of neurophysiology and anatomy are absolute requirements. Furthermore, some knowledge of phonetics and linguistics or a little music theory are highly desirable extras. We have been teaching hearing for many years, and have always lamented that, although one can find good books on acoustics, or on the mathematics of signal processing, the physiology of the ear, psychoacoustics, speech, or on music, so far no single book pulls all of these different aspects of hearing together into a single, integrated introductory text. We hope that this book will help fill this important gap.

We wrote this book with an advanced undergraduate readership in mind, aiming mostly at students in biological or medical sciences, audiology, psychology, neuroscience, or speech science. We assumed that our readers may have little or no prior knowledge of physical acoustics, mathematics, linguistics, or speech science, and any relevant background from these fields will therefore be explained as we go along. However, this is first and foremost a book about brain function, and we have assumed that our readers will be familiar with some basic concepts of neurophysiology and neuroanatomy, perhaps because they have taken a first-year university course on the subject. If you are uncertain about what action potentials, synapses, and dendrites are, or where in your head you might reasonably expect to find the cerebral cortex or the thalamus, then you should read a concise introductory neuroscience text before reading this book. At the very least, you might want to look through a copy of "Brain Facts," a very concise and highly accessible neuroscience primer available free of charge on the Web site of the Society for Neuroscience (www.sfn.org).

The book is divided into eight chapters. The first two provide essential background on physical acoustics and the physiology of the ear. In the chapters that follow, we have consciously avoided trying to "work our way up the ascending auditory pathway" structure by structure. Instead, in chapters 3 to 6, we explore the neurobiology behind four aspects of hearing—namely, the perception of pitch, the processing of speech, the localization of sound sources, and the perceptual separation of sound mixtures.

The final two chapters delve into the development and plasticity of the auditory system, and briefly discuss contemporary technologies aimed at treating hearing loss, such as hearing aids and cochlear implants.

The book is designed as an entirely self-contained text, and could be used either for self-study or as the basis of a short course, with each chapter providing enough material for approximately two lectures. An accompanying Web site with additional materials can be found at www.auditoryneuroscience.com. These supplementary materials include sound samples and demonstrations, animations and movie clips, color versions of some of our illustrations, a discussion forum, links, and other materials, which students and instructors in auditory neuroscience may find instructive, entertaining, or both.

1 Why Things Sound the Way They Do

We are very fortunate to have ears. Our auditory system provides us with an incredibly rich and nuanced source of information about the world around us. Listening is not just a very useful, but also often a very enjoyable activity. If your ears, and your auditory brain, work as they should, you will be able to distinguish thousands of sounds effortlessly—running water, slamming doors, howling wind, falling rain, bouncing balls, rustling paper, breaking glass, or footsteps (in fact, countless different types of footsteps: the crunching of leather soles on gravel, the tic-toc-tic of stiletto heels on a marble floor, the cheerful splashing of a toddler stomping through a puddle, or the rhythmic drumming of galloping horses or marching armies). The modern world brings modern sounds. You probably have a pretty good idea of what the engine of your car sounds like. You may even have a rather different idea of what the engine of your car *ought to* sound like, and be concerned about that difference. Sound and hearing are also enormously important to us because of the pivotal role they play in human communication. You have probably never thought about it this way, but every time you talk to someone, you are effectively engaging in something that can only be described as a telepathic activity, as you are effectively "beaming your thoughts into the other person's head," using as your medium a form of "invisible vibrations." Hearing, in other words, is the telepathic sense that we take for granted (until we lose it) and the sounds in our environment are highly informative, very rich, and not rarely enjoyable.

If you have read other introductory texts on hearing, they will probably have told you, most likely right at the outset, that "sound is a pressure wave, which propagates through the air." That is, of course, entirely correct, but it is also somewhat missing the point. Imagine you hear, for example, the din of a drawer full of cutlery crashing down onto the kitchen floor. In that situation, lots of minuscule ripples of air pressure will be radiating out from a number of mechanically excited metal objects, and will spread outwards in concentric spheres at the speed of sound, a breathless 340 m/s (about 1,224 km/h or 760 mph), only to bounce back from the kitchen walls and ceiling, filling, within only a few milliseconds, all the air in the kitchen with a complex pattern of tiny, ever changing ripples of air pressure. Fascinating as it may be to try to visualize all these wave patterns, these sound waves certainly do not describe what we "hear" in the subjective sense.

The mental image your sense of hearing creates will not be one of delicate pressure ripples dancing through the air, but rather the somewhat more alarming one of several pounds of sharp knives and forks, which have apparently just made violent and unexpected contact with the kitchen floor tiles. Long before your mind has had a chance to ponder any of this, your auditory system will already have analyzed the sound pressure wave pattern to extract the following useful pieces of information: that the fallen objects are indeed made of metal, not wood or plastic; that there is quite a large number of them, certainly more than one or two; that the fallen metal objects do not weigh more than a hundred grams or so each (i.e., the rampaging klutz in our kitchen has indeed spilled the cutlery drawer, not knocked over the cast iron casserole dish); as well as that their impact occurred in our kitchen, not more than 10 meters away, slightly to the left, and not in the kitchen of our next door neighbors or in a flat overhead.

That our auditory brains can extract so much information effortlessly from just a few "pressure waves" is really quite remarkable. In fact, it is more than remarkable, it is astonishing. To appreciate the wonder of this, let us do a little thought experiment and imagine that the klutz in our kitchen is in fact a "compulsive serial klutz," and he spills the cutlery drawer not once, but a hundred times, or a thousand. Each time our auditory system would immediately recognize the resulting cacophony of sound: "Here goes the cutlery drawer again." But if you were to record the sounds each time with a microphone and then look at them on an oscilloscope or computer screen, you would notice that the sound waves would actually look quite different on each and every occasion.

There are infinitely many different sound waves that are all recognizable as the sound of cutlery bouncing on the kitchen floor, and we can recognize them even though we hear each particular cutlery-on-the-floor sound only once in our lives. Furthermore, our prior experience of hearing cutlery crashing to the floor is likely to be quite limited (cutlery obsessed serial klutzes are, thankfully, a very rare breed). But even so, most of us have no difficulty imagining what cutlery crashing to floor would sound like. We can even imagine how different the sound would be depending on whether the floor was made of wood, or covered in linoleum, or carpet, or ceramic tiles.

This little thought experiment illustrates an important point that is often overlooked in introductory texts on hearing. Sound and hearing are so useful because *things make sounds, and different things make different sounds.* Sound waves carry valuable clues about the physical properties of the objects or events that created them, and when we listen we do not seek to sense vibrating air for the sake of it, but rather we hope to learn something about the sound *sources*, that is, the objects and events surrounding us. For a proper understanding of hearing, we should therefore start off by learning at least a little bit about how sound waves are created in the first place, and how the physical properties of sound sources shape the sounds they make.

1.1   Simple Harmonic Motion—Or, Why Bells Go "Bing" When You Strike Them

Real-world sounds, like those we just described, are immensely rich and complex. But in sharp contrast to these "natural" sounds, the sounds most commonly used in the laboratory to study hearing are by and large staggeringly dull. The most common laboratory sound by far is the sine wave pure tone, a sound that most nonscientists would describe, entirely accurately, as a "beep"—but not just any beep, and most certainly not an interesting one. To be a "pure" tone, the beep must be shorn of any "contaminating" feature, be completely steady in its amplitude, contain no "amplitude or frequency modulations" (properties known as *vibrato* to the music lover) nor any harmonics (overtones) or other embellishing features. A pure tone is, indeed, so bare as to be almost "unnatural": pure tones are hardly ever found in everyday sound-scapes, be they manmade or natural.

You may find this puzzling. If pure tones are really quite boring and very rare in nature (and they are undeniably both), and if hearing is about perceiving the real world, then why are pure tones so widely used in auditory research? Why would anyone think it a good idea to test the auditory system mostly with sounds that are neither common nor interesting? There are, as it turns out, a number of reasons for this, some good ones (or at least they seemed good at the time) and some decidedly less good ones. And clarifying the relationship between sinusoidal pure tones and "real" sounds is in fact a useful, perhaps an essential, first step toward achieving a proper understanding of the science of hearing. To take this step we will need, at times, a mere smidgen of mathematics. Not that we will expect you, dear reader, to do any math yourself, but we will encourage you to bluff your way along, and in doing so we hope you will gain an intuitive understanding of some key concepts and techniques. Bluffing one's way through a little math is, in fact, a very useful skill to cultivate for any sincere student of hearing. Just pretend that you kind of know this and that you only need a little "reminding" of the key points. With that in mind, let us confidently remind ourselves of a useful piece of applied mathematics that goes by the pleasingly simple and harmonious name of *simple harmonic motion*. To develop an intuition for this, let us begin with a simple, stylized object, a mass-spring system, which consists of a lump of some material (any material you like, as long as it's not weightless and is reasonably solid) suspended from an elastic spring, as shown in figure 1.1. (See the book's Web site for an animated version of this figure.)

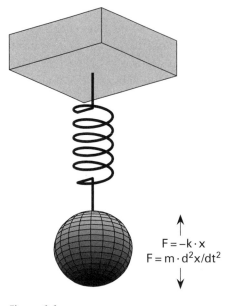

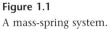

$$F = -k \cdot x$$
$$F = m \cdot d^2x/dt^2$$

Figure 1.1
A mass-spring system.

Let us also imagine that this little suspended mass has recently been pushed, so that it now travels in a downward direction. Let us call this the *x* direction. Now is an excellent time to start pretending that we were once quite good at school math and physics, and, suitably reminded, we now recall that masses on the move are inert, that is, they have a tendency to keep on moving in the same direction at the same speed until something forces them to slow down or speed up or change direction. The force required to do that is given by Newton's second law of motion, which states that force equals mass times acceleration, or $F = m \cdot a$.

Acceleration, we further recall, is the rate of change of velocity ($a = dv/dt$) and velocity is the rate of change of position ($v = dx/dt$). So we can apply Newton's second law to our little mass as follows: It will continue to travel with constant velocity dx/dt in the *x* direction until it experiences a force that changes its velocity; the rate of change in velocity is given by $F = m \cdot d^2x/dt^2$. (By the way, if this is getting a bit heavy going, you may skip ahead to the paragraph beginning "In other words...." We won't tell anyone you skipped ahead, but note that bluffing your way in math takes a little practice, so persist if you can.) Now, as the mass travels in the *x* direction, it will soon start to stretch the spring, and the spring will start to pull against this stretch with a force given by Hooke's law, which states the pull of the spring is proportional to how far it is stretched, and it acts in the opposite direction of the stretch (i.e., $F = -k \cdot x$, where k is the spring constant, a proportionality factor that is large for strong, stiff springs and small for soft, bendy ones; the minus sign reminds us that the force is in a direction that opposes further stretching).

So now we see that, as the mass moves inertly in the x direction, there soon arises a little tug of war, where the spring will start to pull against the mass' inertia to slow it down. The elastic force of the spring and the inertial force of the mass are then, in accordance with Newton's third law of motion, equal in strength and opposite in direction, that is, $-k \cdot x = m \cdot d^2x/dt^2$. We can rearrange this equation using elementary algebra to $d^2x/dt^2 = -k/m \cdot x$ to obtain something that many students of psychology or biology would rather avoid, as it goes by the intimidating name of *second-order differential equation*. But we shall not be so easily intimidated. Just note that this equation only expresses, in mathematical hieroglyphics, something every child playing with a slingshot quickly appreciates intuitively, namely, that the harder one pulls the mass in the slingshot against the elastic, the harder the elastic will try to accelerate the mass in the opposite direction. If that rings true, then deciphering the hieroglyphs is not difficult. The acceleration d^2x/dt^2 is large if the slingshot has been stretched a long way ($-x$ is large), if the slingshot elastic is stiff (k is large), and if the mass that needs accelerating is small (again, no surprise: You may remember from childhood that large masses, like your neighbor's garden gnomes, are harder to catapult at speed than smaller masses, like little pebbles).

But what does all of this have to do with sound? This will become clear when we quickly "remind" ourselves how one solves the differential equation $d^2x/dt^2 = -k/m \cdot x$. Basically, here's how mathematicians do this: they look up the solution in a book, or get a computer program for symbolic calculation to look it up for them, or, if they are very experienced, they make an intelligent guess and then check if it's true. Clearly, the solution must be a function that is proportional to minus its own second derivative (i.e., "the rate of change of the rate of change" of the function must be proportional to minus its value at each point). It just so happens that sine and cosine functions, pretty much uniquely, possess this property. Look at the graph of the cosine function that we have drawn for you in figure 1.2, and note that, at zero, the cosine has a value of 1, but is flat because it has reached its peak, and has therefore a slope of 0. Note also that the −sine function, which is also plotted in gray, has a value of 0 at zero, so here the slope of the cosine happens to be equal to the value of −sine. This is no coincidence. The same is also true for $\cos(\pi/2)$, which happens to have a value of 0 but is falling steeply with a slope of −1, while the value of $-\sin(\pi/2)$ is also −1. It is, in fact, true everywhere. The slope of the cosine is minus the sine, and the slope of minus sine is minus the cosine. Sine waves, uniquely, describe the behavior of mass-spring systems, because they are everywhere proportional to minus their own second derivative [$d^2 \cos(t)/dt^2 = -\cos(t)$] and they therefore satisfy the differential equation that describes the forces in a mass-spring system.

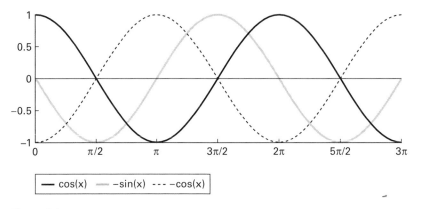

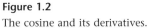

Figure 1.2
The cosine and its derivatives.

In other words, and this is the important bit, *the natural behavior for any mass-spring system is to vibrate in a sinusoidal fashion.* And given that many objects, including (to get back to our earlier example) items of cutlery, have both mass and a certain amount of springiness, it is perfectly natural for them, or parts of them, to enter into "simple harmonic motion," that is, to vibrate sinusoidally. Guitar or piano strings, bicycle bells, tuning forks, or xylophone bars are further familiar examples of everyday mass-spring systems with obvious relevance to sound and hearing. You may object that sinusoidal vibration can't really be the "natural way to behave" for all mass-spring systems, because, most of the time, things like your forks and knives do not vibrate, but sit motionless and quiet in their drawer, to which we would reply that a sinusoidal vibration of zero amplitude is a perfectly fine solution to our differential equation, and no motion at all still qualifies as a valid and natural form of simple harmonic motion.

So the natural behavior (the "solution") of a mass-spring system is a sinusoidal vibration, and written out in full, the solution is given by the formula $x(t) = x_0 \cdot cos(t \cdot \sqrt{(k/m)} + \varphi_0)$, where x_0 is the "initial amplitude" (i.e., how far the little mass had been pushed downward at the beginning of this little thought experiment), and φ_0 is its "initial phase" (i.e., where it was in the cycle at time zero). If you remember how to differentiate functions like this, you can quickly confirm that this solution indeed satisfies our original differential equation. Alternatively, you can take our word for it. But we would not be showing you this equation, or have asked you to work so hard to get to it, if there weren't still quite a few very worthwhile insights to gain from it. Consider the $cos(t \cdot \sqrt{(k/m)})$ part. You may remember that the cosine function goes through one full cycle over an angle of 360°, or 2π radians. So the mass-spring system has swung through one full cycle when $t \cdot \sqrt{(k/m)}$ equals 2π. It follows that the period (i.e., the time taken for one cycle of vibration) is $T = 2\pi/\sqrt{(k/m)}$. And you may recall that the frequency (i.e., the number of cycles per unit time) is equal to 1 over the period, so $f = \sqrt{(k/m)}/2\pi$.

Translated into plain English, this tells us that our mass-spring system has a preferred or natural frequency at which it wants to oscillate or vibrate. This is known as the system's resonance (or resonant) frequency, and it is inversely proportional to the square root of its mass and proportional to the square root of its stiffness. If this frequency lies within the human audible frequency range (about 20–20,000 cycles/s, or Hz), then we may hear these vibrations as sound. Although you may, so far, have been unaware of the underlying physics, you have probably exploited these facts intuitively on many occasions. So when, to return to our earlier example, the sounds coming from our kitchen tell us that a box full of cutlery is currently bouncing on the kitchen floor, we know that it is the cutlery and not the saucepans because the saucepans, being much heavier, would be playing much lower notes. And when we increase the tension on a string while tuning a guitar, we are, in a manner of speaking, increasing its "stiffness," the springlike force with which the string resists being pushed sideways. And by increasing this tension, we increase the string's resonance frequency.

Hopefully, this makes intuitive sense to you. Many objects in the world around us are or contain mass-spring systems of some type, and their resonant frequencies tell us something about the objects' physical properties. We mentioned guitar strings and metallic objects, but another important, and perhaps less obvious example, is the resonant cavity. Everyday examples of resonant cavities might include empty (or rather air-filled) bottles or tubes, or organ pipes. You may know from experience that when you very rapidly pull a cork out of a bottle, it tends to make a "plop" sound, and you may also have noticed that the pitch of that sound depends on how full the bottle is. If the bottle is almost empty (of liquid, and therefore contains quite a lot of air), then the plop is much deeper than when the bottle is still quite full, and therefore contains very little air. You may also have amused yourself as a kid by blowing over the top of a bottle to make the bottle "whistle" (or you may have tried to play a pan flute, which is much the same thing), and noticed that the larger the air-filled volume of the bottle, the lower the sound.

Resonant cavities like this are just another version of mass-spring systems, only here both the mass and the spring are made of air. The air sitting in the neck of the bottle provides the mass, and the air in the belly of the bottle provides the "spring." As you pull out the cork, you pull the air in the neck just below the cork out with it. This decreases the air pressure in the belly of the bottle, and the reduced pressure provides a spring force that tries to suck the air back in. In this case, the mass of the air in the bottle neck and the spring force created by the change in air pressure in the bottle interior are both very small, but that does not matter. As long as they are balanced to give a resonant frequency in the audible range, we can still produce a clearly audible sound. How large the masses and spring forces of a resonator are depends a lot on its geometry, and the details can become very complex; but in the simplest case, the resonant frequency of a cavity is inversely proportional to the square root of its volume, which is why small organ pipes or drums play higher notes than large ones.

Again, these are facts that many people exploit intuitively, even if they are usually unaware of the underlying physics. Thus, we might knock on an object made of wood or metal to test whether it is solid or hollow, listening for telltale low resonant frequencies that would betray a large air-filled resonant cavity inside the object. Thus, the resonant frequencies of objects give us valuable clues to the physical properties, such as their size, mass, stiffness, and volume. Consequently, it makes sense to assume that a "frequency analysis" is a sensible thing for an auditory system to perform.

We hope that you found it insightful to consider mass-spring systems, and "solve" them to derive their resonant frequency. But this can also be misleading. You may recall that we told you at the beginning of this chapter that pure sine wave sounds hardly ever occur in nature. Yet we also said that mass-spring systems, which are plentiful in nature, should behave according to the equation $x(t) = x_0 \cdot \cos(t \cdot \sqrt{k/m} + \varphi_0)$; in other words, they should vibrate sinusoidally at their single preferred resonance frequency, $f = \sqrt{k/m}/2\pi$, essentially forever after they have been knocked or pushed or otherwise mechanically excited. If this is indeed the case, then pure tone–emitting objects should be everywhere. Yet they are not. Why not?

1.2   Modes of Vibration and Damping—Or Why a "Bing" Is Not a Pure Tone

When you pluck a string on a guitar, that string can be understood as a mass-spring system. It certainly isn't weightless, and it is under tension, which gives it a springlike stiffness. When you let go of it, it will vibrate at its resonant frequency, as we would expect, but that is not the only thing it does. To see why, ask yourself this: How can you be sure that your guitar string is indeed just one continuous string, rather than two half strings, each half as long as the original one, but seamlessly joined. You may think that this is a silly question, something dreamt up by a Zen master to tease a student. After all, each whole can be thought of as made of two halves, and if the two halves are joined seamlessly, then the two halves make a whole, so how could this possibly matter? Well, it matters because each of these half-strings weighs half as much and is twice as stiff as the whole string, and therefore each half-string will have a resonance frequency that is twice as high as that of the whole string.

When you pluck your guitar string, you make it vibrate and play its note, and the string must decide whether it is to vibrate as one whole or as two halves; if it chooses the latter option, the frequency at which it vibrates, and the sound frequency it emits, will double! And the problem doesn't end there. If we can think of a string as two half-strings, then we can just as easily think of it as three thirds, or four quarters, and so forth. How does the string decide whether to vibrate as one single whole or to exhibit this sort of "split personality," and vibrate as a collection of its parts? Well, it doesn't. When faced with multiple possibilities, strings will frequently go for them all, all at the same time, vibrating simultaneously as a single mass-spring system, as well as two half mass systems, and as three thirds, and as four quarters, and so on. This behavior is known as "modes of vibration" of the string, and it is illustrated schematically in figure 1.3, as well as in an animation that can be found on the book's Web site.

Due to these modes, a plucked guitar string will emit not simply a pure tone corresponding to the resonant frequency of the whole string, but a mixture that also contains overtones of twice, three, four, or n times that resonant frequency. It will, in other words, emit a complex tone—"complex" not in the sense that it is complicated, but that it is made up of a number of frequency components, a mixture of harmonically related tones that are layered on top of each other. The lowest frequency component, the resonant frequency of the string as a whole, is known as the fundamental frequency, whereas the frequency components corresponding to the resonance of the half, third, fourth strings (the second, third, and fourth modes of vibration) are called the "higher harmonics." The nomenclature of harmonics is a little confusing, in that some authors will refer to the fundamental frequency as the "zeroth harmonic," or F_0, and the first harmonic would therefore equal twice the fundamental frequency, the second harmonic would be three times F_0, and the nth harmonic would be $n + 1$ times F_0. Other authors number harmonics differently, and consider the fundamental

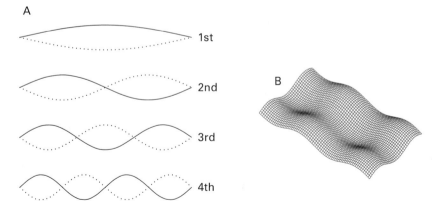

Figure 1.3
(A) The first four modes of vibration of a string. (B) A rectangular plate vibrating in the fourth mode along its length and in the third mode along its width.

to be also the first harmonic, so that the nth harmonic has a frequency of n times F_0. We shall adhere to the second of these conventions, not because it is more sensible, but because it seems a little more commonly used.

Although many physical objects such as the strings on an instrument, bells, or xylophone bars typically emit complex tones made up of many harmonics, these harmonics are not necessarily present in equal amounts. How strongly a particular harmonic is represented in the mix of a complex tone depends on several factors. One of these factors is the so-called initial condition. In the case of a guitar string, the initial condition refers to how, and where, the string is plucked. If you pull a guitar string exactly in the middle before you let it go, the fundamental first mode of vibration is strongly excited, because we have delivered a large initial deflection just at the first mode's "belly." However, vibrations in the second mode vibrate around the center. The center of the string is said to be a node in this mode of vibration, and vibrations on either side of the node are "out of phase" (in opposite direction); that is, as the left side swings down the right side swings up.

To excite the second mode we need to deflect the string asymmetrically relative to the midpoint. The initial condition of plucking the string exactly in the middle does not meet this requirement, as either side of the midpoint is pulled and then released in synchrony, so the second mode will not be excited. The fourth and sixth modes, or any other even modes will not be excited either, for the same reason. In fact, plucking the string exactly in the middle excites only the odd modes of vibration, and it excites the first mode more strongly than progressively higher odd modes. Consequently, a guitar string plucked in the middle will emit a sound with lots of energy at the fundamental, decreasing amounts of energy at the third, fifth, seventh … harmonics, and no energy at all at the second, fourth, sixth… harmonics. If, however, a guitar string is plucked somewhere near one of the ends, then even modes may be excited, and higher harmonics become more pronounced relative to the fundamental. In this way, a skilled guitarist can change the timbre of the sound and make it sound "brighter" or "sharper."

Another factor affecting the modes of vibration of an object is its geometry. The geometry of a string is very straightforward; strings are, for all intents and purposes, one-dimensional. But many objects that emit sounds can have quite complex two- and three-dimensional shapes. Let us briefly consider a rectangular metal plate, which is struck. In principle, a plate can vibrate widthwise just as easily as it can vibrate along its length. It could, for example, vibrate in the third mode along its width and in the fourth mode along its length, as is schematically illustrated in figure 1.3B. Also, in a metal plate, the stiffness stems not from an externally supplied tension, as in the guitar string, but from the internal tensile strength of the material.

Factors like these mean that three-dimensional objects can have many more modes of vibration than an ideal string, and not all of these modes are necessarily harmonically related. Thus, a metal plate of an "awkward" shape might make a rather dissonant, unmelodious "clink" when struck. Furthermore, whether certain modes are possible can depend on which points of the plate are fixed, and which are struck. The situation becomes very complicated very quickly, even for relatively simple structures such as flat, rectangular plates. For more complicated three-dimensional structures, like church bells, for example, understanding which modes are likely to be pronounced and how the interplay of possible modes will affect the overall sound quality, or timbre, is as much an art as a science.

To illustrate these points, figure 1.4 shows the frequency spectra of a piano note and of the chime of a small church bell. What exactly a frequency spectrum is is explained in greater detail later, but at this point it will suffice to say that a frequency spectrum tells us how much of a particular sinusoid is present in a complex sound. Frequency spectra are commonly shown using units of decibel (dB). Decibels are a

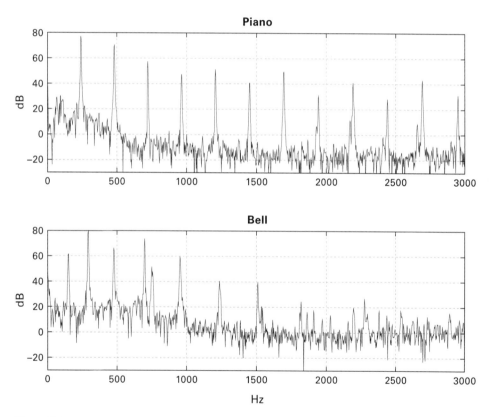

Figure 1.4
Frequency spectra of a piano and a bell, each playing the note B_3 (247 Hz).

logarithmic unit, and they can be a little confusing, which is why we will soon say more about them.

To read figure 1.4, all you need to know is that when the value of the spectrum at one frequency is 20 dB greater than that at another, the amplitude at that frequency is ten times larger, but if the difference is 40 dB, then the amplitude is one hundred times greater, and if it is 60 dB, then it is a whopping one thousand times larger. The piano and the bell shown in figure 1.4 both play the musical note B$_3$ (more about musical notes in chapter 3). This note is associated with a fundamental frequency of 247 Hz, and after our discussion of modes of vibration, you will not be surprised that the piano note does indeed contain a lot of 247-Hz vibration, as well as frequencies that are integer multiples of 247 (namely, 494, 741, 988, 1,235, etc.). In fact, frequencies that are not multiples of 247 Hz (all the messy bits below 0 dB in figure 1.4) are typically 60 dB, that is, one thousand times smaller in the piano note than the string's resonant frequencies. The spectrum of the bell, however, is more complicated. Again, we see that a relatively small number of frequencies dominate the spectrum, and each of these frequency components corresponds to one of the modes of vibration of the bell. But because the bell has a complex three-dimensional shape, these modes are not all exact multiples of the 247-Hz fundamental.

Thus, real objects do not behave like an idealized mass-spring system, in that they vibrate in numerous modes and at numerous frequencies, but they also differ from the idealized model in another important respect. An idealized mass-spring system should, once set in motion, carry on oscillating forever. Luckily, real objects settle down and stop vibrating after a while. (Imagine the constant din around us if they didn't!) Some objects, like guitar strings or bells made of metal or glass, may continue ringing for several seconds, but vibrations in many other objects, like pieces of wood or many types of plastic, tend to die down much quicker, within just a fraction of a second. The reason for this is perhaps obvious. The movement of the oscillating mass represents a form of kinetic energy, which is lost to friction of some kind or another, dissipates to heat, or is radiated off as sound. For objects made of highly springy materials, like steel bells, almost all the kinetic energy is gradually emitted as sound, and as a consequence the sound decays relatively slowly and in an exponential fashion. The reason for this exponential decay is as follows.

The air resistance experienced by a vibrating piece of metal is proportional to the average velocity of the vibrating mass. (Anyone who has ever ridden a motorcycle appreciates that air resistance may appear negligible at low speeds but will become considerable at higher speeds.) Now, for a vibrating object, the average speed of motion is proportional to the amplitude of the vibration. If the amplitude declines by half, but the frequency remains constant, then the vibrating mass has to travel only half as far on each cycle, but the available time period has remained the same, so it need move only half as fast. And as the mean velocity declines, so does the air resistance that provides the breaking force for a further reduction in velocity. Consequently, some small but constant fraction of the vibration amplitude is lost on each cycle—the classic conditions for exponential decay. Vibrating bodies made of less elastic materials may experience a fair amount of internal friction in addition to the air resistance, and this creates internal "damping" forces, which are not necessarily proportional to the amplitude of the vibration. Sounds emitted by such objects therefore decay much faster, and their decay does not necessarily have an exponential time course.

By way of example, look at figure 1.5, which shows sound waves from two musical instruments: one from a wooden castanet, the other from a metal glockenspiel bar. Note that the time axes for the two sounds do not cover the same range. The wooden castanet is highly damped, and has a decay constant of just under 30 ms (i.e., the sound takes 30 ms to decay to $1/e$ or about 37% of its maximum amplitude). The metal glockenspiel, in contrast, is hardly damped at all, and the decay constant of its vibrations is just under 400 ms, roughly twenty times longer than that of the castanet.

Thus, the speed and manner with which a sound decays gives another useful cue to the properties of the material an object is made of, and few people would have any

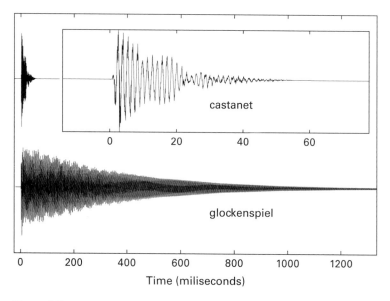

Figure 1.5
A rapidly decaying (castanet) and a slowly decaying (glockenspiel) sound. The castanet sound is plotted twice, once on the same time axis as the glockenspiel, and again, in the inset, with a time axis that zooms in on the first 70 ms.

difficulty using it to distinguish the sound of a copper bar from that of bar made of silver, even though some research suggests that our ability to use these cues is not as good as it perhaps ought to be (Lutfi & Liu, 2007).

We hope the examples in this section illustrate that objects in our environment vibrate in complex ways, but these vibrations nevertheless tell us much about various physical properties of the object, its weight, its material, its size, and its shape. A vibrating object pushes and pulls on the air around it, causing vibrations in the air which propagate as sound (we will look at the propagation of sound in a little more detail later). The resulting sound is hardly ever a pure tone, but in many cases it will be made up of a limited number of frequencies, and these are often harmonically related. The correspondence between emitted frequencies and physical properties of the sound source is at times ambiguous. Low frequencies, for example, could be either a sign of high mass or of low tension. Frequency spectra are therefore not always easy to interpret, and they are not quite as individual as fingerprints; but they nevertheless convey a lot of information about the sound source, and it stands to reason that one of the chief tasks of the auditory system is to unlock this information to help us judge and recognize objects in our environment. Frequency analysis of an emitted sound is the first step in this process, and we will return to the idea of the auditory system as a frequency analyzer in a number of places throughout this book.

1.3 Fourier Analysis and Spectra

In 1822, the French mathematician Jean Baptiste Joseph Fourier posited that any function whatsoever can be thought of as consisting of a mixture of sine waves,[1] and to this day we refer to the set of sine wave components necessary to make up some signal as the signal's Fourier spectrum. It is perhaps surprising that, when Fourier came up with his idea, he was not studying sounds at all. Instead, he was trying to calculate the rate at which heat would spread through a cold metal ring when one end of it was placed by a fire. It may be hard to imagine that a problem as arcane and prosaic as heat flow around a metal ring would be sufficiently riveting to command the attention of a personality as big as Fourier's, a man who twenty-four years earlier had assisted Napoleon Bonaparte in his conquests, and had, for a while, been governor of lower Egypt. But Fourier was an engineer at heart, and at the time, the problem of heat flow around a ring was regarded as difficult, so he had a crack at it. His reasoning must have gone something like this: "I have no idea what the solution is, but I have a hunch that, regardless of what form the solution takes, it must be possible to express it as a sum of sines and cosines, and once I know that I can calculate it." Reportedly, when he first presented this approach to his colleagues at the French Academy of Sciences, his presentation was met by polite silence and incomprehension. After all, positing a sum of sinusoids as a solution was neither obviously correct, nor obviously helpful. But no one dared challenge him as he was too powerful a figure—a classic case of "proof by intimidation."

In the context of sounds, however, which, as we have learned, are often the result of sinusoidal, simple harmonic motion of mass-spring oscillators, Fourier's approach has a great deal more immediate appeal. We have seen that there are reasons in physics why we would expect many sounds to be quite well described as a sum of sinusoidal frequency components, namely, the various harmonics. Fourier's bold assertion that it ought to be possible to describe *any* function, and by implication also any variation in air pressure as a function of time (i.e., *any* sound), seems to offer a nice, unifying approach. The influence of Fourier's method on the study of sound and hearing has consequently been enormous, and the invention of digital computers and efficient algorithms like the fast Fourier transform have made it part of the standard toolkit for the analysis of sound. Some authors have even gone so far as to call the ear itself a "biological Fourier analyzer." This analogy between Fourier's mathematics and the workings of the ear must not be taken too literally though. In fact, the workings of the ear only vaguely resemble the calculation of a Fourier spectrum, and later we will introduce better engineering analogies for the function of the ear. Perhaps this is just as well, because Fourier analysis, albeit mathematically very elegant, is in many respects also quite unnatural, if not to say downright weird. And, given how influential Fourier analysis remains to this day, it is instructive to pause for a moment to point out some aspects of this weirdness.

The mathematical formula of a pure tone is that of a sinusoid (figure 1.6). To be precise, it is $A \cdot \cos(2\pi \cdot f \cdot t + \varphi)$. The tone oscillates sinusoidally with amplitude A, and goes through one full cycle of 2π radians f times in each unit of time t. The period of the pure tone is the time taken for a single cycle, usually denoted by either a capital T or the Greek letter τ (tau), and is equal to the inverse of the frequency $1/f$.

The tone may have had its maximal amplitude A at time 0, or it may not, so we allow a "starting phase parameter," φ, which we can use to shift the peaks of our sinusoid along the time axis as required. According to Fourier, we can describe any sound we like by taking a lot of sine wave equations like this, each with a different

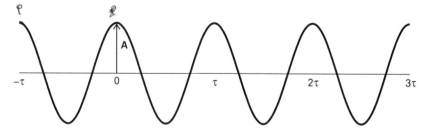

Figure 1.6
A pure tone "in cosine phase" (remember that $\cos(0) = 1$).

frequency f, and if we pick for each f exactly the right amplitude A and the right phase φ, then the sum of these carefully picked sine waves will add up exactly to our arbitrary sound.

The sets of values of A and φ required to achieve this are known as the sound's amplitude spectrum and phase spectrum, respectively. (Amplitude spectra we have encountered previously in figure 1.4, which effectively plotted the values of A for each of the numerous pure tone components making up the sound of a piano or a bell. Phase spectra, that is, the values of φ for each frequency component, are, as we will see, often difficult to interpret and are therefore usually not shown.) Note, however, that, expressed in this mathematically rigorous way, each sine wave component is defined for all times t. Time 0 is just an arbitrary reference on the time axis; it is not in any real sense the time when the sound starts. The Fourier sine wave components making up the sound have no beginning and no end. They must be thought of as having started at the beginning of time and continuing, unchanging, with constant amplitude and total regularity, until the end of time. In that important respect, these mathematically abstract sine waves could not be more unlike "real" sounds. Most real sounds have clearly defined onsets, which occur when a sound source becomes mechanically excited, perhaps because it is struck or rubbed. And real sounds end when the oscillations of the sound source decay away. When exactly sounds occur, when they end, and how they change over time are perceptually very important to us, as these times give rise to perceptual qualities like rhythm, and let us react quickly to events signaled by particular sounds. Yet when we express sounds mathematically in terms of a Fourier transform, we have to express sounds that start and end in terms of sine waves that are going on forever, which can be rather awkward.

To see how this is done, let us consider a class of sounds that decay so quickly as to be almost instantaneous. Examples of this important class of "ultra-short" sounds include the sound of a pebble bouncing off a rock, or that of a dry twig snapping. These sound sources are so heavily damped that the oscillations stop before they ever really get started. Sounds like this are commonly known as "clicks." The mathematical idealization of a click, a deflection that lasts only for one single, infinitesimally short time step, is known as an impulse (or sometimes as a delta-function). Impulses come in two varieties, positive-going "compression" clicks (i.e., a very brief upward deflection or increase in sound pressure) or negative-going "rarefactions" (a transient downward deflection or pressure decrease).

Because impulses are so short, they are, in many ways, a totally different type of sound from the complex tones that we have considered so far. For example, impulses are not suitable for carrying a melody, as they have no clear musical pitch. Also, thinking of impulses in terms of sums of sine waves may seem unnatural. After all, a click is too short to go through numerous oscillations. One could almost say that the defining characteristic of a click is the predominant absence of sound: A click is a click only because there is silence both before and immediately after it. How are we to produce this silence by adding together a number of "always on" sine waves of the form $A \cdot \cos(2\pi \cdot f \cdot t + \varphi)$? The way to do this is not exactly intuitively obvious: We have to take an awful lot of such sine waves (infinitely many, strictly speaking), all of different frequency f, and get them to cancel each other out almost everywhere. To see how this works, consider the top panel of figure 1.7, which shows ten sine waves of frequencies 1 to 10 Hz superimposed. All have amplitude 1 and a starting phase of 0.

What would happen if we were to add all these sine waves together? Well at time $t = 0$, each has amplitude 1 and they are all in phase, so we would expect their sum to have amplitude 10 at that point. At times away from zero, it is harder to guess what the value of the sum would be, as the waves go out of phase and we therefore have to expect cancellation due to destructive interference. But for most values of t, there appear to be as many lines above the x-axis as below, so we might expect a lot of cancellation, which would make the signal small. The middle panel in figure 1.7 shows what the sum of the ten sine waves plotted in the top panel actually looks like, and it confirms our expectations. The amplitudes "pile up" at $t = 0$ much more than elsewhere. But we still have some way to go to get something resembling a real impulse. What if we keep going, and keep adding higher and higher frequencies? The bottom

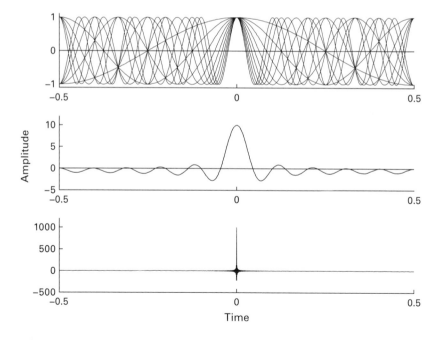

Figure 1.7
Making an impulse from the superposition of a large number of sine waves.

panel shows what we get if we sum cosines of frequencies 1 to 1,000. The result is a great deal more clicklike, and you may begin to suspect that if we just kept going and added infinitely many cosines of ever-increasing frequency, we would eventually, "in the limit" as mathematicians like to say, get a true impulse.

Of course, you may have noticed that, if we approximate a click by summing n cosines, its amplitude is n, so that, in the limit, we would end up with an infinitely large but infinitely short impulse, unless, of course, we scaled each of the infinitely many cosines we are summing to be infinitely small so that their amplitudes at time 0 could still add up to something finite. Is this starting to sound a little crazy? It probably is. "The limit" is a place that evokes great curiosity and wonder in the born mathematician, but most students who approach sound and hearing from a biological or psychological perspective may find it a slightly confusing and disconcerting place. Luckily, we don't really need to go there.

Real-world clicks are very short, but not infinitely short. In fact, the digital audio revolution that we have witnessed over the last few decades was made possible only by the realization that one can be highly pragmatic and think of time as "quantized"; in other words, we posit that, for all practical purposes, there is a "shortest time interval" of interest, know as the "sample interval." The shortest click or impulse, then, lasts for exactly one such interval. The advantage of this approach is that it is possible to think of any sound as consisting of a series of very many such clicks—some large, some small, some positive, some negative, one following immediately on another. For human audio applications, it turns out that if we set this sample period to be less than about 1/40,000 of a second, a sound that is "sampled" in this manner is, to the human ear, indistinguishable from the original, continuous-time sound wave.[2] Figure 1.8 shows an example of a sound that is "digitized" in this fashion.

Each constituent impulse of the sound can still be thought of as a sum of sine waves (as we have seen in figure 1.7). And if any sound can be thought of as composed of many impulses, and each impulse in turn can be composed of many sine waves, then it follows that any sound can be made up of many sine waves. This is not exactly a

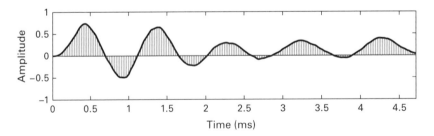

Figure 1.8
One period of the vowel /a/ digitized at 44.1 kHz.

formal proof of Fourier's theorem, but it will do for our purposes. Of course, to make up some arbitrary sound digitally by fusing together a very large number of scaled impulses, we must be able to position each of the constituent impulses very precisely in time. But if one of these impulses is now to occur at precisely some time $t = x$, rather than at time 0 as in figure 1.7, then the sine waves making up that particular impulse must now all cancel at time 0, and pile up at time x. To achieve this, we have to adjust the "phase term" φ in the equation of each sine wave component of that impulse. In other words, at time $t = x$, we need $A \cdot \cos(2\pi \cdot f \cdot t + \varphi)$ to evaluate to A, which means $\cos(2\pi \cdot f \cdot x + \varphi)$ must equal 1, and therefore $(2\pi \cdot f \cdot x + \varphi)$ must equal 0. To achieve that, we must set the phase φ of each sine component to be exactly equal to $-2\pi \cdot f \cdot x$.

Does this sound a little complicated and awkward? Well, it is, and it illustrates one of the main shortcomings of representing sounds in the frequency domain (i.e., as Fourier spectra): Temporal features of a sound become encoded rather awkwardly in the "phase spectrum." A sound with a very simple time domain description like "click at time $t = 0.3$," can have a rather complicated frequency domain description such as: "sine wave of frequency $f = 1$ with phase $\varphi = -1.88496$ plus sine wave of frequency $f = 2$ with phase $\varphi = -3.76991$ plus sine wave of frequency $f = 3$ with phase $\varphi = -5.654867$ plus ..." and so on. Perhaps the most interesting and important aspect of the click, namely, that it occurred at time $t = 0.3$, is not immediately obvious in the click's frequency domain description, and can only be inferred indirectly from the phases. And if we were to consider a more complex natural sound, say the rhythm of hoof beats of a galloping horse, then telling which hoof beat happens when just from looking at the phases of the Fourier spectrum would become exceedingly difficult. Of course, our ears have no such difficulty, probably because the frequency analysis they perform differs in important ways from calculating a Fourier spectrum.

Both natural and artificial sound analysis systems get around the fact that time disappears in the Fourier spectrum by working out short-term spectra. The idea here is to divide time into a series of "time windows" before calculating the spectra. This way, we can at least say in which time windows a particular acoustic event occurred, even if it remains difficult to determine the timing of events inside any one time window. As we shall see in chapter 2, our ears achieve something that vaguely resembles such a short-term Fourier analysis through a mechanical tuned filter bank. But to understand the ear's operation properly, we first must spend a little time discussing time windows, filters, tuning, and impulse responses.

1.4 Windowing and Spectrograms

As we have just seen, the Fourier transform represents a signal (i.e., a sound in the cases that interest us here) in terms of potentially infinitely many sine waves that last, in principle, an infinitely long time. But infinitely long is inconveniently long for most practical purposes. An important special case arises if the sound we are interested in is periodic, that is, the sound consists of a pattern that repeats itself over and over. Periodic sounds are, in fact, a hugely important class of acoustic stimuli, so much so that chapter 3 is almost entirely devoted to them. We have already seen that sounds that are periodic, at least to a good approximation, are relatively common in nature. Remember the case of the string vibrating at its fundamental frequency, plus higher harmonics, which correspond to the various modes of vibration. The higher harmonics are all multiples of the fundamental frequency, and while the fundamental goes through exactly one cycle, the harmonics will go through exactly two, three, four, ... cycles. The waveform of such periodic sounds is a recurring pattern, and, we can therefore imagine that for periodic sounds time "goes around in circles," because the same thing happens over and over again. To describe such periodic sounds, instead of a full-fledged Fourier transform with infinitely many frequencies, we only need a "Fourier series" containing a finite number of frequencies, namely, the fundamental plus all its harmonics up to the highest audible frequency. Imagine we record the sound of an instrument playing a very clean 100-Hz note; the spectrum of any one 10-ms period of that sound would then be the same as that of the preceding and the following period, as these are identical, and with modern computers it is easy to calculate this spectrum using the discrete Fourier transform.

But what is to stop us from taking *any* sound, periodic or not, cutting it into small, say 10-ms wide, "strips" (technically known as time windows), and then calculating the spectrum for each? Surely, in this manner, we would arrive at a simple representation of how the distribution of sound frequencies changes over time. Within any one short time window, our spectral analysis still poorly represents temporal features, but we can easily see when spectra change substantially from one window to the next, making it a straightforward process to localize features in time to within the resolution afforded by a single time window. In principle, there is no reason why this cannot be done, and such windowing and short-term Fourier analysis methods are used routinely to calculate a sound's *spectrogram*. In practice, however, one needs to be aware of a few pitfalls.

One difficulty arises from the fact that we cannot simply cut a sound into pieces any old way and expect that this will not affect the spectrum. This is illustrated in figure 1.9. The top panel of the figure shows a 10-ms snippet of a 1-kHz tone, and its amplitude spectrum. A 1-kHz tone has a period of 1 ms, and therefore ten cycles of the tone fit exactly into the whole 10–ms-wide time window. A Fourier transform considers this 1-kHz tone as the tenth harmonic of a 100-Hz tone—100 Hz because the total time window is 10 ms long, and this duration determines the period of the fundamental frequency assumed in the transform. The Fourier amplitude spectrum of the 1-kHz tone is therefore as simple as we might expect of a pure tone snippet: It contains only a single frequency component. So where is the problem?

Well, the problem arises as soon as we choose a different time window, one in which the window duration is no longer a multiple of the period of the frequencies we wish to analyze. An example is shown in the second row of figure 1.9. We are still dealing with the same pure tone snippet, but we have now cut a segment out of it by imposing a rectangular window on it. The window function is shown in light gray. It is simply equal to 0 at all the time points we don't want, and equal to 1 at all the time points we do want. This rectangular window function is the mathematical description of an on/off switch. If we multiply the window function with the sound at each time point then, we get 0 times sound equals 0 during the off period, and 1 times sound equals sound in the on period. You might think that if you have a 1-kHz pure tone, simply switching it on and off to select a small segment for frequency analysis, should not alter its frequency content. You would be wrong.

Cast your mind back to figure 1.7, which illustrated the Fourier transform of a click, and in which we had needed an unseemly large number of sine waves just to cancel

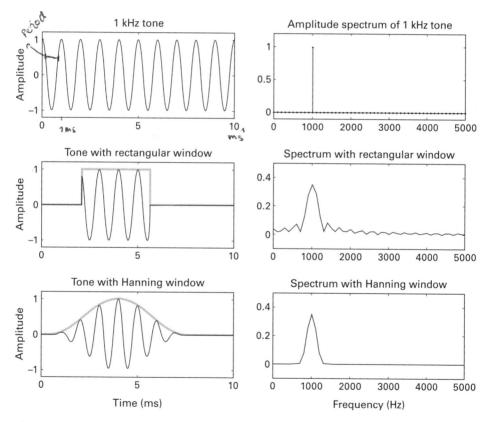

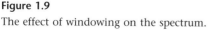

Figure 1.9
The effect of windowing on the spectrum.

the sound off where we didn't want it. Something similar happens when we calculate the Fourier transform of a sine wave snippet where the period of the sine wave is not a multiple of the entire time window entered into the Fourier analysis. The abrupt onset and the offset create discontinuities, that is, "sudden sharp bends" in the waveform, and from the point of view of a Fourier analysis, discontinuities are broadband signals, made up of countless frequencies. You might be forgiven for thinking that this is just a bit of mathematical sophistry, which has little to do with the way real hearing works, but that is not so. Imagine a nerve cell in your auditory system, which is highly selective to a particular sound frequency, say a high frequency of 4,000 Hz or so. Such an auditory neuron should not normally respond to a 1,000-Hz tone, *unless* the 1-kHz tone is switched on or off very suddenly. As shown in the middle panel of figure 1.9, the onset and offset discontinuities are manifest as "spectral splatter," which can extend a long way up or down in frequency, and are therefore "audible" to our hypothetical 4-kHz cell.

This spectral splatter, which occurs if we cut a sound wave into arbitrary chunks, can also plague any attempt at spectrographic analysis. Imagine we want to analyze a so-called frequency-modulated sound. The whining of a siren that starts low and rises in pitch might be a good example. At any one moment in time this sound is a type of complex tone, but the fundamental shifts upward. To estimate the frequency content at any one time, cutting the sound into short pieces and calculating the spectrum for each may sound like a good idea, but if we are not careful, the cutting itself is likely to introduce discontinuities that will make the sound appear a lot more broadband than it really is. These cutting artifacts are hard to avoid completely, but some relatively simple tricks help alleviate them considerably. The most widely used trick is to avoid sharp cutoffs at the onset and offset of each window. Instead of rectangular windows, one uses ramped windows, which gently fade the sound on and off. The engineering mathematics literature contains numerous articles discussing the advantages and disadvantages of ramps with various shapes.

The bottom panels of figure 1.9 illustrate one popular type, the Hanning window, named after the mathematician who first proposed it. Comparing the spectra obtained with the rectangular window and the Hanning window, we see that the latter has managed to reduce the spectral splatter considerably. The peak around 1 kHz is perhaps still broader than we would like, given that in this example we started off with a pure 1-kHz sine, but at least we got rid of the ripples that extended for several kilohertz up the frequency axis. Appropriate "windowing" is clearly important if we want to develop techniques to estimate the frequency content of a sound. But, as we mentioned, the Hanning window shown here is only one of numerous choices. We could have chosen a Kaiser window, or a Hamming window, or simply a linear ramp with a relatively gentle slope. In each case, we would have got slightly different results, but, and this is the important bit, any of these would have been a considerable improvement over the sharp onset of the rectangular window. The precise choice of window function is often a relatively minor detail, as long as the edges of the window consist of relatively gentle slopes rather than sharp edges.

The really important take-home message, the one thing you should remember from this section even if you forget everything else, is this: If we want to be able to resolve individual frequencies accurately, then we must avoid sharp onset and offset discontinuities. In other words, we must have sounds (or sound snippets created with a suitably chosen analysis window) that fade on and off gently—or go on forever, but that is rarely a practical alternative. Sharp, accurate frequency resolution requires gentle fade-in and fade-out, which in turn means that the time windows cannot be very short. This constraint relates to a more general problem, the so-called time-frequency trade-off.

Let us assume you want to know exactly when in some ongoing soundscape a frequency component of precisely 500 Hz occurs. Taking on board what we have just said, you record the sound and cut it into (possibly overlapping) time windows for Fourier analysis, taking care to ramp each time window on and off gently. If you want the frequency resolution to be very high, allowing great spectral precision, then the windows have to be long, and that limits your *temporal* precision. Your frequency analysis might be able to tell you that a frequency very close to 500 Hz occurred somewhere within one of your windows, but because each window has to be fairly long, and must have "fuzzy," fading edges in time, determining exactly when the 500-Hz frequency component started has become difficult. You could, of course, make your window shorter, giving you greater temporal resolution. But that would reduce your frequency resolution. This time-frequency trade-off is illustrated in figure 1.10, which shows a 3-kHz tone windowed with a 10-ms, 5-ms, or 1-ms-wide Hanning window, along with the corresponding amplitude spectrum.

Clearly, the narrower the window gets in time, the greater the precision with which we can claim what we are looking at in figure 1.10 happens at time $t = 5$ ms, and not before or after; but the spectral analysis produces a broader and broader peak, so it is increasingly less accurate to describe the signal as a 3-kHz pure tone rather than a mixture of frequencies around 3 kHz.

This time-frequency trade-off has practical consequences when we try to analyze sounds using spectrograms. Spectrograms, as mentioned earlier, slide a suitable window across a sound wave and calculate the Fourier spectrum in each window to estimate how the frequency content changes over time. Figure 1.11 shows this for the castanet sound we had already seen in figure 1.5 (p. 13). The spectrogram on the left was calculated with a very short, 2.5-ms-wide sliding Hanning window, that on the right with a much longer, 21-ms-wide window. The left spectrogram shows clearly that the sound started more or less exactly at time $t = 0$, but it gives limited frequency resolution. The right spectrogram, in contrast, shows the resonant frequencies of the

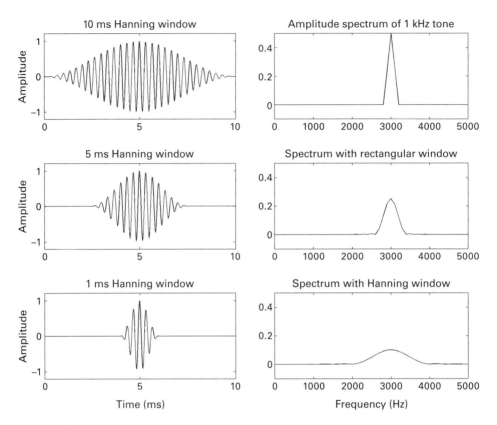

Figure 1.10
The time-frequency trade-off: Short temporal analysis windows give high temporal precision but poor spectral resolution.

castanet in considerably greater detail, but is much fuzzier about when exactly the sound started.

The trade-off between time and frequency resolution is not just a problem for artificial sound analysis systems. Your ears, too, would ideally like to have both very high temporal resolution, telling you exactly when a sound occurred, and very high frequency resolution, giving you a precise spectral fingerprint, which would help you identify the sound source. Your ears do, however, have one little advantage over artificial sound analysis systems based on windowed Fourier analysis spectrograms. They can perform what some signal engineers have come to call multiresolution analysis.

To get an intuitive understanding of what this means, let us put aside for the moment the definition of frequency as being synonymous with sine wave component,

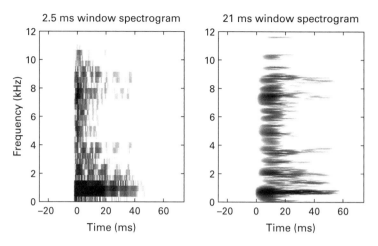

Figure 1.11
Spectrograms of the castanet sound plotted in figure 1.5, calculated with either a short (left) or long (right) sliding Hanning window.

and instead return to the "commonsense" notion of a frequency as a measure of how often something happens during a given time period. Let us assume we chose a time period (our window) which is 1 s long, and in that period we counted ten events of interest (these could be crests of a sound wave, or sand grains falling through an hour glass, or whatever). We would be justified to argue that, since we observed ten events per second—not nine, and not eleven—the events happen with a frequency of 10 Hz. However, if we measure frequencies in this way, we would probably be unable to distinguish 10-Hz frequencies from 10.5-Hz, or even 10.9-Hz frequencies, as we cannot count half events or other event fractions. The 1-s analysis window gives us a frequency resolution of about 10% if we wanted to count events occurring at frequencies of around 10 Hz. But if the events of interest occurred at a higher rate, say 100 Hz, then the inaccuracy due to our inability to count fractional events would be only 1%. The precision with which we can estimate frequencies in a given, fixed time window is greater if the frequency we are trying to estimate is greater.

We could, of course, do more sophisticated things than merely count the number of events, perhaps measuring average time intervals between events for greater accuracy, but that would not change the fundamental fact that *for accurate frequency estimation, the analysis windows must be large compared to the period of the signal whose frequency we want to analyze.* Consequently, if we want to achieve a certain level of accuracy in our frequency analysis, we need very long time windows if the frequencies are likely to be very low, but we can get away with much shorter time windows if we can expect the frequencies to be high. In standard spectrogram (short-term Fourier) analysis, we would have to choose a single time window, which is long enough to be suitable for the lowest frequencies of interest. But our ears work like a mechanical filter bank, and, as we shall see, they can operate using much shorter time windows when analyzing higher frequency sounds than when analyzing low ones. To get a proper understanding of how this works, we need to brush up our knowledge of filters and impulse responses.

1.5   Impulse Responses and Linear Filters

To think of an impulse as being made up of countless pure-tone frequency components, each of identical amplitude, as we have seen in figure 1.7, is somewhat strange, but it can be useful. Let us get back to the idea of a simple, solid object, like a bell, a piece of cutlery, or a piece of wood, being struck to produce a sound. In striking the object, we deliver an impulse: At the moment of impact, there is a very brief pulse of force. And, as we have seen in sections 1.1 and 1.2, the object responds to this force pulse by entering into vibrations. In a manner of speaking, when we strike the object we deliver to it all possible vibration frequencies simultaneously, in one go; the object responds to this by taking up some of these vibration frequencies, but it does not vibrate at all frequencies equally. Instead, it vibrates strongly only at its own resonance frequencies. Consequently, we can think of a struck bell or tuning fork as a sort of *mechanical frequency filter*. The input may contain all frequencies in equal measure, but only resonant frequencies come out. Frequencies that don't fit the object's mechanical tuning properties do not pass.

We have seen, in figure 1.5, that tuning forks, bells, and other similar objects are damped. If you strike them to make them vibrate, their impulse response is an exponentially decaying oscillation. The amplitude of the oscillation declines more or less rapidly (depending on the damping time constant), but in theory it should never decay all the way to zero. In practice, of course, the amplitude of the oscillations will soon become so small as to be effectively zero, perhaps no larger than random thermal motion and in any case too small to detect with any conceivable piece of equipment. Consequently, the physical behavior of these objects can be modeled with great accuracy by so-called *finite impulse response filters* (FIRs).[3] Their impulse responses are said to be finite because their ringing does not carry on for ever. FIRs are *linear systems*. Much scientific discussion has focused on whether, or to what extent, the ear and the auditory system themselves might usefully be thought of as a set of either mechanical or neural linear filters. Linearity and nonlinearity are therefore important notions that recur in later chapters, so we should spend a moment familiarizing ourselves with these ideas. The defining feature of a linear system is a *proportionality relationship* between input and output.

Let us return to our example of a guitar string: If you pluck a string twice as hard, it will respond by vibrating with twice the amplitude, and the sound it emits will be correspondingly louder, but it will otherwise sound much the same. Because of this proportionality between input and output, if you were to plot a graph of the force F with which you pluck the string against the amplitude A of the evoked vibration, you would get a *straight line graph*, hence the term "linear." The graph would be described by the equation $A = F \cdot p$, where p is the proportionality factor which our linear system uses as it converts force input into vibration amplitude output. As you can hopefully appreciate from this, the math for linear systems is particularly nice, simple, and familiar, involving nothing more than elementary-school arithmetic. The corner shop where you bought sweets after school as a kid was a linear system. If you put twice as many pennies in, you got twice as many sweets out. Scientists, like most ordinary people, like to avoid complicated mathematics if they can, and therefore tend to like linear systems, and are grateful that Mother Nature arranged for so many natural laws to follow linear proportionality relationships. The elastic force exerted by a stretched spring is proportional to how far the spring is stretched, the current flowing through an ohmic resistor is proportional to the voltage, the rate at which liquid leaks out of a hole at the bottom of a barrel is proportional to the size of the hole, the amplitude of the sound pressure in a sound wave is proportional to the amplitude of the vibration of the sound source, and so on.

In the case of FIR filters, we can think of the entire impulse response as a sort of extension of the notion of proportional scaling in a way that is worth considering a little further. If we measure the impulse response (i.e., the ping) that a glass of water makes when it is tapped lightly with a spoon, we can predict quite easily and accurately what sound it will make if it is hit again, only 30% harder. It will produce very much the same impulse response, only scaled up by 30%. There is an important caveat, however: *Most things in nature are only approximately linear, over a limited range of inputs.* Strike the same water glass very hard with a hammer, and instead of getting a greatly scaled up but otherwise identical version of the previous ping impulse response, you are likely to get a rather different, crunch and shatter sort of sound, possibly with a bit of a splashing mixed in if the glass wasn't empty. Nevertheless, over a reasonably wide range of inputs, and to a pretty good precision, we can think of a water glass in front of us as a linear system. Therefore, to a good first-order approximation, if we know the glass' impulse response, we know all there is to know about the glass, at least as far as our ears are concerned.

The impulse response will allow us to predict what the glass will sound like in many different situations, not just if it is struck with a spoon, but also, for example, if it was rubbed with the bow of a violin, or hit by hail. To see how that works, look at figure 1.12, which schematically illustrates impulses and impulse responses. The middle panels show a "typical" impulse response of a resonant object, that is, an

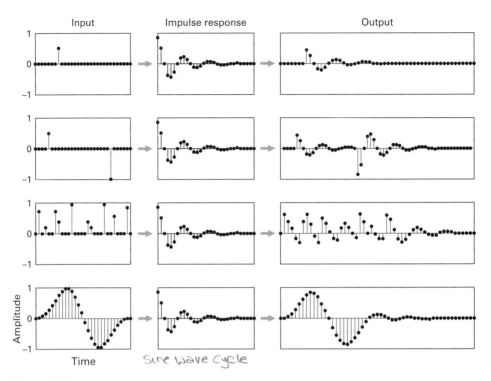

Figure 1.12
Outputs (right panels) that result when a finite impulse response filter (middle panels) is excited with a number of different inputs (left panels).

exponentially decaying oscillation. To keep the figure easy to read, we chose a very short impulse response (of a heavily damped object) and show the inputs, impulse response, and the outputs as discrete, digitized, or sampled signals, just as in figure 1.8.

In the top row of figure 1.12, we see what happens when we deliver a small, slightly delayed impulse to that filter (say a gentle tap with a spoon on the side of a glass). After our recent discussion of impulse responses and linearity, you should not find it surprising that the "output," the evoked vibration pattern, is simply a scaled, delayed copy of the impulse response function. In the second row, we deliver two impulses to the same object (we strike it twice in succession), but the second impulse, which happens after a slightly larger delay, is delivered from the other side, that is, the force is delivered in a negative direction. The output is simply a *superposition* of two impulse responses, each scaled and delayed appropriately, the second being "turned upside-down" because it is scaled by a negative number (representing a force acting in the opposite direction). This should be fairly intuitive: Hit a little bell twice in quick succession, and you get two pings, the second following, and possibly overlapping with, the first.

In the second row example, the delay between the two pulses is long enough for the first impulse response to die down to almost nothing before the second response starts, and it is easy to recognize the output as a superposition of scaled and delayed-impulse responses. But impulses may, of course, come thick and fast, causing impulse responses to overlap substantially in the resulting superposition, as in the example in the third row. This shows what might happen if the filter is excited by a form of "shot noise," like a series of hailstones of different weights, raining down on a bell at rapid but random intervals. Although it is no longer immediately obvious, the output is still simply a superposition of lots of copies of the impulse response, each scaled and delayed appropriately according to each impulse in the input. You may notice that, in this example, the output looks fairly periodic, with positive and negative values alternating every eight samples or so, even though the input is rather random (noisy) and has no obvious periodicity at eight samples. The periodicity of the output does, of course, reflect the fact that the impulse response, a damped sine wave with a period of eight, is itself strongly periodic. Put differently, since the period of the output is eight samples long, this FIR filter has a resonant frequency which is eight times slower than (i.e., one-eighth of) the sample frequency. If we were to excite such an FIR filter with two impulses spaced four samples apart, then the output, the superposition of two copies of the impulse response starting four samples apart, would be subject to destructive interference, the peaks in the second impulse response are canceled to some extent by the troughs in the first, which reduces the overall output.

If, however, the input contains two impulses exactly eight samples apart, then the output would benefit from constructive interference as the two copies of the impulse response are superimposed with peak aligned with peak. If the input contains impulses at various, random intervals, as in the third row of figure 1.12, then the constructive interference will act to amplify the effect of impulses that happen to be eight samples apart, while destructive interference will cancel out the effect of features in the input that are four samples apart; in this manner, the filter selects out intervals that match its own resonant frequency. Thus, hailstones raining down on a concrete floor (which lacks a clear resonance frequency) will sound like noise, whereas the same hailstones raining down on a bell will produce a ringing sound at the bell's resonant frequency. The bell selectively amplifies (filters) its own resonant frequencies out of the frequency mixture present in the hailstorm input.

In the fourth row of figure 1.12, we consider one final important case. Here, instead of delivering a series of isolated impulses to the filter, we give it a sine wave cycle as input. This is a bit like, instead of striking a water glass with a spoon, we were to push a vibrating tuning fork against it. The onset and offset of the sine wave were smoothed off with a Hanning window. The frequency of the sine wave of the input (one-twentieth of the sample rate) is quite a bit slower than the resonant frequency of the filter (one-eighth of the sample rate). What is hopefully quite obvious is that the output is again a sine whose frequency closely matches that of the input.

This illustrates a very important property of linear systems. Linear filters cannot introduce new frequency components; they can only scale each frequency component of the input up or down, and change its phase by introducing delays. Linear systems are therefore said to be sine wave in—sine wave out. Conversely, if we observe that a particular system responds to sine inputs with sine outputs that match the input frequency, then we would take that as an indication that the system is linear. And this holds true even if the input is a mixture of several sine waves. In that case, the output of the linear filter will also be a frequency mixture, and the relative amplitudes of the various frequency components may have changed dramatically, but there will be no components at frequencies that were not present in the input. (Nonlinear filters, in contrast, will quite commonly introduce frequencies into the output signal that weren't there in the input!)

Because we had ramped the sine wave input on and off gently with a Hanning window, the frequency content of this sine cycle is narrow, and contains very little energy at frequencies besides one-twentieth of the sample rate. This input therefore cannot excite the resonant frequency of the linear filter, and, unlike in the hailstones example in the third row, oscillations with a period of eight samples are not apparent in the output. The impulse response of the filter itself, however, has a very sharp onset, and this sharp onset makes its frequency response somewhat broadband. The input frequency of one-twentieth of the sample rate can therefore pass through the filter, but it does lose some of its amplitude since it poorly matches the filter's resonant frequency. If the impulse response of the filter had a gentler onset, its frequency response might well be narrower, and it would attenuate (i.e., reduce the amplitude of) frequencies that are further from its own resonant frequency more strongly.

In fact, filters with suitably chosen impulse responses can become quite highly selective for particular frequencies. We illustrate this in figure 1.13, which shows what happens when a frequency-modulated signal, a so-called FM sweep, is filtered through a so-called gamma-tone filter. A gamma-tone is simply a sinusoid that is windowed (i.e., ramped on and off) with a gamma function. The only thing we need to know about gamma functions for the purposes of this book is that they can take the shape of a type of skewed bell, with a fairly gentle rise and an even gentler decay. Gamma-tone filters are of some interest to hearing researchers because, as we will see in chapter 2, suitably chosen gamma-tone filters may provide a quite reasonable first-order approximation to the mechanical filtering with which the cochlea of your inner ear analyzes sound. So, if we filter a signal like an FM sweep with a gamma-tone filter, in a manner of speaking, we see the sound through the eyes of a point on the basilar

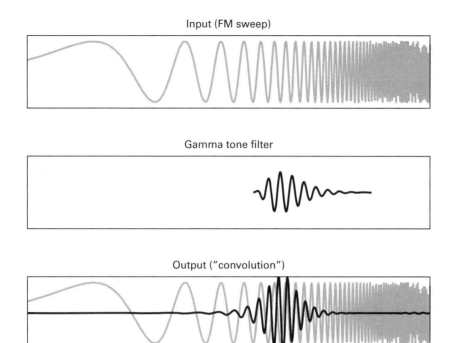

Figure 1.13
An FM sweep filtered by a gamma-tone filter.

membrane of your inner ear (more about that in the next chapter, and apologies for the mixed metaphor).

When we say the input to the filter is frequency modulated, we simply mean that its frequency changes over time. In the example shown in the top panel of figure 1.13, the frequency starts off low but then increases. We made the signal in this example by computer, but you might encounter such frequency modulation in real-world sounds, for example, if you plucked the string on a guitar and then, while the string is still vibrating, either run your finger down the string along the fret board, making the vibrating part of the string effectively shorter, or if you wind up the tension on the string, increasing its effective stiffness.

When we compare the gamma-tone filter in figure 1.13 with the wave-form of the FM sweep, it should be reasonably obvious that the resonant frequency of the gamma-tone filter matches the frequency of the FM sweep in some places, but not in others. In fact, the match between these frequencies starts off and ends up very poor (the frequency of the FM sweep is initially far too low and eventually far too high), but somewhere just over halfway through the frequency of the FM sweep matches that of the filter rather well. And because the gamma-tone is gently ramped on and off, we expect its frequency bandwidth to be quite narrow, so as the FM sweep is filtered through the gamma-tone filter, we expect to see very little in the output at times where the frequencies do not match. These expectations are fully borne out in the third panel of figure 1.13, which shows the output of the gamma-tone filter, plotted as a thick black line superimposed on the original FM sweep input plotted in gray. Frequencies other than those that match the filter's resonance characteristics are strongly suppressed.

It is not difficult to imagine that, if we had a whole series of such gamma-tone filters, each tuned to a slightly different frequency and arranged in order, we could use the resulting gamma-tone filter bank to carry out a detailed frequency analysis of incoming sounds and calculate something very much like a spectrogram on the fly simply by passing the sounds through all the filters in parallel as they come in. As it happens, we are all equipped with such filter banks. We call them "ears," and we will look at their functional organization in greater detail in the next chapter. But first we need to add a few brief technical notes to conclude this section, and we shall see how what we have just learned about filters and impulse responses can help us understand voices. We also need to say a few things about the propagation of sound waves through air.

First, the technical notes. Calculating the output of an FIR filter by superimposing a series of scaled and delayed copies of the impulse response is often referred to as calculating the *convolution* of the input and the impulse responses. Computing convolutions is sometimes also referred to as convolving. If you look up "convolution," you will most likely be offered a simple mathematical formula by way of definition, something along the lines of "the convolution $(f * g)(t)$ of input f with impulse response g equals $\Sigma(g(t - \tau) \cdot f(\tau))$ over all τ." This is really nothing but mathematical shorthand for the process we have described graphically in figure 1.12. The $g(t - \tau)$ bit simply means we take copies of the impulse response, each delayed by a different delay τ (tau), and we then scale each of these delayed copies by the value of the input that corresponds to that delay [that's the "$\cdot f(\tau)$" bit], and then superimpose all these scaled and delayed copies on top of one another, that is, we sum them all up (that's what the "Σ over all τ" means).

One thing that might be worth mentioning in passing is that convolutions are commutative, meaning that if we convolve a waveform f with another waveform g, it does not matter which is the input and which is the impulse response. They are interchangeable and swapping them around would give us the same result: $(f * g)(t) = (g * f)(t)$.

Another thing worth mentioning is that making computers calculate convolutions is quite straightforward, and given that so many real-world phenomena can be quite adequately approximated by a linear system and therefore described by impulse responses, convolution by computer allows us to simulate all sorts of phenomena or situations. Suppose, for example, you wanted to produce a radio crime drama, and it so happens that, according to the scriptwriter, the story line absolutely must culminate in a satanic mass that quickly degenerates into a violent shootout, all taking place right around the altar of the highly reverberant acoustic environment of Oxford's Christ Church cathedral. To ensure that it sounds authentic, you asked the Dean of Christ Church for permission to record the final scene inside the cathedral, but somehow he fails to be convinced of the artistic merit of your production, and declines to give you permission. But recorded in a conventional studio, the scene sounds flat. So what do you do?

Well, acoustically speaking, Christ Church cathedral is just another linear system, with reverberations, echoes, and resonances that can easily be captured entirely by its impulse response. All you need to do is make one decent "impulse" inside the cathedral. Visit the cathedral at a time when few visitors are around, clap your hands together hard and, using a portable recorder with a decent microphone, record the sound that is produced, with all its reverberation. Then use a computer to convolve the studio recorded drama with the canned Christ Church impulse response, and presto, the entire scene will sound as if it was recorded inside the cathedral. Well, almost. The cathedral's impulse response will vary depending on the location of both the sound receiver and the source—the clapping hands—so if you want to create a completely accurate simulation of acoustic scenes that take place in, or are heard from, a variety of positions around the cathedral, you may need to record separate impulse responses for each combination of listener and sound source position. But passable simulations of reverberant acoustic environments are possible even with entirely artificial impulse responses derived on computer models. (See the book's Web site, auditoryneuroscience.com, for a demonstration.)

Or imagine you wanted to make an electronic instrument, a keyboard that can simulate sounds of other instruments including the violin. You could, of course, simply record all sorts of notes played on the violin and, when the musician presses the key on the keyboard, the keyboard retrieves the corresponding note from memory and plays it. The problem with that is that you do not know in advance for how long the musician might want to hold the key. If you rub the bow of a violin across a string it pulls the string along a little, then the string jumps, then it gets pulled along some more, then it jumps again a little, and so on, producing a very rapid and somewhat irregular saw-tooth force input pattern. Such a saw-tooth pattern would not be difficult to create by computer on the fly, and it can then be convolved with the strings' impulse responses, that is, sounds of the strings when they were plucked, to simulate the sound of bowed strings. Of course, in this way you could also simulate what it would sound like if objects were "bowed" that one cannot normally bow, but for which one can either record or simulate impulse responses: church bells, plastic bottles, pieces of furniture, and so on. Convolution is thus a surprisingly versatile little tool for the computer literate who enjoy being scientifically or artistically creative.

1.6 Voices

One very widespread class of natural sounds, which is much easier to understand now that we have discussed impulse responses and convolutions, is voices. Given their central role in spoken words, song, and animal communication, voices are a particularly important class of sounds, and like many other sounds that we have discussed already, voices too are a kind of pulse-resonance sound. When humans or other mammals vocalize, they tighten a pair of tissue flaps known as vocal folds across their airways (the larynx), and then exhale to push air through the closed vocal folds. The vocal folds respond by snapping open and shut repeatedly in quick succession, producing a series of rapid clicks known as "glottal pulses." These glottal pulses then "ring" through a series of resonant cavities, the vocal tract , which includes the throat, the mouth, and the nasal sinuses. (Look for a video showing human vocal folds in action on the book's Web site.) When we speak, we thus effectively convolve a glottal pulse train with the resonant filter provided by our vocal tract, and we can change our voice, in rather different and interesting ways, either by changing the glottal pulse train or by changing the vocal tract.

First, let us consider the glottal pulse train, and let us assume for simplicity that we can approximate this as a series of "proper" impulses at very regular intervals. Recall from figure 1.7 that any impulse can be thought of as a superposition of infinitely many sine waves, all of the same amplitude but different frequency, and with their phases arranged in such a way that they all come into phase at the time of the impulse but at no other time. What happens with all these sine waves if we deal not with one click, but with a series of clicks, spaced at regular intervals?

Well, each click is effectively its own manifestation of infinitely many sine waves, but if we have more than one click, the sine waves of the individual clicks in the click train will start to interfere, and that interference can be constructive or destructive. In fact, the sine components of the two clicks will have the same phase if the click interval happens to be an integer (whole number) multiple of the sine wave period, in other words if exactly one or two or three or n periods of the sine wave fit between the clicks. The top panel of figure 1.14 may help you appreciate that fact. Since these sine waves are present, and in phase, in all clicks of a regular click train of a fixed interval, they will interfere constructively and be prominent in the spectrum of the click train. However, if the click interval is 1/2, or 3/2, or 5/2, ... of the sine period, then the sine components from each click will be exactly out of phase, as is shown in the bottom panel of figure 1.14, and the sine components cancel out.

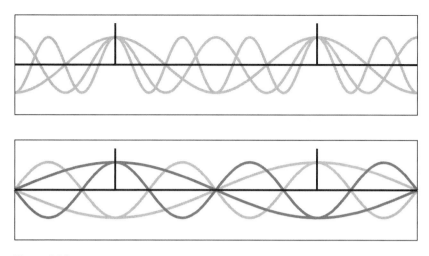

Figure 1.14
Sine components of click trains interfere constructively when the sine period is an integer multiple of the click interval, but not otherwise.

The upshot of this is that a regular, periodic click train is effectively a type of sound that we have already encountered in section 1.2, namely, a type of complex tone, made up of a fundamental frequency and an infinite number of higher harmonics, all of equal amplitude. The periods of the harmonics are equal to 1/1, 1/2, 1/3, ... 1/n of the click interval, and their frequencies are accordingly multiples of the fundamental. Consequently, the closer the clicks are spaced in time, the wider apart the harmonics are in frequency.

All of this applies to glottal pulse trains, and we should therefore not be surprised that the spectrogram of voiced speech sounds exhibits many pronounced harmonics, reaching up to rather high frequencies. But these glottal pulse trains then travel through the resonators of the vocal tract. Because the resonant cavities of the throat, mouth, and nose are linear filters, they will not introduce any new frequencies, but they will raise the amplitude of some of the harmonics and suppress others.

With this in mind, consider the spectrogram of the vowel /a/, spoken by a male adult, shown in figure 1.15. The spectrogram was generated with a long time window, to resolve the harmonics created by the glottal pulse train, and the harmonics are clearly visible as spectral lines, every 120 Hz or so. However, some of the harmonics are much more pronounced than others. The harmonics near 700 to 1,200 Hz are particularly intense, while those between 1,400 and 2,000 Hz are markedly weaker, and then we see another peak at around 2,500 Hz, and another at around 3,500 Hz. To a first approximation, we can think of each of the resonators of the vocal tract as a band pass filter with a single resonant frequency. These resonant frequencies are

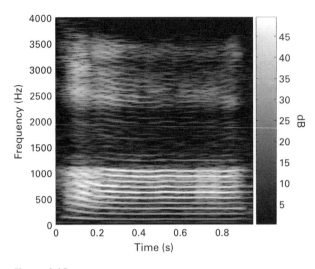

Figure 1.15
Spectrogram of the vowel "a."

known as "formants," and those harmonics that lie close to the formant frequencies
will be scaled up relative to the others, which leads to the peaks we have just observed.

One important feature of our voice is that it gives us independent control of the
harmonic and the formant frequencies. We change the harmonic frequencies by
putting more or less tension on our vocal folds. The higher the tension, the faster the
glottal pulse train, which leads to a higher fundamental frequency and more widely
spaced harmonics, and the voice is perceived as higher pitched. We control the
formant frequencies by moving various parts of our vocal tract, which are commonly
referred to as "articulators," and include the lips, jaws, tongue, and soft palate. Moving
the articulators changes the size and shape of the resonance cavities in the vocal tract,
which in turn changes their resonant frequencies, that is, the formants.

Altering the formants does not affect the pitch of the speech sound, but its timbre,
and therefore its "type" may change quite dramatically; for example, we switch
between /o/- and /a/-like vowels simply by widening the opening of our lips and jaw.
Thus, we control which vowel we produce by changing the formant frequencies, and
we control the pitch at which we speak or sing a vowel by changing the harmonic
frequencies. This can be seen quite clearly in figure 1.16, which shows spectrograms
of the words "hot," "hat," "hit," and "head," spoken by different native speakers of
British English, one with a high-pitched, childlike voice (top row) and then again in
a lower-pitched voice of an adult female (bottom row). (A color version of that figure,
along with the corresponding sound recordings, can be found on the "vocalizations
and speech" section of the book's Web site.)

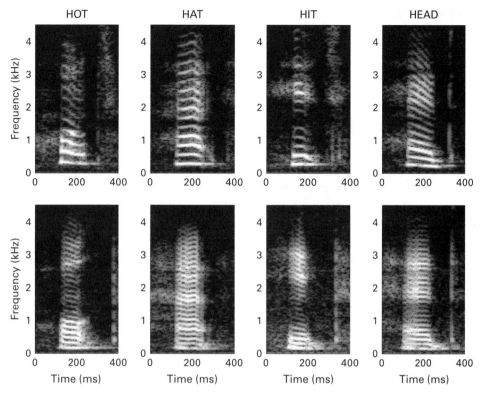

Figure 1.16

Spectrograms of the words "hot," "hat," "hit," and "head," spoken in a high-pitched (top row) and a low-pitched (bottom row) voice.

The vowels in the spoken words are readily apparent in the "harmonic stacks" that mark the arrival of the glottal pulse train, and the spacing of the harmonics is clearly much wider in the high-pitched than in the low-pitched vowels. The fact that, in some of the sounds, the harmonics aren't exactly horizontal tells us that the pitch of these vowels was not perfectly steady (this is particularly noticeable in the high-pitched "hot" and "head"). Where exactly the formants are in these vowels is perhaps not quite so readily apparent to the unaided eye. (Formants are, in fact, easier to see in spectrograms that have short time windows, and hence a more blurred frequency resolution, but then the harmonics become hard to appreciate.) But it is nevertheless quite clear that, for example, in the /i/ sounds the harmonics around 500 Hz are very prominent, but there is little sound energy between 800 and 2000 Hz, until another peak is reached at about 2,300 Hz, and another near 3,000 Hz. In contrast, in the /a/ vowels, the energy is much more evenly distributed across the frequency range, with peaks perhaps around 800, 1,800, and 2,500 Hz, while the /o/ sound has a lot of energy at a few hundred hertz, up to about 1,100 Hz, then much less until one reaches another smaller peak at 2,500 Hz.

Of course, there is more to the words "hot," "hat," "hit," and "head" than merely their vowels. There are also the consonants "h" at the beginning and "t" or "d" at the end. Consonants can be subdivided into different classes depending on a number of criteria. For example, consonants can be "voiced" or "unvoiced". If they are voiced, the vocal folds are moving and we would expect to see harmonics in their spectrogram. The "h" and the "t" in "hot," "hat," "hit," and "heat" are unvoiced, the vocal chords are still. So what generates the sounds of these unvoiced consonants? Most commonly, unvoiced consonants are generated when air is squeezed through a narrow opening in the airways, producing a highly turbulent flow, which sets up random and therefore noisy vibration patterns in the air.

In speaking the consonant "h," the air "rubs" as it squeezes through a narrow opening in the throat. Students of phonetics, the science of speech sounds, would therefore describe this sound as a glottal (i.e., throat produced) fricative (i.e., rubbing sound), in this manner describing the place and the mode of articulation. The "t" is produced by the tongue, but unlike in pronouncing the "h," the airway is at first blocked and then the air is released suddenly, producing a sharp sound onset characteristic of a "plosive" stop consonant. Plosives can be, for example, "labial," that is, produced by the lips as in "p" or "b"; or they can be "laminal-dental," that is, produced when the tip of the tongue, the lamina, obstructs and then releases the airflow at the level of the teeth, as in "t" or "d"; or they can be velar, that is, produced at the back of the mouth when the back of the tongue pushes against the soft palate, or velum, as in "k."

The mouth and throat area contains numerous highly mobile parts that can be reconfigured in countless different ways, so the number of possible speech sounds is rather large. (See the "vocalization and speech" section of the book's Web site for links to x-ray videos showing the human articulators in action.) Cataloguing all the different speech sounds is a science in itself, known as articulatory phonetics. We shall not dwell on this any further here, except perhaps to point out a little detail in figure 1.16, which you may have already noticed. The "h" fricative at the beginning of each word is, as we have just described, the result of turbulent airflow, hence noisy, hence broadband; that is, it should contain a very wide range of frequencies. But the frequencies of this consonant are subjected to resonances in the vocal tract just as much as the harmonics in the vowel. And, indeed, if you look carefully at the place occupied by the "h" sounds in the spectrograms of figure 1.16 (the region just preceding the vowel), you can see that the "h" sound clearly exhibits formants, but these aren't so much the formants of the consonant "h" as the formants of the vowel that is about to follow! When we pronounce "hot" or "hat," our vocal tract already assumes the configuration of the upcoming vowel during the "h," imparting the formants of the following vowel onto the preceding consonant. Consequently, there is, strictly speaking, really no such thing as the sound of the consonant "h," because the "h" followed by an "o" has really quite a different spectrum from that of an "h" that is followed by an "a."

This sort of influence of the following speech sound onto the preceding sound is sometimes referred to as "coarticulation" or "assimilation" in the phonetic sciences, and it is much more common than you might think. In your personal experience, an "h" is an "h"; you know how to make it, you know what it sounds like. Recognizing an "h" is trivially easy for your auditory system, despite the fact that, in reality, there are many different "h" sounds. This just serves to remind us that there is a lot more to hearing than merely accurately estimating frequency content, and for people trying to build artificial speech recognizers, such phenomena as coarticulation can be a bit of a headache.

1.7   Sound Propagation

So far, we have looked almost exclusively at vibration patterns in a variety of sound sources. Developing some insights into how sounds come about in the first place is an essential, and often neglected, aspect of the auditory sciences. But, of course, this is only the beginning. We can hear the sound sources in our environment only if their vibrations are somehow physically coupled to the vibration-sensitive parts of our ears. Most commonly, this coupling occurs through the air.

Air is capable of transmitting sound because it has two essential properties: inert mass and stiffness or elasticity. You may not think of air as either particularly massive or particularly elastic, but you probably do know that air does weigh something (about 1.2 g/L at standard atmospheric pressure), and its elasticity you can easily verify if you block off the end of a bicycle pump and then push down the piston. As the air becomes compressed, it will start to push back against the piston, just as if it were a spring. We can imagine the air that surrounds us as being made up of small "air masses," each linked to its neighboring masses through spring forces that are related to air pressure. This is a useful way of conceptualizing air, because it can help us develop a clear image of how sound waves propagate. A medium made of small masses linked by springs will allow disturbances (e.g., small displacements at one of the edges) to travel through the medium from one mass to the next in a longitudinal wave pattern. How this works is illustrated in figure 1.17, as well as in a little computer animation which you can find on the book's Web site.

Figure 1.17 shows the output of a computer simulation of a sound source, represented by the black rectangle to the left, which is in contact with an air column, represented by a row of air masses (gray circles) linked by springs (zigzag lines). At first (top row), the source and the air masses are at rest, but then the sound source

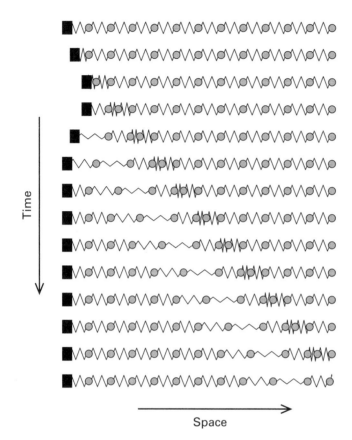

Figure 1.17
A longitudinal wave propagating through a medium of inert masses coupled via elastic springs.
See the book's Web site for an animated version.

briefly lurches a bit to the right, and then returns to its initial position. The rightward movement compresses the spring that links it to the neighboring air mass. That, in turn, causes this air mass to be accelerated rightwards, but because the mass has a small inertia, its movement lags somewhat behind that of the sound source. As the mass immediately to the right of the sound source starts moving rightward, it compresses the spring linking it to the next mass along, which in turn accelerates that mass rightward, and so on and so on. As the sound source returns to its original position, it will start to stretch the spring linking it to the neighboring mass, which in time will pull that mass back to its original position. This stretch also propagates along the air column; thus, while each air mass is first pushed one way it is then pulled the other, so that it ends up where it started. There are thus essentially four phases to the propagating sound wave: first, a compression, followed by a forward displacement, followed by a rarefaction (or stretch, in our spring analogy), followed by a backward (return) displacement. Sound waves therefore consist of displacement waves as well as pressure waves, but the displacement wave lags behind the pressure wave by a quarter of a cycle, and the final net displacement of the air is zero. (Sound is not a wind).

To generate figure 1.17, we got a computer to apply Hooke's law to work out all the spring forces, and then to use Newton's second law to calculate the acceleration of each inert air mass in turn and update the positions of the masses accordingly at each time step. Figure 1.17 illustrates quite nicely how the simple interaction of Hooke's law and Newton's second law allows for a movement of a sound source to be translated into a "disturbance" in the local air pressure (the spring forces), which then propagates through a column of air away from the source. It is essentially that mechanism which links the surfaces of all the sound sources in your environment to your eardrum. And in doing so, it replicates the vibration patterns of the sound sources quite accurately. The forward movement of the source gave rise to a compression of corresponding size, while the return to the original position created a corresponding rarefaction. This simple correspondence is handy, because it means that we can, to a pretty good first approximation, assume that everything we have learned in previous sections about the vibration patterns of different types of sound sources will be faithfully transmitted to the eardrum.

Of course, this phenomenon of longitudinal propagation of waves is not limited to air. Any material that possesses inert mass and at least some springlike elasticity is, in principle, capable of propagating sound waves. Consequently, dolphins can use their lower jaws to pick up sound waves propagated through water, while certain species of toads, or even blind mole rats, appear to be able to collect sound waves conducted through the ground. But different substrates for sound propagation may be more or less stiff, or more or less heavy, than air, and these differences will affect the speed at which sound waves travel through that substrate. We mentioned earlier that the displacement of the first air mass in figure 1.17 lags somewhat behind the displacement of the sound source itself. The movement of the sound source first has to compress the spring, and the spring force then has to overcome the inertia of the first mass. Clearly, if the spring forces are quite large and the masses only small, then the time lag will not be very great.

Materials with such comparatively large internal spring forces are said to have a high acoustic impedance. The acoustic impedance is defined as the amount of pressure (i.e., spring force) required to achieve a given particle velocity. The speed of sound is high in materials that have a high acoustic impedance but a low density (essentially high spring forces and low masses). For air at ambient pressures and temperature, the speed of sound works out to about 343 m/s (equivalent to 1,235 km/h or 767 mph). The precise value depends on factors such as humidity, atmospheric pressure, and temperature, because these may affect the mass density and the elastic modulus (i.e., the springiness) of the air. For water, which is heavier but also much, much stiffer than air, the speed of sound is more than four times larger, at about 1,480 m/s (5,329 km/h or 3,320 mph).

In a number of ways, the longitudinal wave propagation shown in figure 1.17 is, of course, a somewhat oversimplified model of real sound waves. For example, in our idealized model, sound waves propagate without any loss of energy over infinite distances. But you know from experience that sounds are quieter if the sound source is further away. Two factors contribute to this. The first, and often the less important reason, is that in real physical media, sound waves tend to dissipate, which simply means that the coordinated motion of air masses will start to become disorganized and messy, gradually looking less and less like a coherent sound wave and increasingly like random motion; that is, the sound will slowly turn into heat. Interestingly, high-frequency sounds tend to dissipate more easily than low-frequency ones, so that thunder heard from a great distance will sound like a low rumble, even though the same sound closer to the source would have been more of a sharp "crack," with plenty of high-frequency energy. Similarly, ultrasonic communication and echolocation sounds such as those used by mice or bats tend to have quite limited ranges. A mouse would find it difficult to call out to a mate some twenty yards away, something that most humans can do with ease.

The second, and usually major factor contributing to the attenuation (weakening) of sounds with distance stems from the fact that most sound sources are not linked to just a single column of spring-linked masses, as in the example in figure 1.17, but are instead surrounded by air. We really should think more in terms of a three-dimensional lattice of masses with spring forces acting up and down, forward and backward, as well as left and right. And as we mentioned earlier, the springs in our model represent air pressure gradients, and you may recall that pressure will push from the point where the pressure is greater *in all directions* where pressure is lower. Consequently, in a three-dimensional substrate, a sound wave that starts at some point source will propagate outward in a circular fashion in all directions. You want to imagine a wavefront a bit like that in figure 1.17, but forming a spherical shell that moves outward from the source.

Now, this spherical shell of the propagating sound wave does, of course, get larger and larger as the sound propagates, just like the skin of a balloon gets larger as we continue to inflate it. However, all the mechanical energy present in the sound wave was imparted on it at the beginning, when the sound source accelerated the air masses in its immediate neighborhood. As the sound wave propagates outward in a sphere, that initial amount of mechanical energy gets stretched out over a larger and larger area, much like the skin of a balloon becomes thinner as we inflate it. If the area becomes larger as we move further away from the sound source but the energy is constant, then the amount of energy per unit area must decrease. And since the surface area of a sphere is proportional to the square of its radius (surface = $4 \cdot \pi \cdot r^2$), the sound energy per unit surface area declines at a rate that is inversely proportional to the square of the distance from the source. This fact is often referred to as the *inverse square law*, and it is responsible for the fact that sound sources normally are less loud as we move further away from them.

Of course, the inverse square law, strictly speaking, only holds in the "free field," that is, in places where the sound wave really can propagate out in a sphere in all directions. If you send sound waves down a narrow tube with rigid walls, then you end up with a situation much more like that in figure 1.17, where you are dealing with just a column of air in which the sound amplitude should stay constant and not decline with distance. You may think that this is a severe limitation, because in the real world there are almost always some surfaces that may be an obstacle to sound propagation, for example, the floor! However, if you placed a sound source on a rigid floor, then the sound waves would propagate in hemispheres outwards (i.e., sideways and upward), and the surface area of a hemisphere is still proportional to the square of its radius (the surface is simply half of $4\pi r^2$, hence still proportional to r^2), so the inverse square law would still apply.

If, however, we lived in a world with four spatial dimensions, then sound energy would drop off as a function of $1/r^3$—which would be known as the inverse cube law—and because sound waves would have more directions in which they must spread out, their amplitudes would decrease much faster with distance, so communicating with sound over appreciable distances would require very powerful sound sources. Of course, we cannot go into a world of four spatial dimensions to do the experiment, but we can send sound down "effectively one-dimensional" (i.e., long but thin) tubes. If we do this, then the sound amplitude should decrease as a function of $1/r^0 = 1$, that is, not at all, and indeed people in the 1800s were able to use long tubes with funnels on either end to transmit voices, for example, from the command bridge to the lower decks of a large ship.

Thus, the inverse square law does not apply for sounds traveling in confined spaces, and substantial deviations from the inverse square law are to be expected also in many modern indoor environments. Although three-dimensional, such environments nevertheless contain many sound-reflecting surfaces, including walls and ceilings, which will cause the sound waves to bounce back and forth, creating a complex pattern of overlapping echoes known as reverberations. In such reverberant environments, the sound that travels directly from the source to the receiver will obey the inverse square law, but reflected sound waves will soon add to this original sound.

1.8   Sound Intensity

From our previous discussion of propagating sound waves, you probably appreciate the dual nature of sound: A small displacement of air causes a local change in pressure, which in turn causes a displacement, and so on. But if we wanted to measure how large a sound is, should we concern ourselves with the amplitude of the displacement, or its velocity, or the amplitude of the pressure change, or all three? Well, the displacement and the pressure are linked by linear laws of motion, so if we know one, we ought to be able to work out the other. The microphones used to measure sounds typically translate pressure into voltage, making it possible to read the change of pressure over time directly off an oscilloscope screen. Consequently, acoustical measures of sound amplitude usually concern themselves with the sound pressure only. And you might think that, accordingly, the appropriate thing to do would be to report sound amplitudes simply in units of pressure, that is, force per unit area. While this is essentially correct, matters are, unfortunately, a little more complicated.

The first complication we have to deal with is that it is in the very nature of sounds that the sound pressure always changes, which is very inconvenient if we want to come up with a single number to describe the intensity of a sound. We could, of course, simply use the largest (peak) pressure in our sound wave and report that. Peak measurements are sometimes used, and are perfectly fine if the sound we are trying to characterize is a pure sinusoid, for example, because we can infer all the other amplitudes if we know the peak amplitude. But for other types of sound, peak amplitude measures can be quite inappropriate. Consider, for example, two click trains, each made up of identical brief clicks; but in the first click train the interval between clicks is long, and in the second it is much shorter. Because the clicks are the same in each train, the peak amplitudes for the two trains are identical, but the click train with the longer inter-click intervals contains longer silent periods, and it would not be unreasonable to think it therefore has, in a manner of speaking, less sound in it than the more rapid click train.

As this example illustrates, it is often more appropriate to use measures that somehow average the sound pressure over time. But because sounds are normally made up of alternating compressions and rarefactions (positive and negative pressures), our averaging operation must avoid canceling positive against negative pressure values. The way this is most commonly done is to calculate the root-mean-square (RMS) pressure of the sound wave.

As the name implies, RMS values are calculated by first squaring the pressure at each moment in time, then averaging the squared values, and finally taking the square root. Because the square of a negative value is positive, rarefactions of the air are not canceled against compressions when RMS values are calculated. For sine waves, the RMS value should work out as $1/\sqrt{2}$ (70.71%) of the peak value, but that is true only if the averaging for the RMS value is done over a time period that contains a whole number of half-cycles of the sine wave. In general, the values obtained with any averaging procedure will be, to some extent, sensitive to the choice of time window over which the averaging is done, and the choice of the most appropriate time window will depend on the particular situation and may not always be obvious.

Another factor that can cause great confusion among newcomers to the study of sound (and sometimes even among experts) is that even RMS sound pressure values are almost never reported in units of pressure, like pascals (newtons per square meter) or in bars, but are instead normally reported in bels, or more commonly in tenths of bels, known as decibels (dB). Bels are in many ways a very different beast from the units of measurement that we are most familiar with, like the meter, or the kilogram, or the second. For starters, unlike these other units, a bel is a *logarithmic* unit. What is that supposed to mean?

Well, if we give, for example, the length of a corridor as 7.5 m, then we effectively say that it is 7.5 *times* as long as a well-defined standard reference length known as a meter. If, however, we report an RMS sound pressure as 4 bels (or 40 dB), we're saying that it is 4 *orders of magnitude* (i.e., 4 powers of $10 = 10^4 = 10,000$ times) larger than some standard reference pressure. Many newcomers to acoustics will find this orders of magnitude thinking unfamiliar and at times a little inconvenient. For example, if we add a 20-kg weight to a 40-kg weight, we get a total weight of 60 kg. But if we add, in phase, a 1-kHz pure tone with an RMS sound pressure amplitude of 20 dB to another 1-kHz pure tone with an amplitude of 40 dB, then we do not end up with a tone with a 60-dB amplitude. Instead, the resulting sound pressure would be $\log_{10}(10^4 + 10^2) =$ 4.00432 bels, that is, 40.0432 dB. The weaker of the two sounds, having an amplitude 2 orders of magnitude (i.e., 100 times) smaller than the larger one, has added, in terms of orders of magnitude, almost nothing to the larger sound.

Because decibels, unlike weights or lengths or money, work on a logarithmic scale, adding decibels is a lot more like multiplying sound amplitudes than adding to them, and that takes some getting used to. But the logarithmic nature of decibels is not their only source of potential confusion. Another stems from the fact that decibels are used to express all sorts of logarithmic ratios, not just ratios of RMS sound pressure amplitudes. Unlike meters, which can only be used to measure lengths, and always compare these lengths to a uniquely and unambiguously defined standard length, for decibels there is no uniquely defined type of measurement, nor is there a unique, universally accepted standard reference value. Decibel values simply make an order of magnitude comparison between any two quantities, and it is important to be clear about what is being compared to what.

Decibel values need not relate to sound at all. To say that the sun is about 25.8 dB (i.e., $10^{2.58}$, or roughly 380 times) further away from the earth than the moon is would perhaps be a little unusual, but entirely correct. But surely, at least in the context of sound, can't we safely assume that any decibels we encounter will refer to sound pressure? Well, no. Sometimes they will refer to the RMS pressure, sometimes to peak pressure, but more commonly, acoustical measurements in decibels will refer to the *intensity* or the *level* of a sound. In a context of acoustics, the words "level" and "intensity" can be used interchangeably, and an intensity or level stated in decibels is used, in effect, to compare the *power* (i.e., the energy per unit time) per unit area delivered by each of the two sound waves.

Fortunately, there is a rather simple relationship between the energy of a sound and its RMS sound pressure amplitude, so everything we learned so far about pressure amplitudes will still be useful. You may remember from high school physics that the kinetic energy of a moving heavy object is given by $E = mv^2$, that is, the kinetic energy is proportional to the square of the velocity. This also holds for the kinetic energy of our notional lumps of air, which we had encountered in figure 1.17 and which take part in a longitudinal wave motion to propagate sound. Now, the average velocity of these lumps of air is proportional to the RMS sound amplitude, so the energy levels of the sound are proportional to the *square* of the amplitude. Consequently, if we wanted to work out the intensity y of a particular sound with RMS pressure x in decibels relative to that of another known reference sound whose RMS pressure is x_{ref}, then we would do this using the formula

$$y \ (dB) = 10 \cdot \log_{10}(x^2/x_{ref}^2) = 20 \cdot \log_{10}(x/x_{ref})$$

(The factor of 10 arises because there are 10 dB in a bel. And because $\log(a^2) = 2 \cdot \log(a)$, we can bring the squares in the fraction forward and turn the factor 10 into a factor 20).

You might be forgiven for wondering whether this is not all a bit overcomplicated. If we can use a microphone to measure sound pressure directly, then why should we go to the trouble of first expressing the observed pressure amplitudes as multiples of some reference, then calculating the log to base 10 of that fraction, then finally multiply by 20 to work out a decibel sound intensity value. Would it not be much easier and potentially less confusing to simply state the observed sound pressures amplitudes directly in pascals? After all, our familiar, linear units like the meter and the newton and the gram, for which $4 + 2 = 6$, and not 4.00432, have much to commend themselves. So why have the seemingly more awkward and confusing logarithmic measures in bels and decibels ever caught on?

Well, it turns out that, for the purposes of studying auditory perception, the orders of magnitude thinking that comes with logarithmic units is actually rather appropriate for a number of reasons. For starters, the range of sound pressure levels that our ears can respond to is quite simply enormous. Hundreds of millions of years of evolution during which you get eaten if you can't hear the hungry predators trying to creep up on you have equipped us with ears that are simply staggeringly sensitive. The faintest sound wave that a normal, young healthy human can just about hear has an RMS sound pressure of roughly 20 micropascal (μPa), that is, 20 millionth of a newton per square meter. That is approximately 10 million times less than the pressure of a penny resting on your fingertip! Because an amplitude of 20 μPa is close to the absolute threshold of human hearing, it is commonly used as a reference for sound intensity calculations. Sound levels expressed in decibels relative to 20 μPa are usually abbreviated as *dB SPL*, short for sound pressure level.

The sound level of the quietest audible sounds would therefore be around 0 dB SPL. (These almost inaudibly quiet sounds have an amplitude approximately equal to that of the reference of 20 μPa, so the fraction x/x_{ref} in the formula above would work out to about 1, and the log of 1 is 0.) But if you listen, for example, to very loud rock music, then you might expose your ears to sound levels as high as 120 dB SPL. In other words, the sound energy levels in these very loud sounds are twelve orders of magnitude—1,000,000,000,000-fold (1,000 *billion* times!) larger than those in the quietest audible sounds. Thousand billion-fold increases are well beyond the common experience of most of us, and are therefore not easy to imagine.

Let us try to put this in perspective. A large rice grain may weigh in the order of 0.05 g. If you were to increase that tiny weight a thousand billion-fold, you would end up with a mountain of rice weighing 50,000 tons. That is roughly the weight of ten thousand fully grown African elephants, or one enormous, city-block-sized ocean cruise liner like the *Titanic*. Listening to very loud music is therefore quite a lot like taking a delicate set of scales designed to weigh individual rice grains, and piling one hundred fully loaded jumbo jet airliners onto it. It may sound like fun, but it is not a good idea, as exposure to very loud music, or other very intense sounds for that matter, can easily lead to serious and permanent damage to the supremely delicate mechanics in our inner ears. Just a single, brief exposure to 120 dB SPL sounds may be enough to cause irreparable damage.

Of course, when we liken the acoustic energy at a rock concert to the mass of one hundred jumbo jets, we don't want to give the impression that the amounts of energy entering your eardrums are large. Power amplifiers for rock concerts or public address systems do radiate a lot of power, but only a minuscule fraction of that energy enters the ears of the audience. Even painfully loud sound levels of 120 dB SPL carry really only quite modest amounts of acoustic power, about one-tenth of a milliwatt (mW) per square centimeter. A human eardrum happens to be roughly half a square centimeter in cross section, so deafeningly loud sounds will impart 0.05 mW to it. How much is 0.05 mW? Imagine a small garden snail, weighing about 3 g, climbing vertically up a flower stalk. If that snail can put 0.05 mW of power into its ascent, then it will be able to climb at the, even for a snail, fairly moderate pace of roughly 1.5 mm every second. "Snail-power," when delivered as sound directly to our eardrums, is therefore amply sufficient to produce sounds that we would perceive as deafeningly, painfully loud. If the snail in our example could only propel itself with the power equivalent to that delivered to your eardrum by the very weakest audible sounds, a power 12 orders of magnitude smaller, then it would take the snail over two thousand years to climb just a single millimeter! To be able to respond to such unimaginably small quantities of kinetic energy, our ears indeed have to be almost unbelievably sensitive.

When we are dealing with such potentially very large differences in acoustic energy levels, working with orders of magnitude, in a logarithmic decibel scale, rather than with linear units of sound pressure or intensity, keeps the numbers manageably small. But working with decibels brings further, perhaps more important advantages, as it also more directly reflects the way we subjectively perceive sound intensities or loudness. Our ability to detect changes in the amplitude of a sound is governed by Weber's law—at least to a good approximation.[4] Weber's law states that we can detect changes in a particular quantity, like the intensity of a sound, or the weight of a bag or the length of a pencil, only if that quantity changed by more than a given, fixed percentage, the so-called Weber fraction. For broadband noises of an intensity greater than 30 dB SPL, the Weber fraction is about 10%, that is, the intensity has to increase by at least 10% for us to be able to notice the difference (Miller, 1947).

If the increase required to be able to perceive the change is a fixed proportion of the value we already have, then we might expect that the perceived magnitude might be linked to physical size in an exponential manner. This exponential relationship between physical intensity of a sound and perceived loudness has indeed been confirmed experimentally, and is known as Stevens's law (Stevens, 1972). Perceived loudness is, of course, a subjective measure, and varies to some extent from one individual to another, and for reasons that will become clearer when we consider mechanisms of sound capture and transduction by the ear in the next chapter, the relationship between perceived loudness and the physical intensity of a sound will also depend on its frequency content. Nevertheless, for typical listeners exposed to typical sounds, a growth in sound intensity by 10 dB corresponds approximately to a doubling in perceived loudness. Describing sound intensity in terms of decibels, thus, appears to relate better or more directly to how we subjectively perceive a sound than describing it in terms of sound pressure amplitude. But it is important to note that the link between the physical intensity of a sound and its perceptual qualities, like its perceived loudness, is not always straightforward, and there are a number of complicating factors. To deal with at least a few of them, and to arrive at decibel measures that are more directly related to human auditory performance, several other decibel measures were introduced in addition to dB SPL, which we have already encountered. Some of these, which are quite widely used in the literature, are dBA and dB HL, where HL stands for hearing level.

Let us first look at dBA. As you are probably well aware, the human ear is more sensitive to some frequencies than others. Some sounds, commonly referred to as ultrasounds, with a frequency content well above 20 kHz, we cannot hear at all, although other species of animals, for example, dogs, bats, or dolphins, may be able to hear them quite well. Similarly, certain very low (infrasound) frequencies, below 20 Hz, are also imperceptible to us. We tend to be most sensitive to sounds with frequencies between roughly 1 and 4 kHz. For frequencies much below 1 kHz or well above 4 kHz, our sensitivity declines, and when we reach frequencies either below 20 Hz or above 20 kHz, our sensitivity effectively shrinks to nothing. The function that maps out our sensitivity is known as an audiogram, which is effectively a U-shaped curve with maximal sensitivity (lowest detection thresholds) at frequencies between 1 and 4 kHz. The reason that our ears are more sensitive to some frequencies than others seems to stem from mechanical limitations of the outer and middle ear structures whose job it is to transmit sounds from the outside world to the inner ear. We will look at this in more detail in the next chapter.

One consequence of this U-shaped sensitivity curve is that it introduces a massive frequency dependence in the relationship between the acoustic intensity of a sound and its perceived loudness. A 120-dB SPL pure tone of 1 kHz would be painfully loud, and pose a serious threat of permanent damage to your hearing, while a 120-dB SPL pure tone of 30 kHz would be completely inaudible to you, and would also be much safer. When we try to use physical measures of the intensity of ambient sounds to decide how likely a sound is to cause a nuisance or even a health hazard, we need to take this frequency dependence into account. Noise measurements are therefore usually performed with an "A-weighting-filter," a band-pass filter with a transfer function that approximates the shape of the human audiogram and suppresses high and low frequencies at a rate proportional to the decline in human sensitivity for those frequencies. Determining sound intensity in dBA is therefore equivalent to determining dB SPL, except that the sound is first passed through an A-filter.

The link between physical energy, perceived loudness, and potential to cause noise damage is not straightforward. The use of A-weighting filters is only one of many possible approaches to this problem, and not necessarily the best. Other filter functions have been proposed, which go, perhaps unsurprisingly, by names such as B, C, and D, but also, less predictably, by names like ITU-R 468. Each of these possible weighting functions has its own rationale, and may be more appropriate for some purposes than for others; those who need to measure noise professionally may wish to consult the recent Industrial Standards Organization document ISO 226:2003 for further details. Although A-weighting may not always be the most appropriate method, it remains very commonly used, probably because it has been around for the longest time, and almost all commercially available noise level meters will have A-weighting filters built in.

Like dBA, dB HL also tries to take typical human frequency sensitivity into account, but unlike dBA, it is a clinical, not a physical measure: dB HL measurements are not used to describe sounds, but to describe people. When it is suspected that a patient may have a hearing problem, he or she is commonly sent to have a clinical audiogram test performed. During this test, the patient is seated in a soundproof booth and asked to detect weak pure tones of varying frequencies delivered over headphones.

The measured perceptual thresholds are then expressed as sensitivity relative to the threshold expected in normal, young healthy humans. Thus, a patient with normal hearing will have a sensitivity of 0 dB HL. A result of 10 dB HL at a particular frequency means that the patient requires a sound 10 dB more intense than the average young, healthy listener to detect the sound reliably. The patient's detection threshold is elevated by 10 dB relative to what is "normal." In contrast, patients with exceptionally acute hearing may achieve negative dB HL values. A value of +10 dB HL, though slightly elevated, would still be considered within the normal range. In fact, only threshold increases greater than 20 dB would be classified as hearing loss. Since the normal sound sensitivity range covers 12 orders of magnitude, and because sounds with intensities of 20 dBA or less are terribly quiet, losing sensitivity to the bottom 20 dB seems to make little difference to most people's ability to function in the modern world.

Generally, values between 20 and 40 dB HL are considered diagnostic of mild hearing loss, while 40 to 60 dB HL would indicate moderate, 60 to 90 dB HL severe, and more than 90 dB HL profound hearing loss. Note that hearing levels are usually measured at a number of pure tone frequencies, common clinical practice is to proceed in "octave steps" (i.e., successive frequency doublings) from 125 or 250 Hz to about 8 kHz, and patients may show quite different sensitivities at different frequencies.

Conductive hearing loss, that is, a loss of sensitivity due to a mechanical blockage in the outer or middle ear, tends to present as a mild to moderate loss across the whole frequency range. In contrast, sensorineural hearing loss is most commonly caused by damage to the delicate sensory hair cells in the inner ear, which we discuss in the next chapter, and it is not uncommon for such sensorineural losses to affect the sensitivity to high frequencies much more than to low frequencies. Thus, elderly patients often have mild to moderate losses at 8 kHz but normal sensitivity at frequencies below a few kilohertz, and patients who have suffered noise damage frequently present with focal losses of sensitivity to frequencies around 4 kHz. Why some frequency ranges are more easily damaged than others may become clearer when we study the workings of the inner ear, which is the subject of the next chapter.

2 The Ear

In the previous chapter, we saw how sound is generated by vibrating objects in our environment, how it propagates through an elastic medium like air, and how it can be measured and described physically and mathematically. It is time for us to start considering how sound as a physical phenomenon becomes sound as perception. The neurobiological processes involved in this transformation start when sound is "transduced" and encoded as neural activity by the structures of the ear. These very early stages of hearing are known in considerable detail, and this chapter provides a brief summary.

2.1 Sound Capture and Journey to the Inner Ear

Hearing begins when sound waves enter the ear canal and push against the eardrum The eardrum separates the external (or outer) ear from the middle ear. The purpose of the middle ear, with its system of three small bones, or *ossicles*, known as the *malleus*, *incus*, and *stapes* (Latin for hammer, anvil, and stirrup), is to transmit the tiny sound vibrations on to the cochlea,[1] the inner ear structure responsible for encoding sounds as neural signals. Figure 2.1 shows the anatomical layout of the structures involved.

You might wonder, if the sound has already traveled a potentially quite large distance from a sound source to the eardrum, why would it need a chain of little bones to be transmitted to the cochlea? Could it not cover the last centimeter traveling through the air-filled space of the middle ear just as it has covered all the previous distance? The purpose of the middle ear is not so much to allow the sound to travel an extra centimeter, but rather to bridge what would otherwise be an almost impenetrable mechanical boundary between the air-filled spaces of the external and middle ear and the fluid-filled spaces of the cochlea. The cochlea, as we shall see in greater detail soon, is effectively a coiled tube, enclosed in hard, bony shell and filled entirely with physiological fluids known as perilymph and endolymph, and containing very sensitive neural receptors known as "hair cells." Above the coil of the cochlea in figure 2.1, you can see the arched structures of the three semicircular canals of

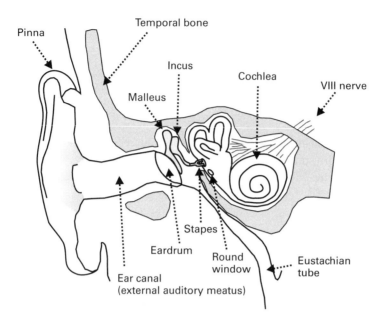

Pinna

Temporal bone

Incus

Cochlea

VIII nerve

Malleus

Stapes

Eardrum

Round
window

Eustachian
tube

Ear canal
(external auditory meatus)

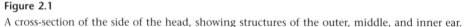

Figure 2.1
A cross-section of the side of the head, showing structures of the outer, middle, and inner ear.

the vestibular system. The vestibular system is attached to the cochlea, also has a bony shell, and is also filled with endolymph and perilymph and highly sensitive hair cells; but the purpose of vestibular system is to aid our sense of balance by collecting information about the direction of gravity and accelerations of our head. It does not play a role in normal hearing and will not be discussed further.

From an acoustical point of view, the fluids inside the cochlea are essentially (slightly salted) water, and we had already mentioned earlier (section 1.7) that the acoustic impedance of water is much higher than that of air. This means, simply put, that water must be pushed much harder than air if the water particles are to oscillate with the same velocity. Consequently, a sound wave traveling through air and arriving at a water surface cannot travel easily across the air-water boundary. The air-propagated sound pressure wave is simply too weak to impart similar size vibrations onto the water particles, and most of the vibration will therefore fail to penetrate into the water and will be reflected back at the boundary. To achieve an efficient transmission of sound from the air-filled ear canal to the fluid-filled cochlea, it is therefore necessary to concentrate the pressure of the sound wave onto a small spot, and that is precisely the purpose of the middle ear. The middle ear collects the sound pressure over the relatively large area of the eardrum (a surface area of about 500 mm^2) and focuses it on the much smaller surface area of the stapes footplate, which is about twenty times smaller. The middle ear thus works a little bit like a thumbtack, collecting pressure over a large area on the blunt, thumb end, and concentrating it on the sharp end, allowing it to be pushed through into a material that offers a high mechanical resistance.

Of course, a thumbtack is usually made of just one piece, but the middle ear contains three bones, which seems more complex than it needs to be to simply concentrate forces. The middle ear is mechanically more complex in part because this complexity allows for the mechanical coupling the middle ear provides to be regulated. For example, a tiny muscle called the stapedius spans the space between the stapes and the wall of the middle ear cavity, and if this muscle is contracted, it reduces the motion of the stapes, apparently to protect the delicate inner ear structures from damage due to very loud sounds.

Sadly, the stapedius muscle is not under our conscious control, but is contracted through an unconscious reflex when we are exposed to continuous loud sounds. And because this stapedius reflex, sometimes called the acoustic reflex, is relatively slow (certainly compared to the speed of sound), it cannot protect us from very sudden loud, explosive noises like gunfire. Such sudden, very intense sounds are therefore particularly likely to damage our hearing. The stapedius reflex is, however, also engaged when we vocalize ourselves, so if you happen to be a gunner, talking or singing to yourself aloud while you prepare to fire might actually help protect your hearing.[2] The stapedius reflex also tends to affect some frequencies more than others, and the fact that it is automatically engaged each time we speak may help explain why most people find their own recorded voice sounds somewhat strange and unfamiliar.

But even with the stapedius muscle relaxed, the middle ear cannot transmit all sound frequencies to the cochlea with equal efficiency. The middle ear ossicles themselves, although small and light, nevertheless have some inertia that prevents them from transmitting very high frequencies. Also, the ear canal, acting a bit like an organ pipe, has its own resonance property. The shape of the human audiogram, the function that describes how our auditory sensitivity varies with sound frequency described in section 1.8, is thought to reflect mostly mechanical limitations of the outer and middle ear.

Animals with good hearing in the ultrasonic range, like mice or bats, tend to have particularly small, light middle ear ossicles. Interesting exceptions to this are dolphins and porpoises, animals with an exceptionally wide frequency range, from about 90 Hz up to 150 kHz or higher. Dolphins therefore can hear frequencies three to four octaves higher than those audible to man. But, then, dolphins do not have an impedance matching problem that needs to be solved by the middle ear. Most of the sounds that dolphins listen to are already propagating through the high-acoustic-impedance environment of the ocean, and, as far as we know, dolphins collect these waterborne sounds not through their ear canals (which, in any event, are completely blocked off by fibrous tissue), but through their lower jaws, from where they are transmitted through the temporal bone to the inner ear.

But for animals adapted to life on dry land, the role of the middle ear is clearly an important one. Without it, most of the sound energy would never make it into the inner ear. Unfortunately, the middle ear, being a warm and sheltered space, is also a cozy environment for bacteria, and it is not uncommon for the middle ear to harbor infections. In reaction to such infections, the blood vessels of the lining of the middle ear will become porous, allowing immune cells traveling in the bloodstream to penetrate into the middle ear to fight the infection, but along with these white blood cells there will also be fluid seeping out of the bloodstream into the middle ear space. Not only do these infections tend to be quite painful, but also, once the middle ear cavity fills up with fluid, it can no longer perform its purpose of providing an impedance bridge between the air-filled ear canal and the fluid-filled cochlea. This condition, known as *otitis media with effusion*, or, more commonly, as glue ear, is one of the most common causes of conductive hearing loss.

Thankfully, it is normally fairly short lived. In most cases, the body's immune system (often aided by antibiotics) overcomes the infection, the middle ear space clears within a couple of weeks, and normal hearing sensitivity returns. A small duct, known as the eustachian tube, which connects the middle ear to the back of the throat, is meant to keep the middle ear drained and ventilated and therefore less likely to harbor bacteria. Opening of the eustachian tube—which occurs, for example, when you yawn—helps to equalize the pressure on either side of the eardrum. If you've ever taken a flight with an upper respiratory tract infection, you are probably all too aware of the painful consequences of not being able to do this when the cabin pressure changes. This is exacerbated in small children, who are much more likely to suffer from glue ear, because the eustachian tube is less efficient at providing drainage in their smaller heads. Children who suffer particularly frequent episodes of otitis media can often benefit from the surgical implantation of a grommet, a tiny piece of plastic tubing, into the eardrum to provide additional ventilation.

When the middle ear operates as it should, it ensures that sound waves are efficiently transmitted from the eardrum through the ossicles to the fluid-filled interior of the cochlea. Figure 2.2 shows the structure of the cochlea in a highly schematic, simplified drawing that is not to scale. For starters, the cochlea in mammals is a coiled structure (see figure 2.1), which takes two and a half turns in the human, but in figure 2.2, it is shown as if it was unrolled into a straight tube. This is fine for our purposes, as the coiling serves only to ensure that the cochlea fits compactly within the temporal bone. The outer wall of the cochlea consists of solid bone, with a membrane lining. The only openings in the hard bony shell of the cochlea are the *oval window*, right under the stapes footplate, and the *round window*, which is situated below. As the stapes vibrates to and fro to the rhythm of the sound, it pushes and pulls on the delicate membrane covering the oval window.

Every time the stapes pushes against the oval window, it increases the pressure in the fluid-filled spaces of the cochlea. Sound travels very fast in water, and the cochlea is a small structure, so we can think of this pressure increase as occurring almost instantaneously and simultaneously throughout the entire cochlea. But because the cochlear fluids are incompressible and almost entirely surrounded by a hard bony shell, these forces cannot create any motion inside the cochlea unless the membrane covering the round window bulges out a little every time the oval window is pushed in, and vice versa. In principle, this can easily happen. Pressure against the oval window can cause motion of a fluid column in the cochlea, which in turn causes motion of the round window.

However, through almost the entire length of the cochlea runs a structure known as the *basilar membrane*, which subdivides the fluid-filled spaces inside the cochlea into upper compartments (the *scala vestibuli* and *scala media*) and lower compartments (the *scala tympani*). The basilar membrane has interesting mechanical properties: It is narrow and stiff at the basal end of the cochlea (i.e., near the oval and round windows), but wide and floppy at the far, apical end. In the human, the distance from the stiff basal to the floppy apical end is about 3.5 cm. A sound wave that wants to travel from the oval window to the round window therefore has some choices to make: It could take a short route (labeled A in figure 2.2), which involves traveling through only small amounts of fluid, but pushing through the stiffest part of the basilar membrane, or it could take a long route (B), traveling through more fluid, to reach a part of the basilar membrane that is less stiff. Or, indeed, it could even travel all the way to the apex, the so-called *helicotrema*, where the basilar membrane ends and the scala vestibuli and scala tympani are joined. There, the vibration would have to travel through no membrane at all. And then there are all sorts of intermediate

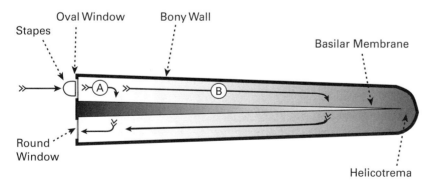

Figure 2.2
Schematic showing the cochlea unrolled, in cross-section. The gray shading represents the inertial gradient of the perilymph and the stiffness gradient of the basilar membrane. Note that these gradients run in opposite directions.

paths, and you might even think that, if this vibration really travels sound wave style, it should not pick any one of these possible paths, but travel down all of them at once.

In principle, that is correct, but just as electrical currents tend to flow to a proportionally greater extent down paths of smaller resistance, most of the mechanical energy of the sound wave will travel through the cochlea along the path that offers the smallest mechanical resistance. If the only mechanical resistance was that offered by the basilar membrane, the choice would be an easy one: All of the mechanical energy should travel to the apical end, where the stiffness of the basilar membrane is low. And low-frequency sounds do indeed predominantly choose this long route. However, high-frequency sounds tend not to, because at high frequencies the long fluid column involved in a path via the apex is itself becoming a source of mechanical resistance, only that this resistance is due to inertia rather than stiffness.

Imagine a sound wave trying to push the oval window in and out, very rapidly, possibly several thousand times a second for a high-frequency tone. As we have already discussed, the sound wave will succeed in affecting the inside of the cochlea only if it can push in and then suck back the cochlear fluids in the scala vestibuli, which in turn pushes and pulls on the basilar membrane, which in turns pushes and pulls on the fluid in the scala tympani, which in turn pushes and pulls on the round window. This chain of pushing and pulling motion might wish to choose a long route to avoid the high mechanical resistance of the stiff basal end of the basilar membrane, but the longer route will also mean that a greater amount of cochlear fluid, a longer fluid column, will have to be accelerated and then slowed down again, twice, on every push and pull cycle of the vibration.

Try a little thought experiment: Imagine yourself taking a fluid-filled container and shaking it to and fro as quickly as you can. First time round, let the fluid-filled container be a small perfume bottle. Second time around, imagine it's a barrel the size of a bathtub. Which one will be easier to shake? Clearly, if you have to try to push and pull heavy, inert fluids forward and backward very quickly, the amount of fluid matters, and less is better. The inertia of the fluid poses a particularly great problem if the vibration frequency is very high. If you want to generate higher-frequency vibrations in a fluid column, then you will need to accelerate the fluid column both harder and more often. A longer path, as in figure 2.2B, therefore presents a greater inertial resistance to vibrations that wish to travel through the cochlea, but unlike the stiffness resistance afforded by the basilar membrane, the inertial resistance does not affect all frequencies to the same extent. The higher the frequency, the greater the extra effort involved in taking a longer route.

The cochlea is thus equipped with two sources of mechanical resistance, one provided by the stiffness of the basilar membrane, the other by inertia of the cochlear fluids, and both these resistances are graded along the cochlea, but they run in opposite directions. The stiffness gradient decreases as we move further away from the oval window, but the inertial gradient increases. We have tried to illustrate these gradients by gray shading in figure 2.2.

Faced with these two sources of resistance, a vibration traveling through the cochlea will search for a "compromise path," one which is long enough that the stiffness has already decreased somewhat, but not so long that the inertial resistance has already grown dramatically. And because the inertial resistance is frequency dependent, the optimal compromise, *the path of overall lowest resistance, depends on the frequency. It is long for low frequencies, which are less affected by inertia, and increasingly shorter for higher frequencies.* Thus, if we set the stapes to vibrate at low frequencies, say a few hundred hertz, we will cause vibrations in the basilar membrane mostly at the apex, a long way from the oval window; but as we increase the frequency, the place of maximal vibration on the basilar membrane shifts toward the basal end. In this manner, each point of the basilar membrane has its own "best frequency," a frequency that will make this point on the basilar membrane vibrate more than any other (see figure 2.3).

This property makes it possible for the cochlea to operate as a kind of mechanical frequency analyzer. If it is furnished with a sound of just a single frequency, then the place of maximal vibration in the basilar membrane will give a good indication of what that frequency is, and if we feed a complex tone containing several frequencies into the cochlea, we expect to see several peaks of maximal excitation, one corresponding to each frequency component in the input signal. (The book's Web site shows

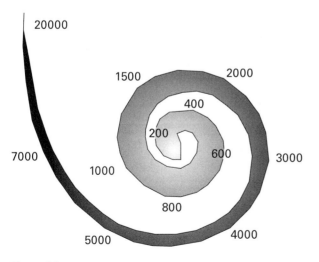

Figure 2.3
Approximate best frequencies of various places along the basilar membrane, in hertz.

several animations illustrating this.) Because of its ability to decompose the frequency content of vibrations arriving at the oval window, the cochlea has sometimes been described as a biological Fourier analyzer. Mathematically, any transformation that decomposes a waveform into a number of components according to how well they match a set of sinusoidal basis functions might be referred to as a Fourier method, and if we understand Fourier methods in quite such broad terms, then the output of the cochlea is certainly Fourier-like. However, most texts on engineering mathematics, and indeed our discussions in chapter 1, tend to define Fourier transforms in quite narrow and precise terms, and the operation of the cochlea, as well as its output, does differ from that of these "standard Fourier transforms" in important ways, which are worth mentioning.

Perhaps the most "standard" of all Fourier methods is the so-called discrete Fourier transform (DFT), which calculates amplitude and phase spectra by projecting input signals onto pure sine waves, which are spaced linearly along the frequency axis. Thus, the DFT calculates exactly one Fourier component for each harmonic of some suitably chosen lowest fundamental frequency. A pure-tone frequency that happens to coincide with one of these harmonics will excite just this one frequency component, and the DFT can, in principle, provide an extremely sharp frequency resolution (although in practice there are limitations, which we had described in section 1.4 under windowing). The cochlea really does nothing of the sort, and it is perhaps more useful to think of the cochlea as a set of mechanical filters. Each small piece of the basilar membrane, together with the fluid columns linking it to the oval and round windows, forms a small mechanical filter element, each with its own resonance frequency, which is determined mostly by the membrane stiffness and the masses of the fluid columns. Unlike the frequency components of a DFT, these cochlear filters are not spaced at linear frequency intervals. Instead, their spacing is approximately logarithmic. Nor is their frequency tuning terribly sharp, and their tuning bandwidth depends on the best (center) frequency of each filter (the equivalent rectangular bandwidth, or ERB, of filters in the human cochlea is, very roughly, 12% of the center frequency, or about one-sixth of an octave, but it tends to be broader for very low frequencies).

We have seen in section 1.5 that if a filter is linear and time invariant, then all we need to know about it is its impulse response. As we shall see in the following sections, the mechanical filtering provided by the cochlea is neither linear, nor is it time invariant. Nevertheless, a set of linear filters can provide a useful first-order approximation of the mechanical response of the basilar membrane to arbitrary sound inputs. A set of filters commonly used for this purpose is the *gamma-tone filter bank*. We have already encountered the gamma-tone filter in figure 1.13. Gamma-tone filters with filter coefficients to match the findings in the human auditory system by researchers like Roy Patterson and Brian Moore have been implemented in Matlab computer code by Malcolm Slaney; the code is freely available and easy to find on the Internet. Figure 2.4

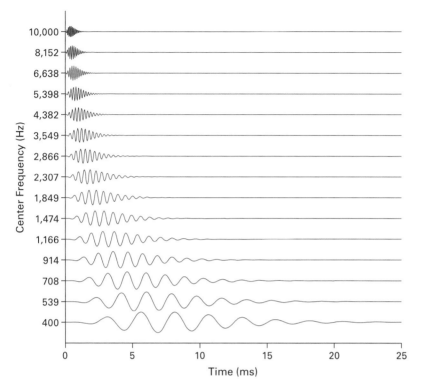

Figure 2.4

A gamma-tone filter bank can serve as a simplified model of the basilar membrane.

shows gamma-tone approximations to the impulse responses of fifteen sites spaced regularly along the basilar membrane between the 400-Hz region near the apex to the 10-kHz region near the base, based on Malcolm Slaney's code. The filters are arranged by best frequency, and the best frequencies of each of the filters are shown along the vertical axis (but note that in this plot, the y-coordinate of each response indicates the amplitude of the basilar membrane vibration, not the frequency).

One thing that is very obvious in the basilar membrane impulse responses shown in figure 2.4 is that the high-frequency impulse responses are much faster than the low-frequency ones, in the sense that they operate over a much shorter time window. If you remember the discussion of the time windows in section 1.5, you may of course appreciate that the length of the temporal analysis window that is required to achieve a frequency resolution of about 12% of the center frequency can be achieved with proportionally shorter time windows as the center frequency increases, which explains why the impulse responses of basal, high-frequency parts of the basilar membrane are shorter than those of the apical, low-frequency parts. A frequency resolution of 12%

of the center frequency does of course mean that, in absolute terms, the high-frequency region of the basilar membrane achieves only a poor spectral resolution, but a high-temporal resolution, while for the low-frequency region the reverse is true.

One might wonder to what extent this is an inevitable design constraint, or whether it is a feature of the auditory system. Michael Lewicki (2002) has argued that it may be a feature, that these basilar membrane filter shapes may in fact have been optimized by evolution, that they form, in effect, a sort of "optimal compromise" between frequency and time resolution requirements to maximize the amount of information that the auditory system can extract from the natural environment. The details of his argument are beyond the scope of this book, and rather than examining the reasons behind the cochlear filter shapes further, we shall look at their consequences in a little more detail.

In section 1.5 we introduced the notion that we can use the impulse responses of linear filters to predict the response of these filters to arbitrary inputs, using a mathematical technique called convolution. Let us use this technique and gamma-tone filter banks to simulate the motion of the basilar membrane to a few sounds, starting with a continuous pure tone.

Figure 2.5A shows the simulated response of a small piece of the basilar membrane near the 1-kHz region to a 1-kHz tone. The best frequencies of the corresponding places on the basilar membrane are plotted on the vertical, y-axis, the gray scale shows

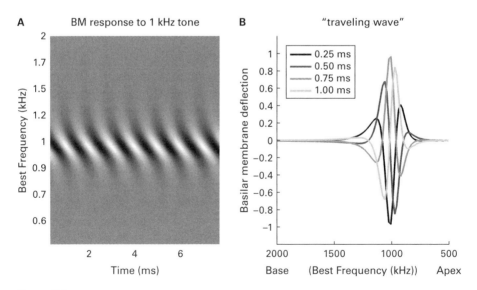

Figure 2.5
Basilar membrane response to a pure tone. Systematic differences in amplitude and time (phase) of the cochlear filters creates a traveling wave.

how far the basilar membrane is deflected from its resting position, and the x-axis shows time. You may recall from our section on filtering that linear filters cannot invent frequencies: Given a sine wave input, they will produce a sine wave output, but the sine wave output may be scaled and shifted in time. The simulated basilar membrane filters behave in just that way too: Each point on the basilar membrane (each row in the left panel of figure 2.5) oscillates at 1 kHz, the input frequency, but those points with best frequencies closest to the input frequency vibrate most strongly, and those with best frequencies far removed from the input frequency vibrate hardly at all. That much you would probably have expected.

But you may also note that the vibrations of the parts of the basilar membrane tuned to frequencies below 1 kHz appear time shifted or delayed relative to those tuned above 1 kHz. This comes about because the mechanical filters that make up the basilar membrane are not all in phase with each other (if you look at figure 2.4, you will see that the impulse responses of the lower-frequency filters rise to their first peak later than those of the high-frequency ones), and this causes the response of the lower-frequency filters to be slightly delayed relative to the earlier ones.

Due to this slight time shift, if you were to look down on the basilar membrane, you would see a traveling wave, that is, it would look as if the peak of the oscillation starts out small at the basal end, grows to reach a maximum at the best frequency region, and then shrinks again. This traveling wave is shown schematically in figure 2.5B. This panel shows snapshots of the basilar membrane deflection (i.e., vertical cuts through figure 2.5A) taken at 0.25-ms intervals, and you can see that the earliest (black) curve has a small peak at roughly the 1.1-kHz point, which is followed 0.25 ms later by a somewhat larger peak at about the 1.05-kHz point (dark gray curve), then a high peak at the 1-kHz point (mid gray), and so on. The peak appears to travel.

The convention (which we did not have the courage to break with) seems to be that every introduction to hearing must mention this traveling wave phenomenon, even though it often creates more confusion than insight among students. Some introductory texts describe the traveling wave as a manifestation of sound energy as it travels along the basilar membrane, but that can be misleading, or at least, it does not necessarily clarify matters. Of course we could imagine that a piece of basilar membrane, having been deflected from its neutral resting position, would, due to its elasticity, push back on the fluid, and in this manner it may help "push it along." The basilar membrane is continuous, not a series of disconnected strings or fibers, so if one patch of the basilar membrane is being pushed up by the fluid below it, it will pull gently on the next patch to which it is attached. Nevertheless, the contribution that the membrane itself makes to the propagation of mechanical energy through the cochlea is likely to be small, so it is probably most accurate to imagine the mechanical vibrations as traveling "along" the membrane only in the sense that they travel mostly *through the fluid next to the membrane* and then *pass through* the basilar membrane as they near the point of lowest resistance, as we have tried to convey in figure 2.2. The traveling wave may then be mostly a curious side effect of the fact that the mechanical filters created by each small piece of basilar membrane, together with the associated cochlear fluid columns, all happen to be slightly out of phase with each other. Now, the last few sentences contained a lot of "perhaps" and "maybe," and you may well wonder, if the traveling wave is considered such an important phenomenon, why is there not more clarity and certainty? But bear in mind that the cochlea is a tiny, delicate structure buried deep in the temporal bone (which happens to be the hardest bone in your body), which makes it very difficult to take precise and detailed measurements of almost any aspect of the operation of the cochlea.

Perhaps the traveling wave gets so much attention because experimental observations of traveling waves on the surface of the basilar membrane, carried out by Georg von Békésy in the 1950s, were among the earliest, and hence most influential, studies into the physiology of hearing, and they won him the Nobel Prize in 1961. They were also useful observations. If the basilar membrane exhibited standing waves, rather than traveling ones, it would indicate that significant amounts of sound energy bounce back from the cochlear apex, and the picture shown in figure 2.2 would need to be revised. The observation of traveling, as opposed to standing, waves therefore provides useful clues as to what sort of mechanical processes can or cannot occur within the cochlea.

But while the traveling wave phenomenon can easily confuse, and its importance may sometimes be overstated, the related notion of *cochlear place coding for frequency,* or *tonotopy*, is undoubtedly an important one. Different frequencies will create maximal vibrations at different points along the basilar membrane, and a mechanism that could measure the maxima in the vibration amplitudes along the length of the cochlea could derive much useful information about the frequency composition of the sound. The basilar membrane is indeed equipped with such a mechanism; it is known as the organ of Corti, and we shall describe its function shortly. But before we do, we should also point out some of the implications and limitations of the mechanical frequency-filtering process of the cochlea.

One very widespread misconception is that there is a direct and causal relationship between cochlear place code and the perception of musical pitch (tone height); that is, if you listen to two pure tones in succession—say first a 1,500-Hz and then a 300-Hz tone—the 300-Hz tone will sound lower *because* it caused maximal vibration at a point further away from the stapes than the 1,500-Hz one did. After our discussion of sound production in chapter 1, you probably appreciate that most sounds, including most "musical" ones with a clear pitch, contain numerous frequency components and will therefore lead to significant vibration on many places along the basilar membrane at once, and trying to deduce the pitch of a sound from where on the basilar membrane vibration amplitudes are maximal is often impossible. In fact, many researchers currently believe that the brain may not even try to determine the pitch of real, complex sounds that way (an animation on the book's Web page showing the response of the basilar membrane to a periodic click train illustrates this).

We will look at pitch perception in much greater detail in chapter 3, but to convey a flavor of some of the issues, and give the reader a better feeling for the sort of raw material the mechanical filtering in the cochlea provides to the brain, we shall turn once more to a gamma-tone filter bank to model basilar membrane vibrations—this time not in response to the perhaps banal 1-kHz pure tone we examined in figure 2.5, but instead to the sound of a spoken word. Figure 2.6 compares the basilar membrane response and the spectrogram of the spoken word "head," which we previously encountered in figure 1.16. You may recall, from section 1.6 in chapter 1, that this spoken word contains a vowel /æ/, effectively a complex tone created by the glottal pulse train, which generates countless harmonics, and that this vowel occurs between two broadband consonants, a fricative /h/ and a plosive /d/. The spacing of the harmonics in the vowel will determine the perceived pitch (or "tone height") of the word. A faster glottal pulse train means more widely spaced harmonics, and hence a higher pitch.

If we make a spectrogram of this vowel using relatively long analysis time windows to achieve high spectral resolution, then the harmonics become clearly visible as stripes placed at regular frequency intervals (left panel of figure 2.6). If we pass the sound instead through a gamma-tone cochlear filter model, many of the higher harmonics largely disappear. The right panel of figure 2.6 illustrates this. Unlike in figure 2.5, which shows basilar membrane displacement at a very fine time resolution, the time resolution here is coarser, and the grayscale shows the logarithm of the RMS

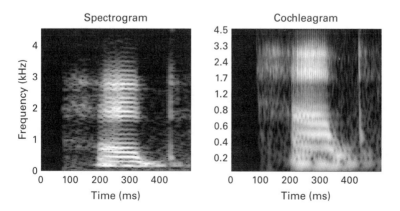

Figure 2.6
Spectrogram of, and basilar membrane response to, the spoken word "head" (compare figure 1.16).

amplitude of the basilar membrane movement at sites with different best frequencies, as shown on the y-axis. (We plot the log of the RMS amplitude to make the output as comparable as possible to the spectrogram, which, by convention, plots relative sound level in dB; that is, it also uses a logarithmic scale). As we already mentioned, the best frequencies of cochlear filters are not spaced linearly along the basilar membrane. (Note that the frequency axes for the two panels in figure 2.6 differ.)

A consequence of this is that the cochlear filters effectively resolve, or zoom in to, the lowest frequencies of the sound, up to about 1 kHz or so, in considerable detail. But in absolute terms, the filters become much less sharp for higher frequencies, so that at frequencies above 1 kHz individual harmonics are no longer apparent. Even at only moderately high frequencies, the tonotopic place code set up by mechanical filtering in the cochlea thus appears to be too crude to resolve the spectral fine structure necessary to make out higher harmonics.[3] The formant frequencies of the speech sound, however, are still readily apparent in the cochlear place code, and the temporal onsets of the consonants /h/ and /t/ also appear sharper in the cochleagram than in the long time window spectrogram shown on the left. In this manner, a cochleagram may highlight different features of a sound from a standard spectrogram with a linear frequency axis and a fixed spectral resolution.

2.2   Hair Cells: Transduction from Vibration to Voltage

As we have seen, the basilar membrane acts as a mechanical filter bank that separates out different frequency components of the incoming sound. The next stage in the auditory process is the conversion of the mechanical vibration of the basilar membrane into a pattern of electrical excitation that can be encoded by sensory neurons in the spiral ganglion of the inner ear for transmission to the brain. As we mentioned earlier, the site where this transduction from mechanical to electrical signals takes place is the organ of Corti, a delicate structure attached to the basilar membrane, as shown in figure 2.7.

Figure 2.7 shows a schematic drawing of a slice through the cochlea, and it is important to appreciate that the organ of Corti runs along the entire length of the basilar membrane. When parts of the basilar membrane vibrate in response to acoustic stimulation, the corresponding parts of the organ of Corti will move up and down together with the membrane. As the inset in figure 2.7 shows, the organ of Corti has a curious, folded structure. In the foot of the structure, the portion that sits directly on the basilar membrane, one finds rows of sensory hair cells. On the modiolar side (the side closer to the modiolus, i.e., the center of the cochlear spiral), the organ of Corti curves up and folds back over to form a little "roof," known as the "tectorial membrane," which comes into close contact with the stereocilia (the hairs) on the

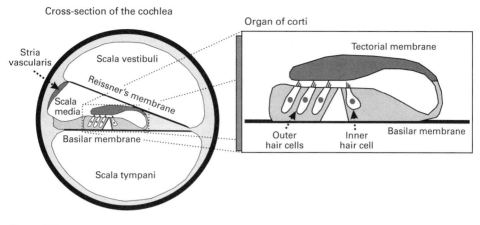

Figure 2.7
Cross-section of the cochlea, and schematic view of the organ of Corti.

sensory hair cells. It is thought that, when the organ of Corti vibrates up and down, the tectorial membrane slides over the top of the hair cells, pushing the stereocilia away from the modiolar side as the organ of Corti is pushed up, and in the opposite direction when it is pushed down.

You may have noticed that the sensory hair cells come in two flavors: inner hair cells and outer hair cells. The inner hair cells form just a single row of cells all along the basilar membrane, and they owe their name to the fact that they sit closer to the modiolus, the center of the cochlea, than the outer hair cells. Outer hair cells are more numerous, and typically form three rows of cells. The stereocilia of the outer hair cells appear to be attached to the tectorial membrane, while those of the inner hair cells may be driven mostly by fluid flowing back and forth between the tectorial membrane and the organ of Corti; however, both types of cells experience deflections of their stereocilia, which reflect the rhythm and the amplitude of the movement of the basilar membrane on which they sit.

Also, you may notice in figure 2.7 that the cochlear compartment above the basilar membrane is divided into two subcompartments, the scala media and the scala vestibuli, by a membrane known as Reissner's membrane. Unlike the basilar membrane, which forms an important and systematically varying mechanical resistance that we discussed earlier, Reissner's membrane is very thin and is not thought to influence the mechanical properties of the cochlea in any significant way. But, although Reissner's membrane poses no obstacle to mechanical vibrations, it does form an effective barrier to the movement of ions between the scala media and the scala vestibuli.

Running along the outermost wall of the scala media, a structure known as the stria vascularis leaks potassium (K^+) ions from the bloodstream into the scala media. As the K^+ is trapped in the scala media by Reissner's membrane above and the upper lining of the basilar membrane below, the K^+ concentration in the fluid that fills the scala media, the endolymph, is much higher than that in the perilymph, the fluid that fills the scala vestibuli and the scala tympani. The stria vascularis also sets up an electrical voltage gradient, known as the endocochlear potential, across the basilar membrane. These ion concentration and voltage gradients provide the driving force behind the transduction of mechanical to electrical signals in the inner ear. Healthy inner ears have an endocochlear potential of about 80 mV or so.

The stereocilia that stick out of the top of the hair cells are therefore bathed in an electrically charged fluid of a high K^+ concentration, and a wealth of experimental evidence now indicates that the voltage gradient will drive K^+ (and some calcium) ions into the hair cells through the stereocilia, but only if the stereocilia are deflected. Each hair cell possesses a bundle of several dozen stereocilia, but the stereocilia in the bundle are not all of the same length. Furthermore, the tips of the stereocilia in each bundle are connected by fine protein fiber strands known as "tip links." Pushing the hair cell bundle toward the longest stereocilium will cause tension on the tip links, while pushing the bundle in the other direction will release this tension. The tip links are thought to be connected, at one or both ends, to tiny ion channels that open in response to stretch on the tip links, allowing K^+ ions to flow down the electrical and concentration gradient from the endolymph into the hair cell. This is illustrated schematically in figure 2.8.

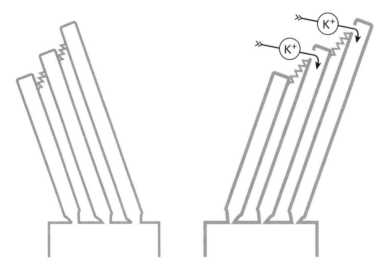

Figure 2.8
Schematic of the hair cell transduction mechanism.

So far, we have discussed hair cell function as if hair cells are all the same, but you already know that there are outer and inner cells, and that some live on high-frequency parts of the basilar membrane and others on low-frequency parts. Do they all function in the same way, or are there differences one ought to be aware of? Let us first consider high- versus low-frequency parts. If you consider the electrical responses shown in figure 2.9 with the tonotopy plot we have seen in figure 2.3, then you may realize that, in real life, most hair cells rarely find the need to switch between AC and DC mode. Hair cells on the basal-most part of the cochlea will, due to the mechanical filtering of the cochlea, experience only high-frequency sounds and should therefore only operate in DC mode.

Well, that is sort of true, but bear in mind that, in nature, high-frequency sounds are rarely continuous, but instead fluctuate over time. A hair cell in the 10-kHz region of the cochlea will be able to encode such amplitude modulations in its membrane potential, but again only to frequencies up to a few kilohertz at most, for the same reasons that a hair cell in the low-frequency regions in the cochlea can follow individual cycles of the sound wave only up to a few kilohertz. Nevertheless, you might wonder whether the hair cells in the high- or low-frequency regions do not exhibit some type of electrical specialization that might make them particularly suitable to operate effectively at their own best frequency.

Hair cells from the inner ear of reptiles and amphibians, indeed, seem to exhibit a degree of electrical tuning that makes them particularly sensitive to certain frequencies (Fettiplace & Fuchs, 1999). But the inner ears of these lower vertebrates differ mechanically from those of mammals, and, so far, no evidence for electrical tuning has been found in mammalian hair cells. Present evidence suggests that the tuning of mammalian hair cells is therefore predominantly or entirely a reflection of the mechanics of the piece of basilar membrane on which they live (Cody & Russell, 1987). But what about differences between outer and inner hair cells? These turn out to be major, and important—so much so that they deserve a separate subsection.

2.3   Outer Hair Cells and Active Amplification

At parties, there are sometimes two types of people: those who enjoy listening to conversation, and those who prefer to dance. With hair cells, it is similar. The job of inner hair cells seems to be to talk to other nerve cells, while that of outer hair cells is to dance. And we don't mean dance in some abstract or figurative sense, but quite literally, in the sense of "moving in tune to the rhythm of the music." In fact, you can find a movie clip showing a dancing hair cell on the Internet. This movie was made in the laboratory of Prof. Jonathan Ashmore, He and his colleagues isolated individual outer hair cells from the cochlea of a guinea pig, fixed them to a patch pipette, and through that patch pipette injected an electrical current waveform of the song "Rock Around the Clock." Under the microscope, one can clearly see that the outer hair cell responds to this electrical stimulation by stretching and contracting rhythmically, following along to the music.

Outer hair cells (OHCs) possess a unique, only recently characterized "motor protein" in their cell membranes, which causes them to shorten every time they are depolarized and lengthen every time they are hyperpolarized. This protein, which has been called "prestin," is not present in inner hair cells or any other cells of the cochlea. The name prestin is very apt. It has the same root as the Italian *presto* for "quick," and prestin is one of the fastest biological motors known to man—much, much faster than, for example, the myosin molecules responsible for the contraction of your muscles. Prestin will not cause the outer hair cells to move an awful lot; in fact, they appear to contract by no more than about 4% at most. But it appears to enable them to carry out these small movements with astounding speed. These small but extremely fast movements do become rather difficult to observe. Most standard video cameras are set up to shoot no more than a few dozen frames a second (they need to be no faster, given that the photoreceptors in the human eye are comparatively slow).

To measure the physiological speed limit of the outer hair cell's prestin motor, therefore, requires sophisticated equipment, and even delivering very fast signals to the OHCs to direct them to move as fast as they can is no easy matter (Ashmore, 2008). Due to these technological difficulties, there is still some uncertainty about exactly how fast OHCs can change length, but we are quite certain they are at least blisteringly, perhaps even stupefyingly fast, as they have been observed to undergo over 70,000 contraction and elongation cycles a second, and some suspect that the OHCs of certain species of bat or dolphin, which can hear sounds of over 100 kHz, may be able to move faster still.

The OHCs appear to use these small but very fast movements to provide a mechanical amplification of the vibrations produced by the incoming sound. Thus, it is thought that, on each cycle of the sound-induced basilar membrane vibration, the OHC's stereocilia are deflected, which causes their membrane to depolarize a little, which causes the cells to contract, which somehow makes the basilar membrane move a little more, which causes their stereocilia to be deflected a little more, creating stronger depolarizing currents and further OHC contraction, and so forth, in a feedforward spiral capable of adding fairly substantial amounts of mechanical energy to otherwise very weak vibrations of the basilar membrane. It must be said, however, that how this is supposed to occur remains rather hazy.

What, for example, stops this mechanical feedback loop from running out of control? And how exactly does the contraction of the hair cells amplify the motion of the basilar membrane? Some experiments suggest that the motility of the OHCs may cause them to "flick" their hair cell bundles (Jia & He, 2005), and thereby pull against the tectorial membrane (Kennedy, Crawford, & Fettiplace, 2005). Indeed, mechanical forces generated by the hair bundles seem to provide the basis for active cochlear amplification in other vertebrate species that lack OHCs. But whether hair bundle movements perform a similar role in mammals, and how they interact with OHC motility, remain areas of active research. Bear in mind that the amplitude of the movement of OHCs is no more than a few microns at most, and they do this work while imbedded in an extremely delicate structure buried deep inside the temporal bone, and you get a sense of how difficult it is to obtain detailed observations of OHCs in action in their natural habitat. It is, therefore, perhaps more surprising how much we already know about the function of the organ of Corti, than that some details still elude us.

One of the things we know with certainty is that OHCs are easily damaged, and animals or people who suffer extensive and permanent damage to these cells are subsequently severely or profoundly hearing impaired, so their role must be critical. And their role is one of mechanical amplification, as was clearly shown in experiments that have measured basilar membrane motion in living cochleas with the OHCs intact and after they were killed off.

These experiments revealed a number of surprising details. Figure 2.10, taken from a paper by Ruggero et al. (1997), plots the mechanical gain of the basilar membrane motion, measured in the cochlea of a chinchilla, in response to pure tones presented at various frequencies and sound levels. The gain is given in units of membrane velocity (mm/s) per unit sound pressure (Pa). Bear in mind that the RMS velocity of the basilar membrane motion must be proportional to its RMS amplitude (if the basilar membrane travels twice as fast, it will have traveled twice as far), so the figure would look much the same if it were plotted in units of amplitude per pressure. We can think of the gain plotted here as the basilar membrane's "exchange rate," as we convert sound pressure into basilar membrane vibration. These gains were measured at the 9-kHz characteristic frequency (CF) point of the basilar membrane, that is, the point which needs the lowest sound levels of a 9-kHz pure tone to produce just measurable vibrations. The curves show the gain obtained for pure-tone frequencies on the x-axis, at various sound levels, indicated to the right of each curve. If this point on the basilar membrane behaved entirely like a linear filter, we might think of its CF as a sort of center frequency of its tuning curve, and would expect gains to drop off on either side of this center frequency.

At low sound levels (5 or 10 dB), this seems to hold, but as the sound level increases, the best frequency (i.e., that which has the largest gains and therefore the strongest response) gradually shifts toward lower frequencies. By the time the sound level reaches 80 dB, the 9-kHz CF point on the basilar membrane actually responds best to frequencies closer to 7 kHz. That is a substantial reduction in preferred frequency, by almost 22%, about a quarter of an octave, and totally unheard of in linear filters. If the cochlea's tonotopy was responsible for our perception of tone height in a direct and straightforward manner, then a piece of music should rise substantially in pitch

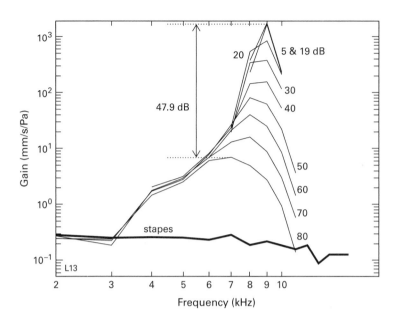

Figure 2.10
Gain of the basilar membrane motion, measured at the 9-kHz characteristic frequency point of
the membrane, in response to tones of various frequencies (shown along the x-axis) at each of
a series of different sound levels (indicated by numbers to the right of each curve).
Adapted from figure 10 of Ruggero et al. (1997) with permission from the Acoustical Society of
America.

if we turn up the volume. That is clearly not the case. Careful psychoacoustical studies
have shown that there are upward pitch shifts with increasing sound intensity, but
they are much smaller than a naïve cochlear place coding hypothesis would lead us
to expect given the nonlinear basilar membrane responses.

   Another striking feature of figure 2.10 is that the gains, the exchange rates applied
as we can convert sound pressure to basilar membrane vibration, are not the same for
weak sounds as they are for intense sounds. The maximal gain for the weakest sounds
tested (5 dB SPL) is substantially greater than that obtained at the loudest sounds tested
(80 dB SPL). Thus, the OHC amplifier amplifies weaker sounds more strongly than
louder sounds, but the amplitude of basilar membrane vibrations nevertheless still
increases monotonically with sound level. In a way, this is very sensible. Loud sounds
are sufficiently intense to be detectable in any event, only the weak sounds need
boosting. Mathematically, an operation that amplifies small values a lot but large
values only a little bit is called a "compressive nonlinearity." A wide range of inputs
(sound pressure amplitudes) is mapped (compressed) onto a more limited range of
outputs (basilar membrane vibration amplitudes).

The OHC amplifier in the inner ear certainly exhibits such a compressive nonlinearity, and thereby helps make the millionfold range of amplitudes that the ear may be experiencing in a day, and which we have described in section 1.8, a little more manageable. This compressive nonlinearity also goes hand in hand with a gain of up to about 60 dB for the weakest audible sounds (you may remember from section 1.8 that this corresponds to approximately a thousandfold increase of the mechanical energy supplied by the sound). This powerful, and nonlinear, amplification of the sound wave by the OHCs is clearly important—we would be able to hear much less well without it, but from a signal processing point of view it is a little awkward.

Much of what we learned about filters in section 1.5, and what we used to model cochlear responses in section 2.1, was predicated on an assumption of linearity, where linearity, you may recall, implies that a linear filter is allowed to change a signal only by applying *constant scale factors* and shifts in time. However, the action of OHCs means that the scale factors are *not* constant: They are larger for small-amplitude vibrations than for large ones. This means that the simulations we have shown in figures 2.4 and 2.5 are, strictly speaking, wrong. But were they only slightly wrong, but nevertheless useful approximations that differ from the real thing in only small, mostly unimportant details? Or are they quite badly wrong?

The honest answer is that, (a) it depends, and (b) we don't really know. It depends, because the cochlear nonlinearity, like many nonlinear functions, can be quite well approximated by a straight line as long as the range over which one uses this linear approximation remains sufficiently small. So, if you try, for example, to model only responses to fairly quiet sounds (say less than 40 dB SPL), then your approximation will be much better than if you want to model responses over an 80- or 90-dB range. And we don't really know because experimental data are limited, so that we do not have a very detailed picture of how the basilar membrane really responds to complex sounds at various sound levels. What we do know with certainty, however, is that the outer hair cell amplifier makes responses of the cochlea a great deal more complicated.

For example, the nonlinearity of the outer hair cell amplifier may introduce frequency components into the basilar membrane response that were not there in the first place. Thus, if you stimulate the cochlea with two simultaneously presented pure tones, the cochlea may in fact produce additional frequencies, known as distortion products (Kemp, 2002). In addition to stimulating inner hair cells, just like any externally produced vibration would, these internally created frequencies may travel back out of the cochlea through the middle ear ossicles to the eardrum, so that they can be recorded with a microphone positioned in or near the ear canal. If the pure tones are of frequencies f_1 and f_2, then distortion products are normally observed at frequencies $f_1 + N(f_2 - f_1)$, where N can be any positive of negative whole number.

These so-called *distortion product otoacoustic emissions* (DPOAEs) provide a useful diagnostic tool, because they occur only when the OHCs are healthy and working as they should. And since, as we have already mentioned, damage to the OHCs is by far the most common cause of hearing problems, otoacoustic emission measurements are increasingly done routinely in newborns or prelingual children in order to identify potential problems early. (Alternatively to DPOAE measurements based on two tones presented at any one time, clinical tests may use very brief clicks to look for transient evoked otoacoustic emissions, or TEOAEs. Since, as we have seen in section 1.3, clicks can be thought of as a great many tones played all at once, distortions can still arise in a similar manner.)

But while cochlear distortions are therefore clinically useful, and they are probably an inevitable side effect of our ears' stunning sensitivity, from a signal processing point of view they seem like an uncalled-for complication. How does the brain know whether a particular frequency it detects was emitted by the sound source, or merely invented by the cochlear amplifier? Distortion products are quite a bit smaller than the externally applied tones (DPOAE levels measured with probe tones of an intensity near 70 dB SPL rarely exceed 25 dB SPL), and large distortion products arise only when the frequencies are quite close together (the strongest DPOAEs are normally seen when $f_2 \approx 1.2 \cdot f_1$). There is certainly evidence that cochlear distortion products can affect responses of auditory neurons even quite high up in the auditory pathway, where they are bound to create confusion, if not to the brain then at least to the unwary investigator (McAlpine, 2004).

A final observation worth making about the data shown in figure 2.10 concerns the widths of the tuning curves. Figure 2.10 suggests that the high gains obtained at low sound levels produce a high, narrow peak, which rides, somewhat offset toward higher frequencies, on top of a low, broad tuning curve, which shows little change of gain with sound level (i.e., it behaves as a linear filter should). Indeed, it is thought that this broad base of the tuning curve reflects the passive, linear tuning properties of the basilar membrane, while the sharp peaks off to the side reflect the active, non-linear contribution of the OHCs. In addition to producing a compressive nonlinearity and shifts in best frequency, the OHCs thus also produce a considerable *sharpening* of the basilar membrane tuning, but this sharpening is again sound-level dependent: For loud sounds, the tuning of the basilar membrane is much poorer than for quiet ones.

The linear gamma-tone filter bank model introduced in figure 2.4 captures neither this sharpening of tuning characteristics for low-level sounds, nor distortion products, nor the shift of responses with increasing sound levels. It also does not incorporate a further phenomenon known as two-tone suppression. Earlier, we invited you to think of each small piece of the basilar membrane, together with its accompanying columns of cochlear fluids and so on, as its own mechanical filter; but as these filters sit side by side on the continuous sheet of basilar membrane, it stands to reason that the behavior of one cochlear filter cannot be entirely independent of those immediately on either side of it. Similarly, the mechanical amplification mediated by the OHCs cannot operate entirely independently on each small patch of membrane. The upshot of this is that, if the cochlea receives two pure tones simultaneously, which are close together in frequency, it cannot amplify both independently and equally well, so that the response to a tone may appear disproportionately small (subject to nonlinear suppression) in the presence of another (Cooper, 1996).

So, if the gamma-tone filter model cannot capture all these well-documented consequences of cochlear nonlinearities, then surely its ability to predict basilar membrane responses to rich, complex, and interesting sounds must be so rough and approximate as to be next to worthless. Well, not quite. The development of more sophisticated cochlear filter models is an area of active research (see, for example, the work by Zilany & Bruce, 2006). But linear approximations to the basilar membrane response provided by a spectrogram or a gamma-tone filter bank remain popular, partly because they are so easy to implement, but also because recordings of neural response patterns from early processing stages of the auditory pathway suggest that these simple approximations are sometimes not as bad as one might perhaps expect (as we shall see, for example, in figure 2.13 in the next section).

2.4 Encoding of Sounds in Neural Firing Patterns

Hair cells are neurons of sorts. Unlike typical neurons, they do not fire action potentials when they are depolarized, and they have neither axons nor dendrites, but they do form glutamatergic, excitatory synaptic contacts with neurons of the spiral ganglion along their lower end. These spiral ganglion neurons then form the long axons that travel through the auditory nerve (also known as the auditory branch of the vestibulocochlear, or VIIIth cranial nerve) to connect the hair cell receptors in the ear to the first auditory relay station in the brain, the cochlear nucleus. The spiral ganglion cell axons are therefore also known as auditory nerve fibers.

Inner and outer hair cells connect to different types of auditory nerve fibers. Inner hair cells connect to the not very imaginatively named type I fibers, while outer hair cells connect to, you guessed it, type II fibers. The type I neurons form thick, myelinated axons, capable of rapid signal conduction, while type II fibers are small, unmyelinated, and hence slow nerve fibers. A number of researchers have been able to record successfully from type I fibers, both extracellularly and intracellularly, so their function is known in considerable detail. Type II fibers, in contrast, appear to be much harder to record from, and very little is known about their role. A number of anatomical observations suggest, however, that the role of type II fibers must be a relatively minor one. Type I fibers aren't just much faster than type II fibers, they also outnumber type II fibers roughly ten to one, and they form more specific connections.

Each inner hair cell is innervated by ten to twenty type I fibers (the numbers seem to vary with the species looked at and may be at the lower end of this range in humans), and each type I fiber receives input from only a single inner hair cell. In this manner, each inner hair cell has a private line consisting of a number of fast nerve fibers, through which it can send its very own observations of the local cochlear vibrations pattern. OHCs connect to only about six type II fibers each, and typically have to share each type II fiber with ten or so other OHCs. The anatomical evidence therefore clearly suggests that information sent by the OHCs through type II fibers will not just be slower (due to lack of myelination) and much less plentiful (due to the relatively much smaller number of axons), but also less specific (due to the convergent connection pattern) than that sent by inner hair cells down the type I fibers.

Thus, anatomically, type II fibers appear unsuited for the purpose of providing the fast throughput of detailed information required for an acute sense of hearing. We shall say no more about them, and assume that the burden of carrying acoustic information to the brain falls squarely on their big brothers, the type I fibers. To carry out this task, type I fibers must represent the acoustic information collected by the inner hair cells as a pattern of nerve impulses. In the previous section, we saw how the mechanical vibration of the basilar membrane is coupled to the voltage across the membrane of the inner hair cell. Synapses in the wall of the inner hair cell sense changes in the membrane voltage with voltage-gated calcium channels, and adjust the rate at which they release the transmitter glutamate according to the membrane voltage. The more their hair cell bundle is deflected toward the tallest stereocilium, the greater the current influx, the more depolarized the membrane voltage, and the greater the glutamate release. And since the firing rate of the type I fibers in turn depends on the rate of glutamate release, we can expect the firing rate of the spiral ganglion cells to reflect the amplitude of vibration of their patch of the basilar membrane.

The more a particular patch of the basilar membrane vibrates, the higher the firing rate of the auditory nerve fibers that come from this patch. Furthermore, the anatomical arrangement of the auditory nerve fibers follows that of the basilar membrane, preserving the tonotopy, the systematic gradient in frequency tuning, described in section 2.1. Imagine the auditory nerve as a rolled-up sheet of nerve fibers, with fibers sensitive to low frequencies from the apical end of the cochlea at the core, and nerve fibers sensitive to increasingly higher frequencies, from increasingly more basal parts of the cochlea, wrapped around this low-frequency center. Thus, the pattern of vibration on the basilar membrane is translated into a neural "rate-place code" in the auditory nerve. As the auditory nerve reaches its destination, the cochlear nuclei, this spiral arrangement unfurls in an orderly manner, and a systematic tonotopy is maintained in many subsequent neural processing stations of the ascending auditory pathway.

Much evidence suggests that the tonotopic rate-place code in the auditory nerve is indeed a relatively straightforward reflection of the mechanical vibration of the basilar

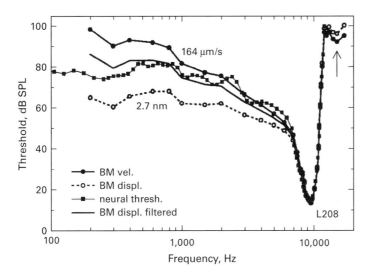

Figure 2.11
Response thresholds of a single auditory nerve fiber (neural thresh) compared to frequency-sound level combinations required to cause the basilar membrane to vibrate with an amplitude of 2.7 nm (BM displ) or with a speed of 164 µm/s (BM vel). The neural threshold is most closely approximated by BM displacement function after high-pass filtering at 3.81 dB/octave (BM displ filtered).
Adapted from Ruggero et al. (2000) with permission from the National Academy of Sciences USA, copyright (2000).

membrane. Consider, for example, figure 2.11, from a study in which Ruggero and colleagues (2000) managed to record both the mechanical vibrations of the basilar membrane and the evoked auditory nerve fiber discharges, using both extracellular recordings in the spiral ganglion and laser vibrometer recordings from the same patch of the basilar membrane. The continuous line with the many small black squares shows the neural threshold curve. Auditory nerve fibers are spontaneously active, that is, they fire even in complete silence (more about that later), but their firing rate increases, often substantially, in the presence of sound.

The neural threshold is defined as the lowest sound level (plotted on the y-axis of figure 2.11) required to increase the firing rate above its spontaneous background level. The auditory nerve fiber is clearly frequency tuned: For frequencies near 9.5 kHz, very quiet sounds of 20 dB SPL or less are sufficient to evoke a measurable response, while at either higher or lower frequencies, much louder sounds are required. The other three lines in the figure show various measures of the mechanical vibration of the basilar membrane. The stippled line shows an isodisplacement contour, that is, it plots the sound levels that were required to produce vibrations of an RMS amplitude of 2.7 nm for each sound frequency. For frequencies near 9.5 kHz, this curve closely matches the neural tuning curve, suggesting that basilar membrane displacements of 2.7 nm or greater are required to excite this nerve fiber. But at lower frequencies, say, below 4 kHz, the isodisplacement curve matches the neural tuning curve less well, and sounds intense enough to produce vibrations with an amplitude of 2.7 nm are no longer quite enough to excite this nerve fiber.

Could it be that the excitation of the auditory nerve fiber depends less on how far the basilar membrane moves, but how fast it moves? The previous discussion of hair cell transduction mechanisms would suggest that what matters is how far the stereocilia are deflected, not how fast. However, if there is any elasticity and inertia in the coupling between the vibration of the basilar membrane and the vibration of the stereocilia, velocities, and not merely the amplitude of the deflection, could start to play a role. The solid line with the small circles shows the isovelocity contour, which connects all the frequency-sound level combinations that provoked vibrations with a mean basilar membrane speed of 164 μm/s at this point on the basilar membrane. At a frequency of 9.5 kHz, the characteristic frequency of this nerve fiber, vibrations at the threshold amplitude of 2.7 nm, have a mean speed of approximately 164 μm/s. The displacement and the velocity curves are therefore very similar near 9.5 kHz, and both closely follow the neural threshold tuning curve. But at lower frequencies, the period of the vibration is longer, and the basilar membrane need not travel quite so fast to cover the same amplitude. The displacement and velocity curves therefore diverge at lower frequencies, and for frequencies above 2 kHz or so, the velocity curve fits the neural tuning curve more closely than the displacement curve.

However, for frequencies below 2 kHz, neither curve fits the neural tuning curve very well. Ruggero and colleagues (2000) found arguably the best fit (shown by the continuous black line) if they assumed that the coupling between the basilar membrane displacement and the auditory nerve fiber somehow incorporated a high-pass filter with a constant roll-off of 3.9 dB per octave. This high-pass filtering might come about if the hair cells are sensitive partly to velocity and partly to displacement, but the details are unclear and probably don't need to worry us here. For our purposes, it is enough to note that there appears to be a close relationship between the neural sensitivity of auditory nerve fibers and the mechanical sensitivity of the cochlea.

You may recall from figure 2.4 that the basilar membrane is sometimes described, approximately, as a bank of mechanical gamma-tone filters. If this is so, and if the firing patterns of auditory nerve fibers are tightly coupled to the mechanics, then it ought to be possible to see the gamma-tone filters reflected in the neural responses. That this is indeed the case is shown in figure 2.12, which is based on auditory nerve fiber responses to isolated clicks recorded by Goblick and Pfeiffer (1969). The responses are from a fiber tuned to a relatively low frequency of approximately 900 Hz, and are shown as peristimulus histograms (PSTHs: the longer the dark bars, the greater the

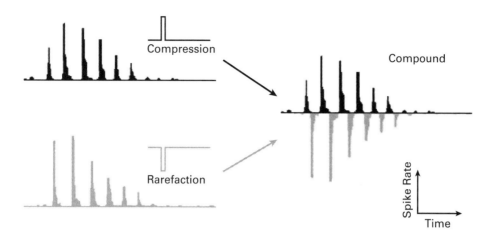

Figure 2.12
Responses of a low-frequency auditory nerve fiber to compression or rarefaction clicks, shown as PSTHs. Basilar membrane ringing causes multiple peaks in the neural discharge in response to a single click. The combined response to compression and rarefaction clicks resembles the impulse response of a gamma-tone filter. Based on data from Goblick and Pfeiffer (1969).

neural firing rate). When stimulated with a click, the 900-Hz region of the basilar membrane should ring, and exhibit the characteristic damped sinusoidal vibrations of a gamma tone. On each positive cycle of the gamma tone, the firing rate of the auditory nerve fibers coming from this patch of the basilar membrane should increase, and on each negative cycle the firing rate should decrease. However, if the resting firing rate of the nerve fiber is low, then the negative cycles may be invisible, because the firing rate cannot drop below zero. The black spike rate histogram at the top left of figure 2.12, recorded in response to a series of positive pressure (compression) clicks, shows that these expectations are entirely born out.

The click produces damped sine vibrations in the basilar membrane, but because nerve fibers cannot fire with negative spike rates this damped sine is half-wave rectified in the neural firing pattern, that is, the negative part of the waveform is cut off. To see the negative part we need to turn the stimulus upside down—in other words, turn compression into rarefaction in the sound wave and vice versa. The gray histogram at the bottom left of figure 2.12 shows the nerve fiber response to rarefaction clicks. Again, we obtain a spike rate function that looks a lot like a half-wave rectified gamma tone, and you may notice that the rarefaction click response is 180° out of phase relative to the compression click response, as it should be if it indeed reflects the negative cycles of the same oscillation. We can recover the negative spike rates that would be observable if neurons could fire less than zero spikes per second if we now flip the rarefaction click response upside down and line it up with the compression click response. This is shown to the right of figure 2.12. The resemblance between the resulting compound histogram and the impulse response waveform of a gamma-tone filter is obvious (compare figure 2.4, p. 59).

So if individual auditory nerve fibers respond approximately like gamma-tone filters, as figure 2.12 suggests, then groups of nerve fibers ought to represent sounds in a manner very much like the cochleagram gamma-tone filter bank we had encountered in figure 2.6 (p. 63). That this is indeed the case is beautifully illustrated by a set of auditory nerve fiber responses recorded by Bertrand Delgutte (1997), and reproduced here in figure 2.13. The nerve fiber responses were recorded in the auditory nerve of an anesthetized cat, and are shown in figure 2.13A as histograms, arranged by each neuron's characteristic frequency, as shown to the left. Below the histograms, in figure 2.13B, you can see the spectrogram of the sound stimulus, the recording of a spoken sentence.

When you compare the spectrogram to the neural responses, you will notice a clear and straightforward relationship between the sound energy and neural firing rate distributions. During the quiet periods in the acoustic stimulus, the nerve fibers fire at some low, spontaneous background rate, but as soon as the stimulus contains appreciable amounts of acoustic energy near the nerve fiber's characteristic frequency, firing rates increase substantially, and the greater the sound intensity, the greater the firing rate increase. The firing rate distribution across this population of auditory nerve fibers has produced a *neurogram* representation of the incoming sounds in the auditory nerve. This neurogram in many ways resembles the short-time spectrogram of the presented speech, and shows formants in the speech sound very clearly.

The neurogram representation in figure 2.13 relies on two basic properties of auditory nerve fibers: first, that they are frequency tuned, and second, that their firing rate increases monotonically with increases in sound level. All of these properties arise simply from the excitatory, synaptic coupling between inner hair cells and auditory nerve fibers. But the synapses linking inner hair cells to auditory nerve fibers appear not to be all the same.

You may recall that each inner hair cell can be connected to as many as twenty type I fibers. Why so many? Part of the answer is probably that more fibers allow a more precise representation of the sound, as encoded in the inner hair cell's membrane voltage. Spike trains are in a sense binary: Nerve fibers, those of the auditory nerve included, are subject to refractory periods, meaning that once they have fired an action potential, they are incapable of firing another for at least 1 ms. Consequently, no neuron can fire at a rate greater than 1 kHz or so, and indeed few neurons appear capable of maintaining firing rates greater than about 600 Hz for any length of time. Consequently, during any short time interval of a millisecond or 2, a nerve fiber either fires an action potential or it does not, which might signal that the sound pressure at the neuron's preferred frequency is large, or that it is not. Of course, if you have several fibers at your

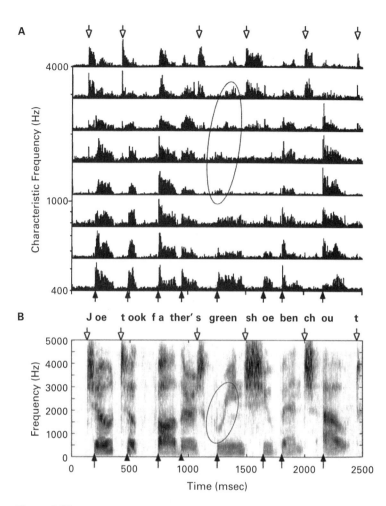

Figure 2.13

(A) Neurogram of the spoken sentence, "Joe took father's green shoe bench out." Poststimulus time histograms of the firing rates of auditory nerve fibers, arranged by each nerve fiber's characteristic frequency. (B) Spectrogram of the spoken sentence shown for comparison. The ellipses are to emphasize that even fine details, like the rapid formant transition in "green," are represented in the dynamic changes of the auditory nerve firing rates.

From Delgutte (1997) with permission from Wiley-Blackwell.

disposal, you can start to send more detailed information. You might, for example, signal that the sound pressure is sort of intermediate, neither very small nor very large, by firing a proportion of the available nerve fibers that corresponds to the strength of the signal. Or you could reserve some nerve fibers exclusively for signaling intense sounds, while others might fire like crazy at the slightest whisper of a sound.

This second option seems to be the one adopted by your auditory nerve. The connections on the modiolar side of the hair cell seem to be less excitable than those facing toward the outside of the cochlear spiral (Liberman, 1982). Nerve fibers connected on the outward-facing side therefore respond even to the quietest sounds, but their firing rates easily saturate, so that at even moderate sound levels of around 30 to 50 dB SPL they fire as fast as they can, and their firing rates cannot increase further with further increases in sound pressure. These highly excitable nerve fibers also have elevated spontaneous firing rates. They fire as many as 20 to 50 spikes or more a second in complete quiet, and they are consequently often referred to as high spontaneous rate fibers. The fibers connected to the inward-facing, modiolar side of the inner hair cells, in contrast, are known either as medium spontaneous rate fibers if they fire less than 18 spikes/s in silence, or as low spontaneous rate fibers, if their spontaneous firing rates are no more than about 1 spike/s. Medium and low spontaneous rate fibers tend not to increase their firing rate above this background rate until sound levels reach at least some 20 to 30 dB SPL, and their responses tend not to saturate until sound levels reach 80 dB SPL or more. The acoustically more sensitive, high spontaneous rate fibers appear to be more numerous, outnumbering the low spontaneous rate fibers by about 4 to 1.

Now, the information that these nerve fibers encode about incoming sounds is, as we had already mentioned, relayed to them from sounds encoded as hair cell membrane potentials via excitatory synapses. You may remember from figure 2.9 that hair cell membrane potentials will encode low frequencies faithfully as analog, AC voltage signals, but for frequencies higher than a few kilohertz, they switch into a DC mode, in which membrane voltage depolarizes with increasing sound level but does not follow individual cycles of the stimulus waveform. This behavior of inner hair cells is also reflected in the firing of the auditory nerve fibers to which they connect. At low frequencies, as the inner hair cell membrane potential oscillates up and down in phase with the incoming sound, the probability of transmitter release at the synapses, and hence the probability of action potential firing of the nerve fiber, also oscillate in step. For low stimulus frequencies, auditory nerve fibers therefore exhibit a phenomenon known as "phase locking," which is illustrated in figure 2.14. (There is also a classic video clip from the University of Wisconsin showing actual recordings of phase locked auditory nerve fiber responses on the book's Web site.)

Figure 2.14 shows a simulation of an extracellular recording of an auditory nerve fiber response (black) to a 100-Hz sine wave (gray). You may observe that the spikes

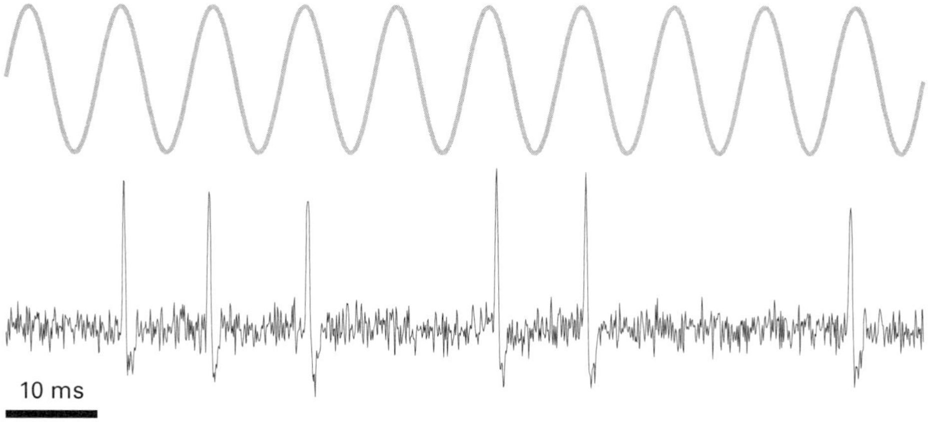

Figure 2.14

Simulation of an auditory nerve fiber recording (black line) in response to a 100-Hz tone (gray line).

tend to occur near the crest of the wave, when the stereocilia of the hair cells are most deflected, the depolarization of the hair cells is greatest, and the rate of neurotransmitter release is maximal. However, it is important to note that this phase locking of the stimulus (i.e., synchronization of the spikes with the crest), the cosine phase, is not a process with clockwork precision. First of all, the spikes do not occur on every crest. This is important if we want to have phase locking but also a spike rate representation of sound intensity. During quiet sounds, a nerve fiber may skip most of the sine wave cycles, but as it gets louder, the fiber skips fewer and fewer cycles, thereby increasing its average firing rate to signal the louder sound. In fact, for very quiet, near-threshold sounds, nerve fibers may not increase their firing rates at all above their spontaneous rate, but merely signal the presence of the sound because their discharges no longer occur at random, roughly Poisson distributed intervals, but achieve a certain regularity due to phase locking. Also note that the spikes are most likely to occur near the crest of the wave, but they are not guaranteed to occur precisely at the top. Action potentials during the trough of the wave are not verboten, they are just less likely.

The phase locking of a nerve fiber response is said to be stochastic, to underline the residual randomness that arises because nerve fibers may skip cycles and because their firing is not precisely time-locked to the crest of the wave. The timing of a single action potential of a single fiber is therefore not particularly informative, but if you can collect enough spikes from a number of nerve fibers, then much can be learned about the temporal fine structure of the sound from the temporal distribution of the spikes. Some authors use the term "volley principle" to convey the idea that, if one nerve fiber skips a particular cycle of sound stimulus, another neighboring nerve fiber may mark it with a nerve impulse. This volley principle seems to make it possible for the auditory nerve to encode temporal fine structure at frequencies up to a few kilohertz, even though no single nerve fiber can fire that fast, and most fibers will have to skip a fair proportion of all wave crests.

There is no evidence at present that auditory nerve fibers use any particularly sophisticated mechanism to take turns in firing phase-locked volleys, but they probably don't need to. Bearing in mind that each inner hair cell connects to ten to twenty nerve fibers, and that the inner hair cells immediately on either side of it must experience virtually identical vibrations, as they sit on more or less the same patch of the basilar membrane, the number of nerve fibers available to provide phase-locked information in any one frequency channel is potentially quite large, perhaps in the hundreds. And there is a lot of evidence that the brain uses the temporal fine structure information conveyed in the spike timing distribution of these fibers in several important auditory tasks, including musical pitch judgments (as we shall see in chapter 3) or the localization of sound sources (as we shall see in chapter 5).

Of course, since phase locking in auditory nerve fibers depends on inner hair cells operating in AC mode, we cannot expect them to phase lock to frequencies or temporal patterns faster than a few kilohertz. That this is, indeed, so has already been demonstrated in auditory nerve fiber recordings conducted many decades ago. Figure 2.15 is based on recordings from an auditory nerve fiber of an anesthetized squirrel monkey, carried out by Rose and colleagues in 1967. Responses to 1,000-, 2,000-, 2,500-, 3,000-, and 4,000-Hz tones are shown. The responses are displayed as period histograms. Period histograms show the number, or the proportion, of action potentials that occur during a particular phase of the stimulus cycle.

In response to the 1,000 Hz sound, the responses were quite obviously phase locked, as a clear majority of spikes happened halfway through the cycle, i.e. ca 180° (π radians) out of phase with the stimulus. (Note that the phase of the stimulus here is determined at the eardrum, and given the phase delays that occur between eardrum and auditory nerve fiber, phase-locked responses need not occur at 0°.) This peak in the period histogram is most obvious in response to the 1,000-Hz tone shown, still quite clear at 2,000 and 2,500 Hz, but definitely on the way out at 3,000 Hz and completely gone at 4,000 Hz.

One thing to point out in the context of figure 2.15 is that it is clearly the frequency content of the sound that determines whether an auditory nerve fiber will phase lock, not the fiber's characteristic frequency. All traces in figure 2.15 show data recorded from one and the same nerve fiber, which happened to have a characteristic frequency of approximately 4,000 Hz. You may be surprised that this 4-kHz fiber, although it is unable to phase lock to tones at its own characteristic frequency, not only clearly responds to 1-kHz sounds, a full two octaves away from its own CF, but also phase

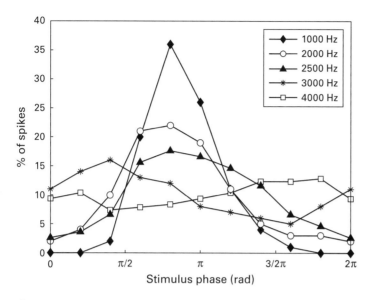

Figure 2.15
Period histograms of responses to pure tones recorded from an auditory nerve fiber in a squirrel monkey. The traces show the proportion of action potentials fired at a particular phase of a pure tone stimulus. The stimulus frequency is indicated in the legend. Based on data collected by Rose et al. (1967).

locks beautifully at these lower frequencies. But bear in mind that the nerve fiber's responses simply reflect both the mechanics of the basilar membrane and the behavior of inner hair cells.

We saw earlier (figure 2.10) that the mechanical tuning of the basilar membrane becomes very broad when stimulated with fairly loud sounds. Consequently, auditory nerve fibers will often happily respond to frequencies quite far removed from their CF, particularly on the lower side, provided these sounds are loud enough. And the AC hair cell responses that are the basis of phase locking appear to occur in similar ways in inner hair cells all along the cochlea. Thus, when we say, on the basis of data like those shown in figure 2.15 and further recordings by many others, that mammals have a phase locking limit somewhere around 3 to 4 kHz, this does not mean that we cannot occasionally observe stimulus-locked firing patterns in neurons that are tuned to frequencies well above 4 kHz. If we stimulate a very sensitive 5-kHz fiber with a very loud 2-kHz tone, we might well observe a response that phase locks to the 2-kHz input. Or we might get high-frequency fibers to phase lock to temporal "envelope patterns," which ride on the high frequencies. Imagine you were to record from a nerve fiber tuned to 10 kHz and present not a single tone, but two tones at once, one of 10 kHz, the other of 10.5 kHz. Since the two simultaneous tones differ in frequency by 500 Hz, they will go in and out of phase with each other 500 times a second, causing rapid cycles of alternating constructive and destructive interference known as "beats." It is a bit as if the 10-kHz tone was switched on and off repeatedly, 500 times a second. Auditory nerve fibers will respond to such a sound, not by phase locking to the 10-kHz oscillation, as that is too high for them, but by phase locking to the 500 Hz beat, the rapid amplitude modulation of this sound. This sort of envelope phase locking to amplitude modulations of a high-frequency signal is thought to be, among other things, an important cue for pitch perception, as we will see in chapter 3.

2.5   Stations of the Central Auditory Pathway

We end this chapter with a whirlwind tour of the main stations of the ascending auditory pathway. The anatomy of the auditory pathway is extraordinarily complicated, and here we will merely offer a very cursory overview of the main processing stations and connections, to orient you and help you embed the discussions in the later chapters in their anatomical context. With that in mind, let us briefly run through the route that acoustic information takes as it travels from the cochlea all the way to the very highest processing centers of your brain.

Upon leaving the cochlea, the auditory nerve fibers join the VIIIth cranial (vestibulocochlear) nerve and enter the cochlear nucleus (CN) in the brainstem. There, they immediately bifurcate. One ascending branch enters the anteroventral cochlear nucleus (AVCN); the other descending branch runs through the posteroventral (PVCN) to the dorsal cochlear nucleus (DCN). Each nerve fiber branch forms numerous synapses with the many distinct types of neurons that populate each of the three subdivisions of the CN. CN neurons come in several characteristic types, which differ in their anatomical location, morphology, cellular physiology, synaptic inputs, and temporal and spectral response properties, as illustrated in figure 2.16.

For example, the AVCN contains so-called spherical and globular bushy cells, which receive a very small number of unusually large, strong, excitatory synapses (the so-called endbulbs of Held) from the auditory nerve fibers. Bushy cells are said to exhibit primary-like responses, which is just a short way of saying that the synaptic coupling between bushy cells and the auditory nerve fibers is so tight that the firing patterns in bushy cells in response to sound are very similar to those in the auditory nerve fibers that drive them. Consequently, they accurately preserve any information carried in the temporal firing patterns of the auditory nerve fibers. Another cell type that can be found in the AVCN and also in the PVCN is the stellate (i.e., star-shaped) cell, which receives convergent inputs from several auditory nerve fibers as well as from other types of neurons. Physiologically, stellate cells of the AVCN are mostly chopper cells, which means they tend to respond to pure-tone stimuli with regular, rhythmic

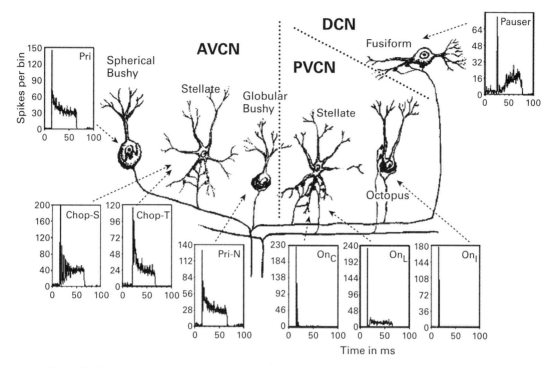

Figure 2.16

Cell types of the cochlear nucleus. Pri, primarylike; Pri-N, primarylike with notch; Chop-S, chopper sustained; Chop-T, chopper transient; On$_C$, onset chopper; On$_L$, onset locker; On$_I$, onset inhibited.

Adapted from original artwork by Prof. Alan Palmer, with kind permission.

bursts, in which the burst frequency appears to be unrelated to that of the tone stimuli. Thus, these neurons do not preserve the timing of their input spikes, but they tend to have narrower frequency tuning, and possibly also a larger dynamic range, than their auditory nerve inputs. This may make them better suited for coding details of the spectral shape of the incoming stimuli.

In the PVCN, one frequently finds onset cells that respond to pure-tone bursts with just a single action potential at the start of the sound. Morphologically, these onset cells are either stellate (with somewhat different intrinsic properties from the choppers), or octopus shaped. They receive convergent input from many auditory nerve fibers and are therefore very broadly frequency tuned. While they mark the onset of pure tones with great accuracy (their response latency jitter is in the range of tens of microseconds), it would nevertheless be misleading to think of the purpose of these cells as only marking the beginning of a sound. In fact, if these cells are stimulated with complex tones, for example, a 300-Hz and a 400-Hz tone played together so that they would beat against each other 100 times a second, then the onset cells would mark not just the beginning of this complex tone, but every beat, with an action potential. These cells may therefore provide much more detail about the time structure of a complex tone than the term "onset cell" would suggest. In contrast, cells in the DCN, which have more complex, pauser-type temporal response patterns and can have a fusiform (or pyramidal) morphology, exhibit responses that are often characterized by being inhibited by some frequencies, as well as excited by others. Thus, while VCN cells may be specialized for processing the temporal structure of sounds, DCN cells may play a particular role in detecting spectral contrasts. To make all of this even more perplexing, the DCN receives, in addition to its auditory inputs, some somatosensory input from the skin. Note that cognoscenti of the cochlear nucleus distinguish further subtypes among the major classes we have just discussed, such as choppertransients or onset-lockers or primary-like with notch, but a detailed discussion of these distinctions is unnecessary at this stage.

The various principal cell types in the CN also send their outputs to different parts of the ascending auditory pathway. The major stations of that pathway are illustrated schematically in figure 2.17. All (or almost all) of the outputs from the CN will eventually reach the first major acoustic processing station of the midbrain, the inferior colliculus (IC), but while most stellate and most DCN cells send axons directly to the IC, the outputs from AVCN bushy cells take an indirect route, as they are first relayed through the superior olivary complex (SOC) of the brainstem. At the olivary nuclei, there is convergence of a great deal of information from the left and right ears, and these nuclei make key contributions to our spatial (stereophonic) perception of sound. We will therefore revisit the SOC in some detail when we discuss spatial hearing in chapter 5.

Axons from the cochlear and superior olivary nuclei then travel along a fiber bundle known as the lateral lemniscus to the IC. On the way, they may or may not send side branches to the ventral, intermediate or dorsal nuclei of the lateral lemniscus (NLL). Note that the paths from CN to the IC are predominantly crossed, and so neurons in the midbrain and cortex tend to be most strongly excited by sounds presented to the opposite, contralateral ear.

The IC itself has a complex organization, with a commissural connection between the left and right IC that allows for yet further binaural interactions within the ascending pathway. There are also numerous interneurons within the IC, which presumably perform all manner of as yet poorly understood operations. The IC is subdivided into several subnuclei. The largest, where most of the inputs from the brainstem arrive, is known as the central nucleus of the IC (ICC), and it is surrounded by the dorsal cortex at the top, the external or lateral nucleus (ICX), and the nucleus of the brachium of the IC (nBIC) at the side. The nBIC sends axons to a gaze control center known as

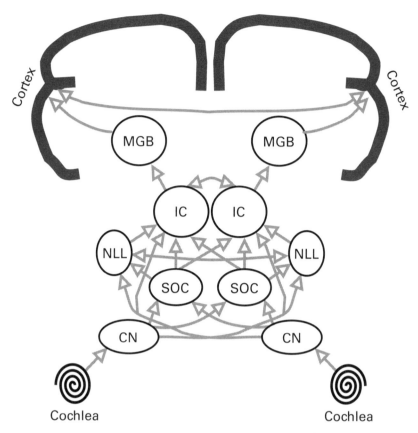

Figure 2.17
Simplified schematic of the ascending auditory pathway. CN, cochlear nuclei; SOC, superior olivary complex; NLL, nuclei of the lateral lemniscus; IC, inferior colliculus; MGB, medial geniculate body.

the superior colliculus (SC), to enable reflexive eye and head movements toward unexpected sounds. However, most of the axons leaving the nuclei of the IC travel through the fiber bundle of the brachium toward the major auditory relay nucleus of the thalamus, the medial geniculate body (MGB). The MGB, too, has several distinct subdivisions, most notably its ventral, dorsal, and medial nuclei. Note that the CN, the SOC, the NLL, as well as the ICC and the ventral division of the MGB all maintain a clear tonotopic organization, that is, neurons within these nuclei are more or less sharply frequency tuned and arranged anatomically according to their characteristic frequency. Thus, in the ICC, for example, neurons tuned to low frequencies are found near the dorsal surface and neurons with progressively higher characteristic frequencies are found at increasingly deeper, more ventral locations. In contrast, the ICX, nBIC, and dorsal division of the MGB lack a clear tonotopic order. Tonotopically organized auditory midbrain structures are sometimes referred to as "lemniscal," and those that lack tonotopic order as "nonlemniscal."

Some thalamic output fibers from the MGB then connect to limbic structures of the brain, such as the amygdala, which is thought to coordinate certain types of emotional or affective responses and conditioned reflexes to sound, but the large majority of fibers from the thalamus head for the auditory cortex in the temporal lobes. The auditory cortical fields on either side are also interconnected via commissural connections through the corpus callosum, providing yet another opportunity for an exchange of information between left and right, and, indeed, at the level of the auditory cortex, the discharge patterns of essentially all acoustically responsive neurons can be influenced by stimuli delivered to either ear.

The auditory cortex, too, is subdivided into a number of separate fields, some of which show relatively clear tonotopic organization, and others less so. Apart from their tonotopy, different cortical fields are distinguished by their anatomical connection patterns (how strong a projection they receive from which thalamic nucleus, and which brain regions they predominantly project to), physiological criteria (whether neurons are tightly frequency tuned or not, respond at short latencies or not, etc.) or their content of certain cell-biological markers, such as the protein parvalbumin. Up to and including the level of the thalamus, the organization of the ascending auditory pathway appears to be fairly stereotyped among different mammalian species. There are some differences; for example, rats have a particularly large intermediate NLL, cats a particularly well-developed lateral superior olivary nucleus, and so on, but cats, rats, bats, and monkeys nevertheless all have a fundamentally similar organization of subcortical auditory structures, and anatomically equivalent structures can be identified without too much trouble in each species. Consequently, the anatomical names we have encountered so far apply equally to all mammals. Unfortunately, the organization of auditory cortical fields may differ from one species of mammal to the next, particularly in second- or third-order areas, and very different names are used to designate cortical fields in different species. We illustrate the auditory cortex of ferrets, cats, and monkeys in figure 2.18. Note that the parcellations shown in figure 2.18 are based in large part on anatomical tract tracer injection and extracellular recording studies, which cannot readily be performed in humans, and our understanding of the organization of human auditory cortex therefore remains fairly sketchy, but we will say a bit more about this in chapter 4 when we discuss the processing of speech sounds.

It may be that some of the fields that go by different names in different species actually have rather similar functions, or common evolutionary histories. For example, both carnivores and primates have two primary cortical areas, which lie side-by-side and receive the heaviest thalamic input; but while these fields are called A1 (primary

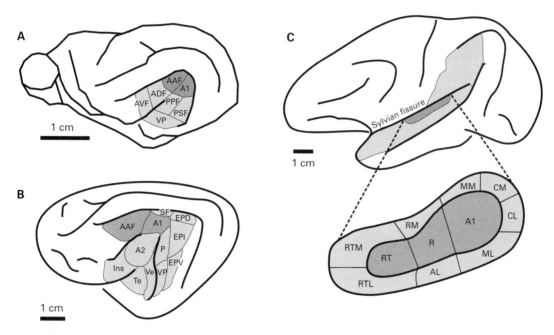

Figure 2.18
Drawings showing identified auditory cortical areas in the ferret (A), the cat (B) and the rhesus macaque (C). Primary areas are shown in dark gray, higher-order (belt and parabelt) areas in light gray.

auditory cortex) and AAF (for anterior auditory field) in carnivores, they are designated as A1 and R in monkeys. To what extent AAF and R are really equivalent is uncertain. Similarly, the cat's posterior auditory field (P, or PAF) shows certain similarities with the monkey's areas CL and CM, but it remains unclear what the homologous regions might be in other species. It is easily possible, perhaps even likely, that there may be quite fundamental differences in the organization of auditory cortex in different species. The cortex is after all the youngest and most malleable part of the brain in evolutionary terms. Thus, the auditory cortex of echolocating bats features a number of areas that appear to be specialized for the processing of echo delays and Doppler shifts for which there is no obvious equivalent in the brain of a monkey.

What seems to be true for all mammals, though, is that one can distinguish primary (or core) and second-order (belt) areas of auditory cortex, and these interact widely with the rest of the brain, including the highest-order cognitive structures, such as prefrontal lobe areas thought to be involved in short-term memory and action planning, or the inframtemporal structures thought to mediate object recognition. To the best of our knowledge, without these very high level cortical areas, we would be unable to recognize the sound of a squealing car tire, or to remember the beginning of a spoken sentence by the time the sentence is concluded, so they, too, are clearly integral parts of the auditory brain.

Our whirlwind tour of the auditory pathway has, thus, finally arrived at the very highest levels of the mammalian brain, but we do not want to leave you with the impression that in this pathway information only flows upwards, from the cochlea toward the cortex. There are also countless neurons relaying information back down, from frontal cortex to auditory cortex, from auditory cortex to each subcortical processing level—particular the MGB and the IC, but also the NLL, the SOC and the CN —and, in turn, from each subcortical station to the auditory nuclei below it. These descending projections even go all the way back to the cochlea. Thus, "olivocochlear bundle" axons originate in the SOC and travel with the VIIIth cranial nerve to synapse either directly with the outer hair cells or on the endings of the auditory nerve fibers that innervate the inner hair cells. This anatomical arrangement indicates that auditory processing does not occur in a purely feedforward fashion. It can incorporate feedback loops on many levels, which make it possible to retune the system on the fly, right down to the level of the mechanics of the cochlea, to suit the particular demands the auditory system faces in different environments or circumstances.

3 Periodicity and Pitch Perception: Physics, Psychophysics, and Neural Mechanisms

The American National Standards Institute (ANSI, 1994) defines pitch as "that auditory attribute of sound according to which sounds can be ordered on a scale from low to high." Thus, pitch makes it possible for us to appreciate melodies in music. By simultaneously playing several sounds with different pitches, one can create harmony. Pitch is also a major cue used to distinguish between male and female voices, or adult and child voices: As a rule, larger creatures produce vocalizations with a lower pitch (see chapter 1). And pitch can help convey meaning in speech—just think about the rising melody of a question ("You really went there?") versus the falling melody of a statement ("You really went there!"); or you may be aware that, in tonal languages like Mandarin Chinese, pitch contours differentiate between alternative meanings of the same word. Finally, pitch also plays less obvious roles, in allowing the auditory system to distinguish between inanimate sounds (most of which would not have pitch) and animal-made sounds (many of which do have a pitch), or to segregate speech of multiple persons in a cocktail party. Pitch therefore clearly matters, and it matters because the high pitch of a child's voice is a quintessential part of our auditory experience, much like an orange-yellow color would be an essential part of our visual experience of, say, a sunflower.

The ANSI definition of pitch is somewhat vague, as it says little about what properties the "scale" is meant to have, nor about who or what is supposed to do the ordering. There is a clear consensus among hearing researchers that the "low" and "high" in the ANSI definition are to be understood in terms of musical notes, and that the ordering is to be done by a "listener." Thus, pitch is a percept that is evoked by sounds, rather than a physical property of sounds. However, giving such a central role to our experience of sound, rather than to the sound itself, does produce a number of complications. The most important complication is that the relationship between the physical properties of a sound and the percepts it generates is not always straightforward, and that seems particularly true for pitch. For example, many different sounds have the same pitch—you can play the same melody with a (computer-generated) violin or with a horn or with an oboe (Sound Example "Melodies and

Timbre" on the book's Web site). What do the many very different sounds we perceive as having the same pitch have in common?

As we tackle these questions, we must become comfortable with the idea that pitch is to be judged by the listener, and the correct way to measure the pitch of a sound is, quite literally, to ask a number of people, "Does this sound high or low to you?," and hope that we get a consistent answer. A complete understanding of the phenomenon of pitch would need to contain an account of how the brain generates subjective experiences. That is a very tall order indeed, and as we shall see, even though the scientific understanding of pitch has taken great strides in recent decades, a large explanatory gap still remains.

But we are getting ahead of ourselves. Even though pitch is ultimately a subjective percept rather than a physical property of sounds, we nevertheless know a great deal about what sort of sounds are likely to evoke particular types of pitch percept. We shall therefore start by describing the physical attributes of sound that seem most important in evoking particular pitches, briefly review psychoacoustics of pitch perception in people and animals, and briefly outline the conventions used for classifying pitches in Western music, before moving on to a discussion of how pitch cues are encoded and processed in the ascending auditory pathway.

3.1 Periodicity Is the Major Cue for Pitch

Probably the most important determinant of the pitch of a sound is its "periodicity." A sound is periodic when it is composed of consecutive repetitions of a single short segment (figure 3.1). The duration of the repeated segment is called the period (abbreviated T). In figure 3.1, the period is 1 s. Sometimes, the whole repeated segment is called the period—we shall use both meanings interchangeably. Only a small number of repetitions of a period are required to generate the perception of pitch (Sound Example "How many repetitions are required to produce pitch?" on the book's Web site). Long periods result in sounds that evoke low pitch, while short periods result in sounds that evoke high pitch.

Periodicity is, however, most often quantified not by the period, but rather by the "fundamental frequency" (F_0 in hertz), which is the number of times the period repeats in 1 s ($F_0 = 1/T$). For example, if the period is 1 ms (1/1,000 s), the fundamental frequency is 1,000 Hz. Long periods correspond to low fundamental frequencies, usually evoking low pitch, while short periods correspond to high fundamental frequencies, usually evoking high pitch. As we will see later, there are a number of important deviations from this rule. However, for the moment we describe the picture in its broad outlines, and we will get to the exceptions later.

This is a good point to correct a misconception that is widespread in neurobiology texts. When describing sounds, the word "frequency" is often used to describe two

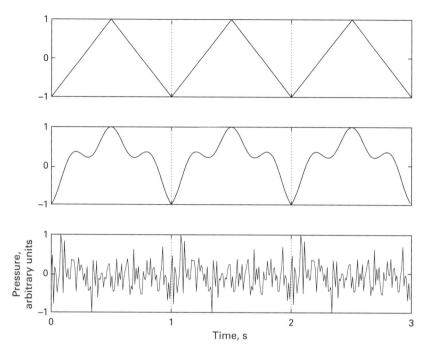

Figure 3.1

Three examples of periodic sounds with a period of 1 s. Each of the three examples consists of a waveform that repeats itself exactly every second.

rather different notions. The first is frequency as a property of pure tones, or a property of Fourier components of a complex sound, as we discussed in chapter 1, section 1.3. When we talk about frequency analysis in the cochlea, we use this notion of frequency, and one sound can contain many such frequency components at once. In fact, we discussed the frequency content of complex sounds at length in chapter 1, and from now on, when we use the terms "frequency content" or "frequency composition," we will always be referring to frequency in the sense of Fourier analysis as described in chapter 1. However, we have now introduced another notion of frequency, which is the fundamental frequency of a periodic sound and the concomitant pitch that such a sound evokes.

Although for pure tones the two notions of frequency coincide, it is important to realize that these notions of frequency generally mean very different things: Pitch is not related in a simple way to frequency content as we defined it in chapter 1. Many sounds with the same pitch may have very different frequency composition, while sounds with fairly similar frequency composition may evoke different pitches. In particular, there is no "place code" for pitch in the cochlea—the place code of the cochlea is for frequency content, not for pitch. In fact, sounds with the same pitch may excite different positions along the cochlea, while sounds with different pitch may excite identical locations along the cochlea. In order to generate the percept of pitch, we need to process heavily the signals from the cochlea and often to integrate information over many cochlear places. We will learn about some of these processes later. For the rest of this chapter, we will use F_0 to signify fundamental frequency.

As a rule, periodic sounds are said to evoke the perception of pitch at their F_0. But what does that mean? By convention, we use the pitch evoked by pure tones as a yardstick with respect to which we judge the pitch evoked by other sounds. In practical terms, this is performed by matching experiments: A periodic sound whose pitch we want to measure is presented alternately with a pure tone. Listeners are asked to change the frequency of the pure tone until it evokes the same pitch as the periodic sound. The frequency of the matching pure tone then serves as a quantitative measure of the pitch of the tested periodic sound. In such experiments, subjects most often set the pure tone so that its period is equal to the period of the test sound (Sound Example "Pitch Matching" on the book's Web site).

At this point, it's time to mention complications that have to be added on top of the rather simple picture presented thus far. As we shall see again and again, every statement about the relationships between a physical characteristic of sounds and the associated perceptual quality will have many cautionary notes attached (often in "fine print"). Here are already a number of such fine print statements:

First, periodic sounds composed of periods that are too long do not evoke pitch at their F_0. They may instead be perceived as a flutter—a sequence of rapidly repeating discrete events—or they may give rise to a sensation of pitch at a value that is different from their period (we will encounter an example later in this chapter). To evoke pitch at the fundamental frequency, periods must be shorter than about 25 ms (corresponding to an F_0 above about 40 Hz). Similarly, if the periods are too short, less than about 0.25 ms (i.e., the F_0 is higher than 4,000 Hz), the perception of pitch seems to deteriorate (Sound Example "The Range of Periods that Evoke Pitch" on the book's Web site). For example, the ability to distinguish between different F_0 values declines substantially, and intervals do not sound quite the same.

Second, as alluded to earlier, many sounds that are not strictly periodic also have pitch. If the periods are absolutely identical, the sound might be called strictly periodic, but it is usually enough for subsequent periods to be similar to each other for the sound to evoke pitch. We therefore don't think of periodicity as an all-or-none property. Rather, sounds may be more or less periodic according to the degree to which successive periods are similar to each other. We shall consider later ways of measuring the amount of periodicity, and relate it to the saliency or strength of the evoked pitch. Sounds that are not strictly periodic but do evoke pitch are typical—human voices are rarely strictly periodic (figure 3.2 and Sound Example "Vowels are not strictly periodic"

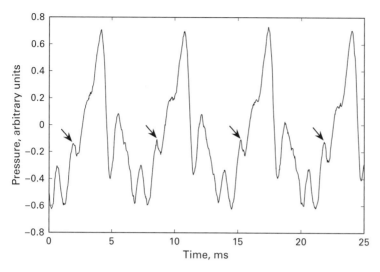

Figure 3.2

Four periods of the vowel /a/ from natural speech. The periods are similar but not identical (note the change in the shape of the feature marked by the arrows between successive periods).

 on the book's Web site)—and the degree of periodicity that is sufficient for evoking pitch can be surprisingly small, as we shall see later. Pitch can even be evoked by presenting a different sound to each ear, each of which, when presented alone, sounds completely random; in those cases, it is the interaction between the sounds in the two ears that creates an internal representation of periodicity that is perceived as pitch.

3.2   The Relationship between Periodicity, Frequency Content, and Pitch

In chapter 1, we discussed Fourier analysis—the expression of any sound as a sum of sine waves with varying frequencies, amplitudes, and phases. In the previous section, we discussed pure tones (another name for pure sine waves) as a yardstick for judging the pitch of a general periodic sound. These are two distinct uses of pure tones. What is the relationship between the two?

To consider this, let us first look at strictly periodic sounds. As we discussed in chapter 1, there is a simple rule governing the frequency representation of such sounds: All their frequency components should be multiples of F_0. Thus, a sound whose period, T, is 10 ms (or 0.01 s, corresponding to a F_0 of 100 Hz as $F_0 = 1/T$) can contain frequency components at 100 Hz, 200 Hz, 300 Hz, and so on, but cannot contain a frequency component at 1,034 Hz. Multiples of F_0 are called harmonics (thus, 100 Hz, 200 Hz, 300 Hz, and so on are harmonics of 100 Hz). The multiplier is called the number, or order, of the harmonic. Thus, 200 Hz is the second harmonic of 100 Hz, 300 Hz is the third harmonic of 100 Hz, and the harmonic number of 1,000 Hz (as a harmonic of 100 Hz) is ten.

It follows that a complex sound is the sum of many pure tones, each of which, if played by itself, evokes a different pitch. Nevertheless, most complex sounds would evoke a single pitch, which may not be related simply to the pitch of the individual frequency components. A simple relationship would be, for example, for the pitch evoked by a periodic sound to be the average of the pitch that would be evoked by its individual frequency components. But this is often not the case: For a sound with a period of 10 ms, which evokes a pitch of 100 Hz, only one possible component, at 100 Hz, has the right pitch. All the other components, by themselves, would evoke the perception of other, higher, pitch values. Nevertheless, when pure tones at 100 Hz, 200 Hz, and so on are added together, the overall perception is that of a pitch at F_0, that is, of 100 Hz.

Next, a periodic sound need not contain all harmonics. For example, a sound composed of 100, 200, 400, and 500 Hz would evoke a pitch of 100 Hz, in spite of the missing third harmonic. On the other hand, not every subset of the harmonics of 100 Hz would result in a sound whose pitch is 100 Hz. For example, playing the "harmonic" at 300 Hz on its own would evoke a pitch at 300 Hz, not at 100 Hz. Also, playing the even harmonics at 200, 400, 600 Hz, and so on, together, would result in a sound whose pitch is 200 Hz, not 100 Hz. This is because 200 Hz, 400 Hz, and 600 Hz, although all harmonics of 100 Hz (divisible by 100), are also harmonics of 200 Hz (divisible by 200). It turns out that, in such cases, it is the largest common divisor of the set of harmonic frequencies that is perceived as the pitch of the sound. In other words, to get a sound whose period is 10 ms, the frequencies of the harmonics composing the sound must all be divisible by 100 Hz, but not divisible by any larger number (equivalently, the periods of the harmonics must all divide 10 ms, but must not divide any smaller number).

Thus, for example, tones at 200 Hz, 300 Hz, and 400 Hz, when played together, create a sound with a pitch of 100 Hz. The fact that you get a pitch of 100 Hz with sounds that do not contain a frequency component at 100 Hz was considered surprising, and such sounds have a name: sounds with a missing fundamental. Such sounds, however, are not uncommon. For example, many small loudspeakers (such as the cheap loudspeakers often used with computers) cannot reproduce frequency components below a few hundred hertz. Thus, deep male voices, reproduced by such loudspeakers, will "miss their fundamental." As long as we consider pitch as the perceptual correlate of periodicity, there is nothing strange about pitch perception with a missing fundamental.

But this rule is not foolproof. For example, adding the harmonics 2,100, 2,200, and 2,300 would produce a sound whose pitch would be determined by most listeners to be about 2,200 Hz, rather than 100 Hz, even though these three harmonics of 100 Hz have 100 as their greatest common divisor, so that their sum is periodic with a period of 10 ms (100 Hz). Thus, a sound composed of a small number of high-order harmonics will not necessarily evoke a pitch percept at the fundamental frequency (Sound Example "Pitch of 3-Component Harmonic Complexes" on the book's Web site).

There are quite a few such exceptions, and they have been studied in great detail by psychoacousticians. Generally, they are summarized by stating that the periodicity as the determinant of pitch has "existence regions": combinations of periodicity and harmonic numbers that would give rise to a perception of pitch at the fundamental frequency. The existence regions of pitch are complex, and their full description will not be attempted here (see Plack & Oxenham, 2005).

What happens outside the existence regions? As you may have noticed if you had a chance to listen to Sound Example "Pitch of 3-Component Harmonic Complexes" on the book's Web site, such a sound does not produce a pitch at its F_0, but it does evoke a pitch that is, in this case, related to its frequency content: This sound would cause the cochlea to vibrate maximally at the location corresponding to 2,100 Hz. There are a number of other sound families like this one, where pitch is determined by the cochlear place that is maximally stimulated. Pitch is notably determined by the cochlear place in cochlear implant users, whose pitch perception is discussed in chapter 8. Some authors would call this type of pitch "place pitch" and differentiate it from the periodicity pitch we discuss here. The important fact is that the extent of the existence regions for periodicity pitch is large, and consequently, for essentially all naturally occurring periodic sounds, the period is the major determinant of pitch.

We already mentioned that there are sounds that are not strictly periodic but are nonetheless sufficiently periodic to evoke a pitch. What about their frequency composition? These sounds will usually have a frequency content that resembles a series of harmonics. Figure 3.3 (Sound Example "Non-Periodic Sounds That Evoke Pitch" on the book's Web site) shows three stimuli with this characteristic. The first is a strictly periodic sound to which white noise is added. The frequency content of this sound is the sum of the harmonic series of the periodic sound and the white noise. Thus, although it is not a pure harmonic series, such a spectrum is considered to be a minor variation on a harmonic series.

The second example comes from a family of stimuli called iterated repeated noise (also called iterated ripple noise, or IRN), which will play an important role later in the chapter. To create such a sound, we take a segment of white noise, and then add to it a delayed repeat of the same noise (i.e., an identical copy of the noise that has been shifted in time by exactly one period). Any leftovers at the beginning and the end of the segment that have had no delayed copies added to them are discarded. This operation can be repeated (iterated) a number of times, hence the name of this family of stimuli. The sound in figure 3.3B was created using eight iteration steps. In

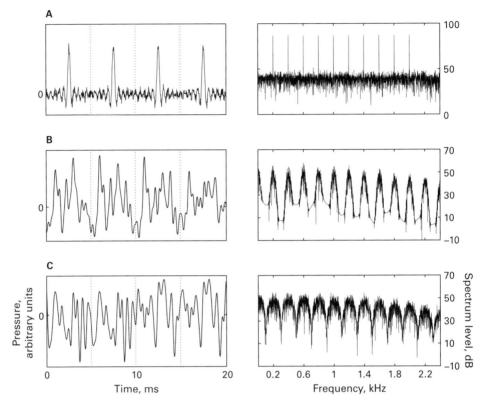

Figure 3.3

Three examples of nonperiodic sounds that evoke a perception of pitch. Each sound is displayed as a time waveform (left) showing four quasi-periods (separated by the dotted lines), and the corresponding long-term power spectrum (right) showing the approximate harmonic structure. All sounds have a pitch of 200 Hz. (A) A harmonic complex containing harmonics 1 to 10 of 200 Hz with white noise. The white noise causes the small fluctuations between the prominent peaks to be slightly different from period to period. (B) Iterated repeated noise with eight iterations [IRN(8)]. The features of the periods vary slowly, so that peaks and valleys change a bit from one period to the next. (C) AABB noise. Here the first and second period are identical, and again the third and fourth periods, but the two pairs are different from each other.

the resulting sound, successive sound segments whose duration is equal to the delay are not identical, but nevertheless share some similarity to each other. We will therefore call them "periods," although strictly speaking they are not. The similarity between periods decreases with increasing separation between them, and disappears for periods that are separated by more than eight times the delay. As illustrated in figure 3.3B, the spectrum of this sound has peaks at the harmonic frequencies. These peaks have a width—the sound contains frequency components away from the exact harmonic frequencies—but the similarity with a harmonic spectrum is clear.

The third example is a so-called AABB noise. This sound is generated by starting with a segment of white noise whose length is the required period. This segment is then repeated once. Then a new white noise segment with the same length is generated and repeated once. A third white noise segment is generated and repeated once, and so on. This stimulus, again, has a partial similarity between successive periods, but the partial similarity in this case consists of alternating episodes of perfect similarity followed by no similarity at all. The spectrum, again, has peaks at the harmonic frequencies, although the peaks are a little wider (figure 3.3C).

These examples suggest that the auditory system is highly sensitive to the similarity between successive periods. It is ready to suffer a fair amount of deterioration in this similarity and still produce the sensation of pitch. This tolerance to perturbations in the periodicity may be related to the sensory ecology of pitch—periodic sounds are mostly produced by animals, but such sounds would rarely be strictly periodic. Thus, a system that requires precise periodicity would be unable to detect the approximate periodicity of natural sounds.

3.3   The Psychophysics of Pitch Perception

Possibly the most important property of pitch is its extreme stability, within its existence region, to variations in other sound properties. Thus, pitch is essentially independent of sound level—the same periodic sound, played at different levels, evokes the same (or very similar) pitch. Pitch is also independent of the spatial location of the sound. Finally, the pitch of a periodic sound is, to a large extent, independent of the relative levels of the harmonics composing it. As a result, different musical instruments, playing sounds with the same periodicity, evoke the same pitch (as illustrated by Sound Example "Melodies and Timbre" on the book's Web site). Once we have equalized loudness, spatial location, and pitch, we call the perceptual quality that still differentiates between sounds timbre. Timbre is related (among other physical cues) to the relative levels of the harmonics. Thus, pitch is (almost) independent of timbre.

Since pitch is used to order sounds along a single continuum, we can try to cut this continuum into steps of equal size. There are, in fact, a number of notions of distance along the pitch continuum. The most important of these is used in music. Consider the distance between 100 Hz and 200 Hz along the pitch scale. What would be the pitch of a sound at the corresponding distance above 500 Hz? A naïve guess would be that 600 Hz is as distant from 500 Hz as 200 Hz is from 100 Hz. This is, however, wrong. Melodic distances between pitches are related not to the frequency difference but rather to the frequency ratio between them. Thus, the frequency ratio of 100 and 200 Hz is 200/100 = 2. Therefore, the sound at the same distance from 500 Hz has a pitch of 1,000 Hz (1,000/500 = 2). Distances along the pitch scale are called intervals, so that the interval between 100 and 200 Hz and the interval between 500 and 1,000 Hz are the same. The interval in both cases is called an octave—an octave corresponds to a doubling of the F_0 of the lower-pitched sound. We will often express intervals as a percentage (There is a slight ambiguity here: When stating an interval as a percentage, the percentage is always relative to the lower F_0): The sound with an F_0 that is 20% above 1,000 Hz would have an F_0 of 1,200 [= 1,000 * (1 + 20/100)] Hz, and the F_0 that is 6% above 2,000 Hz would be 2,120 [= 2,000 * (1 + 6/100)] Hz. Thus, an octave is an interval of 100%, whereas half an octave is an interval of about 41% [this is the interval called "tritone" in classical music, for example, the interval between B and F]. Indeed, moving twice with an interval of 41% would correspond to multiplying the lower F_0 by (1 + 41/100) * (1 + 41/100) ≈ 2. On the other hand, twice the interval of 50% would multiply the lower F_0 by (1 + 50/100) * (1 + 50/100) = 2.25, an interval of 125%, substantially more than an octave.

How well do we perceive pitch? This question has two types of answers. The first is whether we can identify the pitch of a sound when presented in isolation. The capacity to do so is called absolute pitch or perfect pitch (the second name, while still in use, is really a misnomer—there is nothing "perfect" about this ability). Absolute pitch is an ability that is more developed in some people than in others. Its presence depends on a large number of factors: It might have some genetic basis, but it can be developed in children by training, and indeed it exists more often in speakers of tonal languages such as Chinese than in English speakers.

The other type of answer to the question of how well we perceive pitch has to do with our ability to differentiate between two different pitches presented sequentially, an ability that is required in order to tune musical instruments well, for example. The story is very different when sounds with two different pitches are presented simultaneously, but we will not deal with that here. For many years, psychoacousticians have studied the limits of this ability. To do so, they measured the smallest "just noticeable differences" (JNDs) that can be detected by highly trained subjects. Typical experiments use sounds that have the same timbre (e.g., pure tones, or sounds that are combinations of the second, third, and fourth harmonics of a fundamental). One pitch value serves as a reference. The subject hears three tones: The first is always the reference, and the second and third contain another presentation of the reference and another sound with a slightly different pitch in random order. The subject has to indicate which sound (the second or third) is the odd one out. If the subject is consistently correct, the pitch difference between the two sounds is decreased. If an error is made, the pitch difference is increased. The smaller the pitch difference between the two sounds, the more likely it is for the subject to make an error. Generally, there won't be a sharp transition from perfect to chance-level discrimination. Instead, there will be a range of pitch differences in which the subject mostly answers correctly, but makes some mistakes. By following an appropriate schedule of decreases and increases in the pitch of the comparison sound, one can estimate a "threshold" (e.g., the pitch interval that would result in 71% correct responses). Experienced subjects, under optimal conditions, can perceive at threshold the difference between two sounds with an interval of 0.2% (e.g., 1,000 and 1,002 Hz) (Dallos, 1996). This is remarkably small—for comparison, the smallest interval of Western music, the semitone, corresponds to about 6% (e.g., 1,000 and 1,060 Hz), about thirty times larger than the JND of well-trained subjects.

However, naïve subjects generally perform much worse than that. It is not uncommon, in general populations, to find a subject who cannot determine whether two sounds are different even for intervals of 10 or 30% (Ahissar et al., 2006; Vongpaisal & Pichora-Fuller, 2007). The performance in such tasks also depends on some seemingly unimportant factors: For example, discrimination thresholds are higher (worse) if the two sounds to be compared are shifted in frequency from one trial to the next, keeping the interval fixed (the technical term for such a manipulation is "roving"), than if the reference frequency is fixed across trials (Ahissar et al., 2006). Finally, the performance can be improved dramatically with training. The improvement in the performance of tasks such as pitch discrimination with training is called "perceptual learning," and we will say more about this in chapter 7.

In day-to-day life, very accurate pitch discrimination is not critical for most people (musicians are a notable exception). But this does not mean that we cannot rely on pitch to help us perceive the world. Pitch is important for sound segregation—when multiple sounds are present simultaneously, periodic sounds stand out over a background of aperiodic background noise. Similarly, two voices speaking simultaneously with different pitches can be more easily segregated than voices with the same pitch. The role of pitch (and periodicity) in grouping and segregating sounds will be discussed in greater detail in chapter 6.

3.4 Pitch and Scales in Western Music

As an application for the ideas developed in the previous sections, we will now provide a brief introduction to the scales and intervals of Western music. We start by describing the notions that govern the selection of pitch values and intervals in Western music (in other words, why are the strings in a piano tuned the way they are). We then explain how this system, which is highly formalized and may seem rather arbitrary, developed.

We have already mentioned the octave—the interval that corresponds to doubling F_0. Modern Western music is based on a subdivision of the octave into twelve equal intervals, called the semitones, which correspond to a frequency ratio of $2^{1/12} \approx 1.06$ (in our terminology, this is an interval of about 6%). The "notes," that is, the pitches, of this so-called chromatic scale are illustrated in figure 3.4. Notes that differ by exactly one octave are in some sense equivalent (they are said to have the same chroma), and they have the same name. Notes are therefore names of "pitch classes" (i.e., a collection of pitches sharing the same chroma), rather than names of just one particular pitch. The whole system is locked to a fixed reference: the pitch of the so-called middle

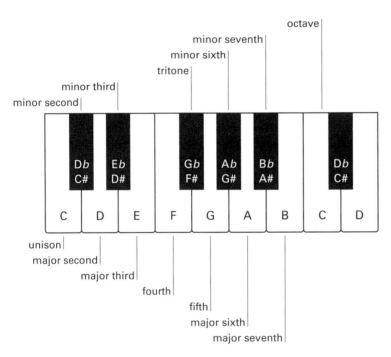

Figure 3.4

The chromatic scale and the intervals of Western music. This is a schematic representation of part of the keyboard of a piano. The keyboard has a repeating pattern of twelve keys, here represented by a segment starting at a C and ending at a D one octave higher. Each repeating pattern comprises seven white keys and five black keys, which lie between neighboring white keys except for the pairs E and F, and B and C. The interval between nearby keys (white and the nearest black key, or two white keys when there is no intermediate black key) is a semitone. The names of the intervals are given with respect to the lower C. Thus, for example, the interval between C and F♯ is a tritone, that between the lower and upper Cs is an octave, and so on.

A, which corresponds to an F_0 of 440 Hz. Thus, for example, the note "A" denotes the pitch class that includes the pitches 55 Hz (often the lowest note on the piano keyboard), 110 Hz, 220 Hz, 440 Hz, 880 Hz, 1,760 Hz, and so on.

The names of the notes that denote these pitch classes are complicated (figure 3.4). For historical reasons, there are seven primary names: C, D, E, F, G, A, and B (in English notation—Germans use the letter H for the note that the English call B, while in many other countries these notes have the entirely different names of do, re, mi, fa, sol, la, and si or ti). The intervals between these notes are 2, 2, 1, 2, 2, and 2 semitones, respectively, giving a total of 11 semitones between C and B; the interval between B and the C in the following octave is again 1 semitone, completing the 12 semitones that form an octave. There are five notes that do not have a primary name: those lying between C and D, between D and E, and so on. These correspond to the black keys on the piano keyboard (figure 3.4), and are denoted by an alteration of their adjacent primary classes. They therefore have two possible names, depending on which of their neighbors (the pitch above or below them) is subject to alteration. Raising a pitch by a semitone is denoted by ♯ (sharp), while lowering it by a semitone is denoted by ♭ (flat). Thus, for example, C♯ and D♭ denote the same pitch class (lying between C and D, one semitone above C and one semitone below D, respectively). Extending this notation, E♯, for example, denotes the same note as F (one semitone above E) and F♭ denotes the same note as E (one semitone below F). Finally, all the intervals in a scale have standard names: For example, the interval of one semitone is also called a minor second; an interval of seven semitones is called a fifth; and an interval of nine semitones is called a major sixth. The names of the intervals are also displayed in figure 3.4.

Although there are twelve pitch classes in Western music, most melodies in Western music limit themselves to the use of a restricted set of pitch classes, called a "scale." A Western scale is based on a particular note (called the key), and it comprises seven notes. There are a number of ways to select the notes of a scale. The most important ones in Western music are the major and the minor scales. The major scale based on C consists of the notes C, D, E, F, G, A, and B, with successive intervals of 2, 2, 1, 2, 2, 2 semitones (the white keys of the piano keyboard). A major scale based on F would include notes at the same intervals: F, G, A, B♭ (since the interval between the third and fourth notes of the scale should be one, not two, semitones), C (two semitones above B♭), D, and E. B♭ is used instead of A♯ due to the convention that, in a scale, each primary name of a pitch class is used once and only once. Minor scales are a bit more complicated, as a number of variants of the minor scales are used—but a minor key will always have an interval of a minor third (instead of a major third) between the base note and the third note of the scale. Thus, for example, the scale of C minor will always contain E♭ instead of E.

Generally, the musical intervals are divided into "consonant" and "dissonant" intervals, where consonant intervals, when played together in a chord, seem to merge together in a pleasant way, while dissonant intervals may sound harsh. Consonant intervals include the octave, the fifth, the third, and the sixth. Dissonant intervals include the second and the seventh.

The most consonant interval is the octave. Its strong consonance may stem from the physics of what happens when two sounds that are an octave apart are played together: All the harmonics of the higher-pitched sound are also harmonics of the lower-pitched one (figure 3.5A). Thus, the combination of these two sounds results in a sound that has the periodicity of the lower-pitched sound. Two such sounds "fuse" together nicely.

In contrast, sounds separated by the dissonant interval of a major second (two semitones apart) do not merge well (figure 3.5C). In particular, many harmonics are relatively close to each other, but very few match exactly. This is important because adding up two pure tones with nearby frequencies causes "beating"—regular changes in sound level at a rate equal to the difference between the two frequencies, which come about as the nearby frequencies alternate between constructive and destructive interference. This causes "roughness" in the amplitude envelope of the resulting sound (Tramo et al., 2001), which can be observed in neural responses. The dissonance of the major second is therefore probably attributable to the perception of roughness it elicits.

What about the interval of a fifth? The fifth corresponds to an interval of 49.8%, which is almost 50%, or a frequency ratio of 3/2. The frequency ratio of 50% is indeed called the perfect fifth. While sounds that are a perfect fifth apart do not fuse quite as well as sounds that are an octave apart, they still merge rather well. They have many harmonics in common (e.g., the third harmonic of the lower sound is the same as the second harmonic of the higher one, figure 3.5B), and harmonics that do not match tend to be far from each other, avoiding the sensation of roughness. Thus, perfect fifths are consonant, and the fifths used in classical music are close enough to be almost indistinguishable from perfect fifths.

However, this theory does not readily explain consonance and dissonance of other intervals. For example, the interval of a perfect fourth, which corresponds to the frequency ratio of 4 to 3 (the ratio between the frequencies of the fourth and third harmonics), is considered as consonant, but would sound dissonant to many modern listeners. On the other hand, the interval of a major third was considered an interval to avoid in medieval music due to its dissonance, but is considered highly consonant in modern Western music. Thus, there is much more to consonance and dissonance than just the physics of the sounds.

All of this may appear rather arbitrary, and to some degree it is. However, the Western scale is really based on a rather natural idea that, when pushed far enough, results in inconsistencies. The formal system described above is the result of the devel-

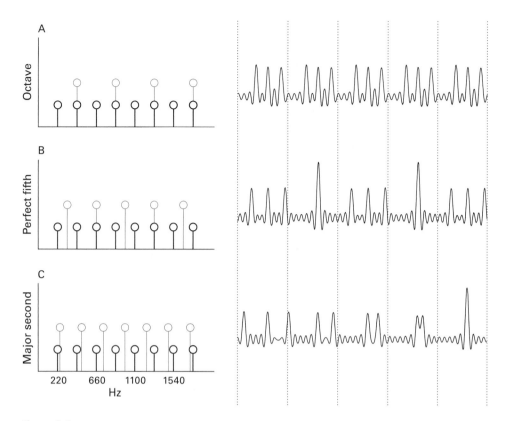

Figure 3.5

A (partial) theory of consonance. A schematic representation of the spectrum (left) and a portion of the waveform (right) of three combinations of two notes. The lower note is always an A on 220 Hz. Its harmonics are plotted in black and half height (left). The dotted lines on the right mark the duration of one period of that lower note. (A) The higher note is also A, an octave above the lower note. Its harmonics (gray full height) match a subset of the harmonics of the lower note, resulting in a sound whose periodicity is that of the lower note (the sound between each pair of successive dotted lines is the same). (B) The higher note is E, a perfect fifth above A. The harmonics of this E are either midway or match exactly harmonics of the lower A. The waveform has a periodicity of 110 Hz (the pattern repeats every two dotted lines on the right). (C) The higher note is B, a major second above A. None of the harmonics match and some of them are rather close to each other. The waveform doesn't show any periodicity within the five periods that are displayed, and in fact its period is outside the existence region of pitch. It has irregular variations of amplitude (almost random location of the high peaks, with this choice of phases). This irregularity presumably results in the perception of dissonant sounds.

opment of this idea over a long period of time in an attempt to solve these inconsistencies, and it reached its final shape only in the nineteenth century.

Consider the C major key, with its seven pitch classes. What motivates the choice of these particular pitches, and not others? The Western scale is based on an interplay between the octave and the perfect fifth, which are considered to be the two most consonant intervals. (To remind the reader, the perfect fifth is the "ideal" interval between, e.g., C and G, with a ratio of 3 to 2, although we have seen that in current practice the fifth is slightly smaller.) The goal of the process we describe next is to create a set of notes that has as many perfect fifths as possible—we would like to have a set of pitches that contains a perfect fifth above and below each of its members. We will see that this is actually impossible, but let's start with the process and see where it fails.

Starting with C, we add G to our set of notes. Note that modern G is not a perfect fifth about C, but we will consider for now the "natural" G, which is. We are going to generate other notes which we will call by their modern names, but which are slightly different from their modern counterparts. The notes we are going to generate are the natural notes, so called because they are going to be generated by using jumps of natural fifths.

Since we want the scale to contain perfect fifths above and below each of its members, we also move one fifth down from C, to arrive at (natural) F, a note with an F_0 of 2/3 that of C. This F is outside the octave starting at our C, so we move one octave up to get to the next higher F, which therefore has an F_0 of 4/3 times that of the C that serves as our starting point. In this manner, we have already generated three of the seven pitch classes of the major scale, C, F, and G, just by moving in fifths and octaves (figure 3.6).

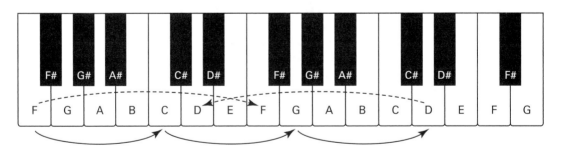

Figure 3.6
The beginning of the cycle of fifths. G is one fifth above C, and D (in the next octave) is one fifth above G. It is shifted down by an octave (dashed arrow). The fifth from F up to C is also displayed here, since F would otherwise not be generated (instead, E♯ is created as the penultimate step in the cycle, and the perfect 4/3 relationship with C would not exist). This F has to be shifted up by an octave in order to generate the F note within the correct range.

The other pitch classes of the major scale can be generated in a similar manner by continued use of perfect fifths and octaves. Moving from G up by one fifth, we get to natural D (at an interval of $3/2 \times 3/2 = 9/4$ above the original C). This interval is larger than an octave ($9/4 > 2$), however, and to get a note in the original octave it has to be transposed by one octave down; in other words, its frequency has to be divided by 2. Thus, the natural D has a frequency that is $9/8$ that of C. The next pitch class to generate is A, a perfect fifth above D (at a frequency ratio of $9/8 \times 3/2 = 27/16$ above C), and then E (at an interval of $27/16 \times 3/2 = 81/32$ above C). This is, again, more than an octave above C, and to get the E within the original octave, we transpose it down by an octave, arriving at an F_0 for natural E, which is $81/64$ that of C. Finally, a perfect fifth above E we get B, completing all the pitch classes of the major scale.

The scale that is generated using this interplay of fifths and octaves is called the natural, or Pythagorean, scale. The pitches of the natural scale are related to each other by ratios that are somewhat different from those determined by the equal-tempered chromatic scale we discussed previously. For example, the interval between E and C in the natural scale corresponds to a ratio of $81/64 \approx 1.266$, whereas the corresponding interval of four semitones is $2^{4/12} \approx 1.260$. Similarly, the interval of a fifth corresponds to seven semitones, so in the modern scale it corresponds to a frequency ratio of $2^{7/12} \approx 1.498$, slightly smaller than $3/2 = 1.5$. Why these differences?

We wanted to have a set of sounds that contains the fifths above and below each of its members. We stopped at natural B, and we already generated the fifth below it (E), but not the fifth above it. So we have to continue the process. Moving up by perfect fifths and correcting by octaves, we generate next the five pitch classes that are still missing (in order F♯, C♯, G♯, D♯, and A♯). However, thereafter the situation becomes less neat. The next pitch class would be E♯, which turns out to be almost, but not quite, equal to F, our starting point (figure 3.6). This pitch class, the thirteenth tone in the sequence, has a F_0, which is $(3/2)^{12}/2^7$ times that of the original F—in other words, it is generated by moving up twelve times by a fifth and correcting seven times with an octave down. However, that frequency ratio is about 1.014 rather than 1. So, we generated twelve pitch classes using motions of fifths and octaves, but the cycle did not quite close at the thirteenth step.

Instruments can still be tuned by the natural scale, but then scales in keys that are far from C (along the cycle of fifths) do not have quite the right intervals, and therefore sound mistuned. On an instrument that is tuned for playing in the natural C major scale, music written in C♯ major will sound out of tune.

The problem became an important issue when, in the seventeenth and eighteenth centuries, composers started to write music in all keys, or even worse, started writing music that moved from one key to another within the same piece. To perform such music in tune, it was necessary to modify the natural scale. A number of suggestions have been made to achieve this. The modern solution consists of keeping octaves exact (doubling F_0), but changing the definition of all other intervals. In particular, the interval of perfect fifth was abandoned for the slightly reduced modern approximation. As a result, twelve fifths became exactly seven octaves, and E♯ became exactly F. The resulting system fulfills our original goal of having a set of pitch classes in which we can go by a fifth above and below each of its members.

Is there any relationship between this story and the perceptual issues we discussed earlier? We encountered two such connections. The first is in the primacy of the octave and the fifth, the two most consonant intervals. The second is in the decision that the difference between E♯ and F was too small, and that the two pitch classes should be treated as equivalent. Interestingly, essentially all formalized musical systems in the world use intervals of about the same size, with the smallest intervals being around half of the semitone. In other words, musical systems tend not to pack many more than twelve steps into the octave—maybe up to twenty-four, but not more than that. This tendency can possibly be traced to perceptual abilities. Music is a form of communication, and therefore requires distinguishable basic components. Thus, the basic steps of any musical scales should be substantially larger than the minimum discrimination threshold. It may well be that this is the reason for the quite constant density of notes in the octave across cultures. The specific selection of pitches for these notes may be justified by other criteria, but is perhaps more arbitrary.

3.5   Pitch Perception by Nonhuman Listeners

In order to study the way the nervous system estimates the pitch of sounds, we will want to use animal models. This raises a crucial issue: Is pitch special for humans, or do other species perceive pitch in a similar way? This is a difficult question. It is impossible to ask animals directly what they perceive, and therefore any answer is by necessity indirect. In spite of this difficulty, a number of studies suggest that many animals do have a perceptual quality similar to pitch in humans.

Thus, songbirds seem to perceive pitch: European starlings (*Sturnus vulgaris*) generalize from pure tones to harmonic complexes with a missing fundamental and vice versa. Cynx and Shapiro (1986) trained starlings to discriminate the frequencies of pure tones, and then tested them on discrimination of complex sounds with the same F_0 but missing the fundamental. Furthermore, the complex sounds were constructed such that use of physical properties other than F_0 would result in the wrong choice. For example, the mean frequency of the harmonics of the high-F_0 sound was lower than the mean frequency of the harmonics of the low-F_0 sound. As a result, if the starlings would have used place pitch instead of periodicity pitch, they would have failed the test.

Even goldfish generalize to some extent over F_0, although not to the same degree as humans. The experiments with goldfish were done in a different way from those with birds. First, the animals underwent classical conditioning to a periodic sound, which presumably evokes a pitch sensation in the fish. In classical conditioning, a sound is associated with a consequence (a mild electric shock in this case). As a result, when the animal hears that sound, it reacts (in this case, by suppressing its respiration for a brief period). Classical conditioning can be used to test whether animals generalize across sound properties. Thus, the experimenter can present a different sound, which shares some properties with the original conditioning stimulus. If the animal suppresses its respiration, it is concluded that the animal perceives the new stimulus as similar to the conditioning stimulus. Using this method, Fay (2005) demonstrated some generalization—for example, the goldfish responded to the harmonic series in much the same way, regardless of whether the fundamental was present or missing. But Fay also noted some differences from humans. For example, IRNs, a mainstay of human pitch studies, do not seem to evoke equivalent pitch percepts in goldfish.

In mammals, it generally seems to be the case that "missing fundamentals are not missed" (to paraphrase Fay, 2005). Heffner and Whitfield (1976) showed this to be true in cats by using harmonic complexes in which the overall energy content shifted down while the missing fundamental shifted up and vice versa (a somewhat similar stratagem to that used by Cynx and Shapiro with starlings); and Tomlinson and Schwarz (1988) showed this in macaques performing a same-different task comparing sounds composed of subsets of harmonics 1–5 of their fundamental. The monkeys had to compare two sounds: The first could have a number of low-order harmonics missing while the second sound contained all harmonics.

Other, more recent experiments suggest that the perceptual quality of pitch in animals is similar but not identical to that evoked in humans. For example, when ferrets are required to judge whether the pitch of a second tone is above or below that of a first tone, their discrimination threshold is large—20% or more—even when the first tone is fixed in long blocks (Walker et al., 2009). Under such conditions, humans will usually do at least ten times better (Ahissar et al., 2006). However, the general trends of the data are similar in ferrets and in humans, suggesting the existence of true sensitivity to periodicity pitch.

Thus, animals seem to be sensitive to the periodicity, and not just the frequency components, of sounds. In this sense, animals can be said to perceive pitch. However, pitch sensation in animals may have somewhat different properties from that in humans, potentially depending more on stimulus type (as in goldfish) or having lower resolution (as in ferrets).

3.6 Algorithms for Pitch Estimation

Since, as we have seen, pitch is largely determined by the periodicity (or approximate periodicity) of the sound, the auditory system has to extract this periodicity in order to determine the pitch. As a computational problem, producing running estimates of the periodicity of a signal turns out to have important practical applications in speech and music processing. It has therefore been studied in great depth by engineers. Here, we will briefly describe some of the approaches that emerged from this research, and in a later section, we will discuss whether these "engineering solutions" correspond to anything that may be happening in our nervous systems when we hear pitch.

As discussed previously, there are two equivalent descriptions of the family of periodic sounds. The "time domain" description notes whether the waveform of the sound is composed of a segment of sound that repeats over and over, in rapid succession. If so, then the pitch the sound evokes should correspond to the length of the shortest such repeating segment. The "frequency domain" description asks whether the frequency content of the sound consists mostly or exclusively of the harmonics of some fundamental. If so, then the pitch should correspond to the highest F_0 consistent with the observed sequence of harmonics. Correspondingly, pitch estimation algorithms can be divided into time domain and frequency domain methods. It may seem overcomplicated to calculate the frequency spectra when the sound waveform is immediately available, but sometimes there are good reasons to do so. For example, noise may badly corrupt the waveform of a sound, but the harmonics may still be apparent in the frequency domain. Possibly more important, as we have seen in chapter 2, the ear performs approximate frequency decomposition; therefore it may seem that a frequency domain algorithm might be more relevant for understanding pitch processing in the auditory system. However, as we will see later in this chapter, time domain methods certainly appear to play a role in the pitch extraction mechanisms used by the mammalian auditory system.

Let us first look at time domain methods. We have a segment of a periodic sound, and we want to determine its period. Suppose we want to test whether the period is 1 ms (F_0 of 1,000 Hz). The thing to do would be to make a copy of the sound, delay the copy by 1 ms, and compare the original and delayed versions—if they are identical, or at least sufficiently similar, then the sound is periodic, with a period of 1 ms. If they are very different, we will have to try again with another delay. Usually, such methods start by calculating the similarity for many different delays, corresponding to many candidate F_0s, and at a second stage select the period at which the correspondence between the original and delayed versions is best.

Although this is a good starting point, there are many details that have to be specified. The most important one is the comparison process—how do we perform it? We shall discuss this in some detail below, since the same issue reappears later in a number of guises. Selecting the best delay can also be quite complicated—several different delays may work quite well, or (not unusual with real sounds) many delays could be equally unsatisfactory. Algorithms often use the rule of thumb that the "best delay" is the shortest delay that is "good enough" according to some criteria that are tweaked by trial and error.

So, how are we to carry out the comparison of the two sounds (in our case, the original and delayed versions of the current bit of sound)? One way would be to subtract one from the other. If they are identical, the difference signal would be zero. In practice, however, the signal will rarely be strictly periodic, and so the difference signal would not be exactly zero. Good candidates for the period would be delays for which the difference signal is particularly small. So we have to gauge whether a particular difference signal is large or small. Just computing the average of the difference signal would not work, since its values are sometimes likely to be positive and sometimes negative, and these values would cancel when averaging. So we should take the absolute value of the differences, or square all differences, to make the difference signal positive, and then average to get a measure of its typical size.

There is, however, a third way of doing this comparison: calculating the correlation between the original and time-shifted signals. The correlation would be maximal when the time shift is 0 ms (comparing the sound with a nonshifted version of itself), and may remain high for other very small shifts. In addition, if the sound is periodic, the correlation will be high again for a time shift that is equal to the period, since the original sound and its shifted version would be very similar to each other at this shift. On the other hand, the correlation is expected to be smaller at other shifts. Thus, periodic sounds would have a peak in the correlation at time shifts equal to the period (or multiples thereof).

Although calculating the correlation seems a different approach from subtracting and estimating the size of the difference signal, the two approaches are actually closely related, particularly when using squaring to estimate the size of the difference signal. In that case, the larger the correlation, the smaller the difference signal would generally be.

While implementation details may vary, the tendency is to call all of these methods, as a family, autocorrelation methods for pitch estimation. The term "autocorrelation" comes from the fact that the comparison process consists of computing the correlation (or a close relative) between a sound and its own shifted versions. It turns out that biological neural networks have many properties that should enable them to calculate autocorrelations. Therefore, the autocorrelation approach is not a bad starting point for a possible neural algorithm. One possible objection against the use of autocorrelations in the brain stems from the delays this approach requires—since the lower limit of pitch is about 40 Hz, the correlation would require generating delays as long as 25 ms. That is a fairly long time relative to the standard delays produced by biological "wetware" (typical neural membrane time constants, conduction velocities, or synaptic delays would result in delays of a few milliseconds, maybe 10 ms), so how neural circuits might implement such long delay lines is not obvious. However, this potential problem can be overcome in various ways (de Cheveigné & Pressnitzer, 2006).

As we discussed previously, a different approach to the extraction of pitch would be to calculate the frequency content of the sound and then analyze the resulting pattern of harmonics, finding their largest common divisor. If we know the pattern of harmonics, there is a neat trick for finding their greatest common divisor. Suppose we want to know whether 1,000 Hz is a candidate F_0. We generate a harmonic "sieve" —a narrow paper strip with holes at 1,000 Hz and its multiples. We put the frequency content of the sound through the sieve, letting only the energy of the frequency components at the holes fall through, and estimate how much of the energy of the sound successfully passed through the sieve. Since only harmonics of 1,000 Hz line up with these holes, if the sound has an F_0 of 1,000 Hz, all of the energy of the sound should be able to pass through this sieve. But if the frequency composition of the sound is poorly matched to the structure of the sieve (for example, if there are many harmonics that are not multiples of 1,000 Hz), then a sizeable proportion of the sound will fail to pass through, indicating that another candidate has to be tested.

As in the autocorrelation method, in practice we start with sieves at many possible F_0s ("harmonic hole spacing"), and test all of them, selecting the best. And again, as in the autocorrelation method, there are a lot of details to consider. How do we estimate the spectra to be fed through the sieves? As we discussed in chapters 1 and 2, the cochlea, while producing a frequency decomposition of a sound, does its calculations in fairly wide frequency bands, and its output may not be directly appropriate for comparison with a harmonic sieve, possibly requiring additional processing before the sieve is applied. How do we select the best candidate sieve out of many somewhat unsatisfactory ones (as would occur with real-world sounds)? How do we measure the amount of energy that is accounted for by each sieve? How "wide" should the holes in the sieve be? These issues are crucial for the success of an implementation of these methods, but are beyond the scope of this book. These methods are generally called harmonic sieve methods, because of the computational idea at their heart.

One major objection to harmonic sieve methods is that the harmonic sieve would have to be assembled from a neural network somewhere in the brain, but it is not immediately obvious how such an object could be either encoded genetically or learned in an unsupervised manner. However, a natural scheme has recently been proposed that would create such sieves when trained with sounds that may not be periodic at all (Shamma & Klein, 2000). Thus, harmonic sieves for pitch estimation could, in principle, be created in the brain.

Let us see how the autocorrelation and the harmonic sieve approaches deal with a difficult case. Consider a sound whose frequency components are 220, 320, and 420 Hz. This sound has a periodicity of 20 Hz, but evokes a pitch at 106 Hz: This is an example of a sound that evokes a pitch away from its F_0.

How would the two approaches explain this discrepancy? Figure 3.7A displays two true periods (50 ms long) of this sound. Strictly speaking, the sound is periodic, with a period of 50 ms, but it has some repeating structure slightly less than every 10 ms (there are ten peaks within the 100-ms segment shown). Figure 3.7B shows the auto-correlation function of this sound. It has a peak at a delay of 50 ms (not shown in figure 3.7B), corresponding to the exact periodicity of 20 Hz. But 20 Hz is below the lower limit of pitch perception, so we can safely assume that the brain does not consider such a long delay. Instead, the evoked pitch should correspond to a high correlation value that would occur at a shorter delay. Indeed, the highest correlation occurs at a delay of 9.41 ms. The delay of 9.41 ms corresponds to a pitch of 106 Hz. Autocorrelation therefore does a good job at identifying the correct pitch.

How would the harmonic sieve algorithm account for the same result? As above, 20 Hz is too low for evoking a pitch. On the other hand, 106 Hz is an approximate

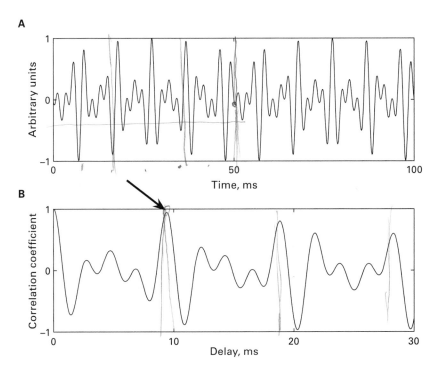

Figure 3.7

A sound composed of partials at 220, 320, and 420 Hz. The sound has a period of 50 ms (F_0 of 20 Hz—two periods are displayed in A), which is outside the existence region for pitch. It evokes a low pitch at 106 Hz, which is due to the approximate periodicity at that rate (note the large peaks in the signal, which are almost, but not quite, the same). Indeed, its autocorrelation func-tion (B) has a peak at 9.41 ms (marked by the arrow).

divisor of all three harmonics: 220/106 = 2.07 (so that 220 Hz is almost the second harmonic of 106 Hz), 320/106 = 3.02, and 420/106 = 3.96. Furthermore, 106 is the best approximate divisor of these three numbers. So the harmonic sieve that best fits the series of frequency components corresponds to a pitch of 106 Hz. This example therefore illustrates the fact that the "holes" in the sieve would need to have some width in order to account for pitch perception!

3.7 Periodicity Encoding in Subcortical Auditory Pathways

We have just seen how one might try to program a computer to estimate the pitch of a sound, but is there any relationship between the engineering methods just discussed and what goes on in your auditory system when you listen to a melody? When discussing this issue, we have to be careful to distinguish between the coding of periodicity (the physical attribute) and coding of pitch (the perceptual quality). The neural circuits that extract or convey information about the periodicity of a sound need not be the same as those that trigger the subjective sensation of a particular pitch. To test whether some set of neurons has any role to play in extracting periodicity, we need to study the relationship between the neural activity and the sound stimuli presented to the listener. But if we want to know what role that set of neurons might play in triggering a pitch sensation, what matters is how the neural activity relates to what the listeners report they hear, not what sounds were actually present. We will focus mostly on the neural encoding for stimulus periodicity, and we briefly tackle the trickier and less well understood question of how the sensation of pitch is generated in the next section.

Periodicity is encoded in the early stations of the auditory system by temporal patterns of spikes: A periodic sound would elicit spike patterns in which many interspike intervals are equal to the period of the sound (we elaborate on this statement later). It turns out that some processes enhance this representation of periodicity in the early auditory system, increasing the fraction of interspike intervals that are equal to the period. However, this is an implicit code—it has to be "read" in order to extract the period (or F_0) of the sound. We will deal with this implicit code first.

The initial representation of sounds in the brain is provided by the activity of the auditory nerve fibers. We cannot hope that periodicity (and therefore pitch) would be explicitly encoded by the firing of auditory nerve fibers. First, auditory nerve fibers represent frequency content (as we discussed in chapter 2), and the relationships between frequency content and periodicity are complex. Furthermore, auditory nerve fibers carry all information needed to characterize sounds, including many dimensions other than pitch. Therefore, the relationship between pitch and the activity pattern of auditory nerve fibers cannot be straightforward.

Nevertheless, the activity pattern of auditory nerve fibers must somehow carry enough information about the periodicity of sounds so that, at some point, brain circuits can extract the pitch. Understanding how periodicity is encoded in the activity of auditory nerve fibers is therefore important in order to understand how further stations of the nervous system would eventually generate the pitch percept.

The key to understanding encoding of periodicity in the auditory nerve is the concept of phase locking—the tendency of fibers to produce spikes at specific points during each period, usually corresponding to amplitude maxima of the motion of the basilar membrane (see chapter 2). As a result, a periodic waveform creates a pattern of spike times that repeats itself (at least on average) on every period of the sound. Thus, the firing patterns of auditory nerve fibers in response to periodic sounds are themselves periodic. If we can read the periodicity of this pattern, we have F_0. As usual, there are a lot of details to consider, the most important of which is that auditory nerve fibers are narrowly tuned; we will consider this complexity later.

How do we find the periodicity of the auditory nerve fiber discharge pattern? When we discussed algorithms for estimating periodicity, we developed the idea of autocorrelation—a process that results in an enhanced representation of the periodicity of a waveform. The same process can be applied to the firing patterns of auditory nerve fibers. Since the waveform of neuronal firings is really a sequence of spikes, the autocorrelation process for auditory nerve fibers has a special character (figure 3.8). This process consists of tallying the number of time intervals between each spike and every other spike in the spike train. If the spike train is periodic, the resulting interval histogram will have a strong representation of the interval corresponding to the period: Many spikes would occur at exactly one period apart, whereas other intervals will be less strongly represented.

The autocorrelation in its pure form is not a very plausible mechanism for extracting periodicity by neurons. For one thing, F_0 tends to vary with time—after all, we use pitch to create melodies—and, at least for humans, the range of periods that evoke pitch is limited. Therefore, using all intervals in a long spike train does not make sense. Practical algorithms for extracting periodicity from auditory nerve firings would always limit both the range of time over which they tally the interspike intervals, and the range of intervals they would consider as valid candidates for the period.

What would be reasonable bounds? A possible clue is the lower limit of pitch, at about 40 Hz. This limit suggests that the auditory system does not look for intervals that are longer than about 25 ms. This might well be the time horizon over which intervals are tallied. Furthermore, we need a few periods to perceive pitch, so the duration over which we would have to tally intervals should be at least a few tens of milliseconds long. While the lower limit of pitch would suggest windows of ~100 ms (4×25 ms), this is, in fact, an extreme case. Most pitches that we encounter are higher—100 Hz (a period of 10 ms) would be considered a reasonably deep male voice—and so a

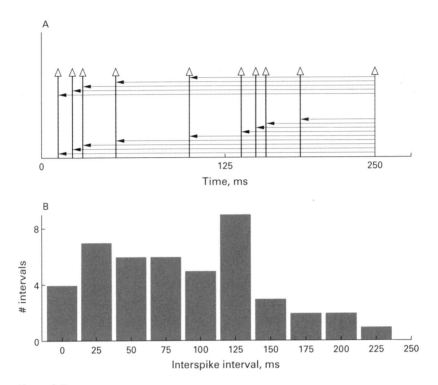

Figure 3.8
Autocorrelation of a spike sequence containing two approximate repeats of the same spike pattern at an interval of 125 ms. (A) The autocorrelation is a tally of all intervals between pairs of spikes. This can be achieved by considering, for each spike, the intervals between it and all preceding spikes (these intervals are shown for two of the spikes). (B) The resulting histogram. The peak at 125 ms corresponds to the period of the spike pattern in A.

40 ms long integration time window may be a practical choice (the window may even be task dependent).

The shortest interval to be considered for pitch is about 0.25 ms (corresponding to a pitch of 4,000 Hz). This interval also poses a problem—auditory nerve fibers have a refractory period of about 1 ms, and anyway cannot fire at sustained rates that are much higher than a few hundred hertz. As a result, intervals as short as 0.25 ms cannot be well represented in the firings of a single auditory nerve fibers. To solve this problem, we would need to invoke the volley principle (chapter 2). In other words, we should really consider the tens of auditory nerve fibers that innervate a group of neighboring inner hair cells, and calculate the autocorrelation of their combined spike trains.

Until this point, we have considered a single nerve fiber (or a homogeneous group of fibers with the same CF), and assumed that the periodicity of the sound is expressed in the firing of that particular fiber. However, this is usually wrong! In fact, many periodic sounds contain a wide range of frequencies. On the other hand, auditory nerve fibers are narrowly tuned—as we have seen in chapter 2, they respond only to a restricted range of frequencies, even if the sound contains many more frequencies. As a specific example, consider the sound consisting of frequency components at 200, 400, and 600 Hz. This sound has an F_0 of 200 Hz, and, at moderate sound levels, it would evoke activity mostly in auditory nerve fibers whose characteristic frequencies are near its component frequencies. Thus, an auditory nerve fiber responding to 200 Hz would be activated by this sound. The bandwidth of the 200-Hz auditory nerve fiber would be substantially less than 200 Hz (in fact, it is about 50 Hz, based on psychophysical experiments). Consequently it would "see" only the 200-Hz component of the sound, not the higher harmonics. We would therefore expect it to fire with a periodicity of 200 Hz, with a repetition of the firing pattern every 5 ms, corresponding to the correct F_0. In a similar way, however, the 400-Hz auditory nerve fiber would respond only to the 400-Hz component of the sound, since its bandwidth would be substantially less than 200 Hz (about 60 Hz). And because it phase locks to a harmonic, not to the fundamental, it would fire with a periodicity of 400 Hz, with a repetition of the firing pattern every 2.5 ms, which corresponds to a wrong periodicity.

The same problem would not occur for higher harmonics. To continue with the same example, the bandwidth of the auditory nerve fibers whose best frequency is 2,000 Hz in humans is believed to be larger than 200 Hz. As a result, if our sound also included harmonics around 2,000 Hz (the tenth harmonic of 200 Hz), auditory nerve fibers around that frequency would hear multiple harmonics. A sound composed of multiple harmonics of 200 Hz would have a periodicity of 200 Hz, and therefore the 2,000-Hz auditory nerve fibers would have a periodic firing pattern with a periodicity of 200 Hz.

This difference between lower and higher harmonics of periodic sounds occurs at all pitch values, and it has a name: The lower harmonics (up to order 6 or so) are called the resolved harmonics, while the higher ones are called unresolved. The difference between resolved and unresolved harmonics has to do with the properties of the auditory system, not the properties of sounds—it is determined by the bandwidth of the auditory nerve fibers. However, as a consequence of these properties, we cannot calculate the right periodicity from the pattern of activity of a single auditory nerve fiber in the range of resolved harmonics. Instead, we need to combine information across multiple auditory nerve fibers. This can be done rather easily. Going back to the previous example, we consider the responses of the 200-Hz fiber as "voting" for a period of 5 ms, by virtue of the peak of the autocorrelation function of its spike train. The 400-Hz fiber would vote for 2.5 ms, but its spike train would also contain intervals of 5 ms (corresponding to intervals of two periods), and therefore the autocorrelation function would have a peak (although possibly somewhat weaker) at 5 ms. The autocorrelation function of the 600-Hz fiber would peak at 1.66 ms (one period), 3.33 ms (two periods), and 5 ms (corresponding to intervals between spikes emitted three periods apart). If we combine all of these data, we see there is overwhelming evidence that 5 ms is the right period.

The discussion we have just gone through might suggest that the pitch of sounds composed of unresolved harmonics may be stronger or more robust than that of sounds composed of resolved harmonics, which requires across-frequency processing to be extracted. It turns out that exactly the opposite happens—resolved harmonics dominate the pitch percept (Shackleton & Carlyon, 1994), and the pitch of sounds composed of unresolved harmonics may not correspond to the periodicity (as demonstrated with Sound Example "Pitch of 3-Component Harmonic Complexes" on the book's Web site). Thus, the across-frequency integration of periodicity information must be a crucial aspect of pitch perception.

A number of researchers have studied the actual responses of auditory nerve fibers to stimuli-evoking pitch. The goal of such experiments was to test whether all the ideas we have been discussing work in practice, with the firing of real auditory nerve fibers. Probably the most complete of these studies were carried by Peter Cariani and Bertrand Delgutte (Cariani & Delgutte, 1996a, b). They set themselves a hard problem: to develop a scheme that would make it possible to extract pitch of a large family of pitch-evoking sounds from real auditory nerve firings. To make the task even harder (but closer to real-life conditions), they decided to use stimuli whose pitch changes with time as well.

Figure 3.9 shows one of the stimuli used by Cariani and Delgutte (Sound Example "Single Formant Vowel with Changing Pitch" on the book's Web site). At each point in time, it was composed of a sequence of harmonics. The fundamental of the harmonic complex varied continuously, initially going up from 80 to 160 Hz and then back again (figure 3.9C). The amplitudes of the harmonics varied in time so that the peak harmonic always had the same frequency (at low F_0, the peak amplitude occurred at a higher-order harmonic, whereas at high F_0 it occurred at a lower-order harmonic; this is illustrated in figure 3.9A and B). The resulting time waveform, at a very compressed time scale, is shown in figure 3.9D. For reasons that may become clear in chapter 4, this stimulus is called a single formant vowel.

Cariani and Delgutte recorded the responses of many auditory nerve fibers, with many different best frequencies, to many repetitions of this sound. They then used a variant of the autocorrelation method to extract F_0. Since F_0 changed in time, it was necessary to tally intervals separately for different parts of the stimulus. They therefore computed separate autocorrelation functions for 20-ms sections of the stimulus, but overlapped these 20-ms sections considerably to get a smooth change of the autocorrelation in time. In order to integrate across many frequencies, Cariani and Delgutte

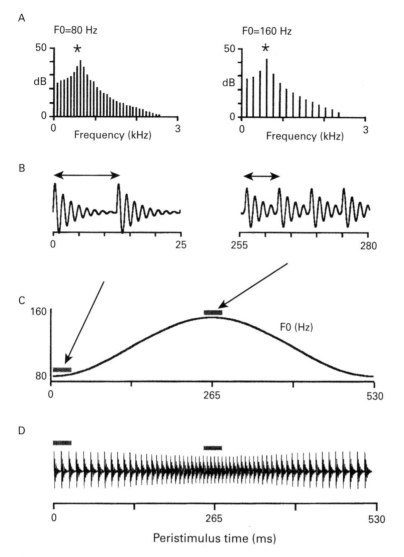

Figure 3.9

The single-formant vowel stimulus with varying pitch used by Cariani and Delgutte. (A) Spectra of the stimulus at its beginning (pitch of 80 Hz) and at its middle (pitch of 160 Hz). At the lower pitch, the harmonics are denser (with a separation of 80 Hz) and at the higher pitch they are less dense (with a separation of 160 Hz). However, the peak amplitude is always at 640 Hz. (B) The time waveform at the beginning and at the middle of the sound, corresponding to the spectra in A. At 80 Hz, the period is 12.5 ms (two periods in the 25-ms segment are displayed in the figure), while at 160 Hz, the period is 6.25 ms, so that in the same 25 ms there are four periods. (C) The pattern of change of the F_0 of the stimulus. (D) The time course of the stimulus, at a highly compressed time scale. The change in pitch is readily apparent as an increase and then a decrease in the density of the peaks.

From Cariani and Delgutte (1996a) with permission from the American Physiological Society.

did almost the simplest thing—they added the time-varying autocorrelation patterns across all the auditory nerve fibers they recorded, except that different frequency regions were weighted differentially to take into account the expected distribution of nerve fiber characteristic frequencies.

The rather complex result of this process is displayed in figure 3.10A. Time through the stimulus is represented along the abscissa, interval durations are along the ordinate, and the values of the time-varying autocorrelation function are displayed in gray level. Let us focus our attention on the abscissa at a certain time (e.g., the small window around 50 ms, marked in figure 3.10A by the two vertical lines with the "B" at the top). This strip is plotted in details in figure 3.10B. This is the autocorrelation function around time 50 ms into the stimulus: the tally of the interspike intervals that occurred around this time in the auditory nerve responses. Clearly, these interspike intervals contain an overrepresentation of intervals around 12.5 ms, which is the pitch period at that moment. Figure 3.10C shows a similar plot for a short window around time 275 ms (when the pitch is highest, marked again in figure 3.10A by two vertical lines with "C" at the top). Again, there is a peak at the period (6.25 ms), although a second peak at 12.5 ms is equal to twice the period. This is one of those cases where it is necessary to make the correct decision regarding the period: Which of these two peaks is the right one? The decision becomes hard if the peak at the longer period is somewhat larger than the peak at the shorter period (for example, because of noise in the estimation process). How much larger should the longer period peak be before it is accepted as the correct period? This is one of the implementation questions that have to be solved to make this process work in practice.

The resulting approach is surprisingly powerful. The time-varying period is tracked successfully (as illustrated by the high density of intervals marked by $1/F_0$ in figure 3.10A). Cariani and Delgutte could account not only for the estimation of the time-varying F_0, but also for other properties of these sounds. Pitch salience, for example, turns out to be related to the size of the autocorrelation peak at the perceived pitch. Larger peaks are generally associated with stronger, or more salient, pitch.

The major conclusion from studies such as that of Cariani and Delgutte is that it is certainly possible to read F_0 from the temporal structure of auditory nerve fiber responses, so there is no magic here—all the information necessary to generate the pitch percept is available to the brain. On the other hand, these studies do not tell us how the brain extracts periodicity or generates the percept of pitch; for that purpose, it is necessary to go higher up into the auditory system.

The auditory nerve fibers terminate in the cochlear nucleus. The cochlear nucleus has multiple cell types, transforming the representation of sounds in the auditory nerve arrays in various ways (chapter 2). When testing these neurons with pitch-evoking stimuli, Ian Winter and his colleagues (2001) found that, as in the auditory nerve, the autocorrelation functions of these neurons have an overrepresentation of

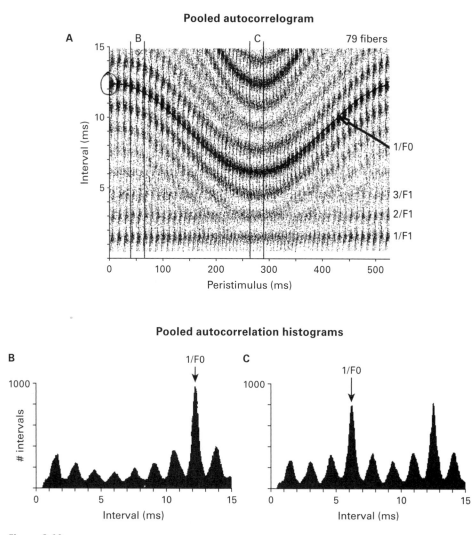

Pooled autocorrelogram

Pooled autocorrelation histograms

Figure 3.10

(A) The time-varying autocorrelation function of Cariani and Delgutte. Time during the stimulus is displayed along the abscissa. At each time along the stimulus, the inter-spike intervals that occurred around that time are tallied and the resulting histogram is displayed along the ordinate. This process was performed for segments of 20 ms, with a substantial amount of overlap. (B) A section of the time-varying autocorrelation function, at the beginning of the sound. Note the single high peak at 12.5 ms. (C) A section of the time-varying autocorrelation function, at the time of the highest pitch. There are two equivalent peaks, one at the correct period and one at twice the period.

From Cariani and Delgutte (1996a) with permission from the American Physiological Society.

the pitch period. However, some of these neurons show an important variation on this theme: The representation of the pitch period was also enhanced in their first-order intervals (those between one spike and the following one). Extracting the periodicity of the sound from the activity of these neurons is therefore easier than extracting it from auditory nerve fibers: Whereas calculating autocorrelations requires measuring all intervals, including those that contain other spikes, counting first-order intervals requires only measuring the times from one spike to the next.

Figure 3.11 illustrates this effect. First-order interspike interval histograms are displayed for an "onset-chopper neuron," one type of neuron found in the ventral cochlear nucleus (VCN). The neuron fires rather regularly even when stimulated with irregular stimuli such as white noise—its interspike intervals have a clear peak at about 10 ms. The neuron was tested with three types of stimuli that evoke pitch: IRN, random phase harmonic complexes (RPH, as in figure 3.1C), and cosine phase harmonic complexes (CPH; these are periodic sounds with a single large peak in their period). CPHs are often used as pitch-evoking stimuli, but they are in a sense extreme. Indeed, in response to CPHs, the neuron fired almost exclusively at the pitch period and its multiples—its spikes were apparently very strongly locked to the large-amplitude peak that occured once during each period of the stimulus. The more interesting tests are therefore the other two stimuli, which do not contain the strong temporal envelope cues that occur in the CPH. Even for these two stimulus types, the interspike interval histograms sometimes contained a sharp peak at the stimulus period. This occurred most clearly when the pitch period was close to 10 ms, which also happened to be the preferred interval for this neuron when stimulated by white noise. Thus, this neuron enhances the representation of the periodicity of pitch-evoking stimuli around its preferred interval.

This turns out to be a rather general finding—many cell types in the cochlear nucleus show such interval enhancement, and for many of them the preferred first-order interspike interval can be observed, for example, in the neuron's response to white noise. The range of best intervals of neurons in the cochlear nucleus is rather wide, covering at least the range from 1 to 10 ms and beyond (1,000 Hz to below 100 Hz).

As we mentioned earlier, the perceived pitch of a sound tends to change very little with change in sound levels. However, many response properties of neurons in the more peripheral parts of the auditory system depend very strongly on sound level. For example, the preferred intervals of onset choppers in the VCN become shorter with

Figure 3.11
First-order interspike intervals of an onset chopper unit in response to noise and to three types of pitch-evoking stimuli with different periods (indicated by the numbers on the right). The first-order intervals are those between a spike and the next one, rather than intervals of all order (as in figure 3.8). This unit represents periods of 8 ms and 11.2 ms well, with weaker representation of shorter and longer periods.
From figure 5 in Winter, Wiegrebe, and Patterson (2001).

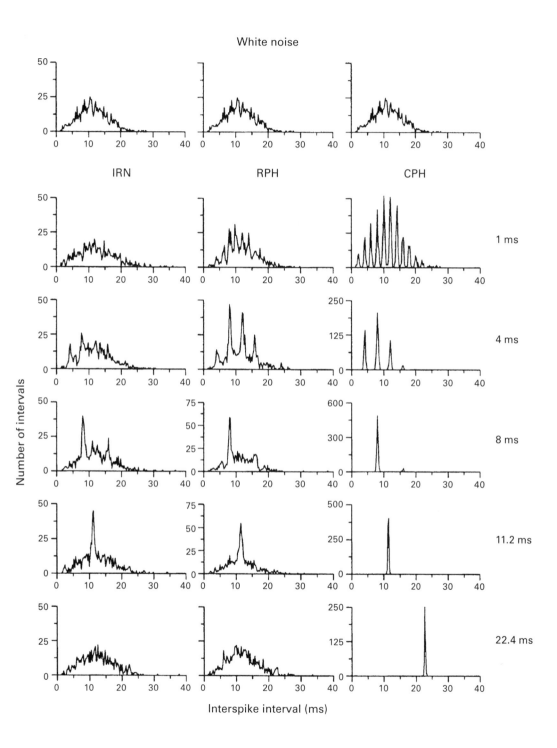

increasing sound level—this is related to the high firing rates of those neurons in response to white noise. Thus, although onset choppers represent periodicity well, they prefer different best periodicities at different sound levels. This makes the readout of the periodicity information from their responses complicated (although not impossible).

However, it turns out that one type of neuron in the VCN, the so-called sustained choppers, shows both an enhancement of the representation of periodicity by first-order interspike intervals and preferred intervals that are essentially independent of sound level. These neurons could be the beginning of a pathway that encodes periodicity in a level-invariant way.

Thus, at the output of the cochlear nucleus, we have neurons that strongly represent F_0 in their temporal firing pattern. This is still not an explicit representation of F_0—we only made it easier for a higher station to extract F_0. In terms of the algorithms we discussed earlier, the all-interval autocorrelation process can be replaced by a simple tallying of the first-order intervals between spikes. While this substantially facilitates the computational problem facing the next stations of the auditory pathways, the crucial step, which is calculating the periodicity itself, has apparently not yet been performed in the VCN.

The cochlear nucleus projects both directly and indirectly to the inferior colliculus (IC). At the level of the IC, the representation of periodicity in terms of the temporal firing patterns appears to be transformed into a firing rate code. IC neurons generally appear less able to phase lock to particular periods with the same vigor and precision as neurons in the VCN. Instead, some neurons in the IC appear to be tuned to specific periodicities—one of these neurons might, for example, respond with high firing rates to sounds with a period of 100 Hz and not respond at all to sounds with a period of 10 Hz or 1,000 Hz (figure 3.12A). An array of such neurons could, in principle, encode periodicity in the same way that the array of auditory nerve fibers encodes frequency content. If this array of "periodicity tuned neurons" was arranged in a systematic manner, the result would be a "periodotopic map" (Schreiner & Langner, 1988). However, many results argue against such an explicit, topographic representation of periodicity in IC.

Figure 3.12 shows the responses of two IC neurons to amplitude-modulated best frequency tones presented with varying sound levels. These stimuli evoke relatively weak pitch (if at all), but nevertheless have been extensively used to study the coding of periodicity in the IC. The modulation frequency (represented along the abscissa) would correspond to the evoked pitch. Figure 3.12A shows the responses of a classical neuron—it has a best modulation frequency at about 60 Hz, and its response at all modulation frequencies grows monotonically with stimulus level.

However, such neurons are not necessarily typical of IC. Most neurons do not have a clear preference for specific modulation rates. Figure 3.12B shows the responses of

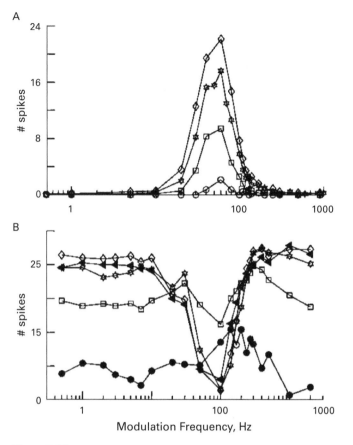

Figure 3.12

The responses of two IC neurons to periodic sounds (SAM complexes). (A) This neuron responds to a narrow range of periods, centered at 60 Hz, and increases its firing rate monotonically with increasing sound level (different symbols). (B) This neuron has a complex pattern of responses as a function of period and sound level.

From figures 5 and 6 in Krishna and Semple (2000) with permission the American Physiological Society.

another neuron. This neuron had a complex pattern of responses as a function of sound level: At low levels it responded weakly with a peak around 100 Hz (filled circles), at intermediate levels it responded to all modulation frequencies without significant selectivity (open squares), and at high sound levels it failed to respond to a restricted set of modulation frequencies while responding to all others (stars, filled triangles, and open diamonds). Thus, a first objection against the presence of a periodotopic map in IC is the finding that IC neurons are far from uniform in their responses to modulation frequencies, and their selectivity to periodic stimuli sometimes depends on irrelevant variables such as sound level. This objection could be surmounted by positing that the representation of the periodicity map is really the role of the classical neurons—like the one shown in figure 3.12A—excluding the neurons with more complex response patterns.

Another major problem with the assumption that a periodotopic map in IC might serve as a neural substrate for pitch perception is that the range of preferred modulation frequencies (and hence, stimulus periods) found in the IC does not correspond to the range of perceived pitches. In a number of species in which these issues have been tested (including cats, gerbils, guinea pigs, and chinchillas), the large majority of IC neurons responds maximally to modulation frequencies below 100 Hz, with a small number of exceptions. Thus, the "pitch axis" would be represented far from uniformly (remember that the note middle A, about the middle of the musical pitch range in humans, has a frequency of 440 Hz), and neurons capable of representing pitch in this manner in the kilohertz range would be very rare indeed.

Finally, more refined tests of IC responses suggest that the selectivity to periodicity of IC neurons may have nothing to do with pitch. Surprisingly, few studies have tested IC neurons with periodic stimuli that evoke a strong pitch percept. Those that have been conducted suggest that IC neurons are sensitive to the periodicity in the envelope of sounds. To see why this is important, consider the sounds in figure 3.13. Both sounds have a period of 10 ms, evoking a pitch of 100 Hz (Sound Example "Periodicity of Sounds and of Envelopes" on the book's Web site). Figure 3.13A displays the waveform of a sound with a single prominent peak in each period, but figure 3.13B displays the waveform of a sound with two prominent peaks in each period (one positive and one negative). Gray lines display the envelope of the two sounds, which measures the overall energy at each moment in time. The envelope of the sound in figure 3.13B has a period of 5 ms, because of the presence of the second peak. When played to IC neurons, sounds such as the one in figure 3.13B evoke responses that correspond to the periodicity of its envelope, rather than to its true periodicity (Shackleton, Liu, & Palmer, 2009).

Thus, the relationship between the representation of periodicity in the IC and pitch is still unclear. It may well be that there is a subset of IC neurons that do encode waveform periodicity, rather than envelope periodicity, but these have not been demonstrated yet.

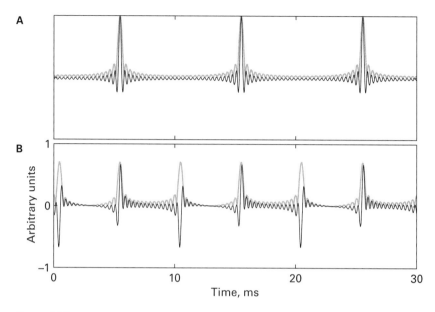

Figure 3.13

A cosine-phase harmonic complex (A) and an alternating-phase harmonic complex (B). In each panel, the waveform is plotted in black, and the envelope in gray. IC neurons respond to the envelope periodicity, and therefore respond to an alternate-phase complex as if it had half the period of the corresponding cosine-phase complex.

3.8   Periodicity Coding in Auditory Cortex

Is there an "explicit" representation of periodicity in the auditory system? It may seem strange to raise this question now, after considering in great detail how pitch might be extracted and represented. But the question is not trivial at all. We cannot exclude the possibility that periodicity is represented only implicitly in the auditory system, in the sense that neural responses in the auditory pathway might never fully separate periodicity from other physical or perceptual qualities of a sound, such as intensity, timbre, or sound source direction. Such an "implicit" representation would not necessarily make it impossible for other, not strictly auditory but rather cognitive or motor areas of the brain to deduce the pitch of a sound if the need arises (similar arguments have been made in the context of so-called motor theories of speech perception).

There is, however, some evidence from imaging experiments (Krumbholz et al., 2003) that parts of the auditory cortex may respond in a "periodicity specific" manner. This experiment used noise stimuli, which metamorphosed from simple, pitchless noise to pitch-evoking but otherwise acoustically similar IRNs (as in figure 3.3B). The transition between noise and IRNs was controlled so that there was no change in bandwidth or sound level. These sounds were played to subjects while the magnetic fields from their brains were recorded. The magnetic fields showed a transient increase just past the change point, resulting in what the authors called pitch onset responses (PORs). These responses increased with pitch strength (related to the number of iterations used to generate the IRNs) and shifted in time with the period—it seems as if the brain had to count a fixed number of periods before it generated the PORs. Finally, magnetoencephalography (MEG) recordings allow some level of localization of the currents that create the fields, and the source of the POR seems to be in auditory cortex (although not necessarily in primary auditory cortex). These results show that human auditory cortex takes notice when periodicity appears or disappears in the ongoing soundscape, but they do not tell us much about how periodicity is represented there.

Before we delve deeper into recent experiments that have tried to shed light on cortical representations of pitch, let us briefly consider what properties such a cortical representation might have. We expect neurons that participate in such representations to be sensitive to periodicity—they should respond to periodic sounds and not (or less) to nonperiodic sounds. We expect their responses to be somehow modulated by periodicity—their rate, or their firing patterns, should be different for different F_0s. These properties are necessary since periodicity is the primary correlate of pitch. In particular, properties such as sound level, timbre, or spatial location should not affect the responses of these neurons, or should affect them in ways that do not impact on their ability to encode periodicity.

However, these properties miss an important feature of pitch—that it is a perceptual, rather than physical, property of sounds. The crucial property of a true pitch representation (in addition to its representation of periodicity) is that it should be able to underpin the listener's perception of pitch. This last, and perhaps most problematic, requirement harks back to a point we made in the opening paragraphs of this chapter, when we pondered the ANSI definition of pitch as an "attribute of sound" that enables listeners to "order sounds on a scale from high to low." If a cortical representation is to underpin the listener's perception, then properties of stimulus-response relationships, such as those we just discussed, are insufficient. Since pitch is a perceptual phenomenon, it is what the listener thought he or she heard, not what the sound actually was, that really matters. A cortical representation of pitch therefore ought to reflect the listener's subjective experience rather than the actual sound. For example, such pitch representation ought to discriminate between pitch values no worse, but also no better, than the listener. Even more important, when asked to make difficult pitch judgments, it should make the same mistakes as the listener on each and every trial.

There is one more property that a pitch representation may have (but is not required to have), and which would make it much easier to find it. Ever since Paul Broca's (who we will meet again in chapter 4) description of a cortical speech area in the 1860s, scientists have been fond of the idea that particular functions might be carried out by neatly localized cortical modules. Such a cortical pitch module would be particularly neat if it featured a topographic (periodotopic) map. However, the existence of a specialized pitch area, or indeed of a topographic pitch map within it, is by no means a necessity, as one could also envisage a distributed cortical pitch network whose constituent neurons are spread out over potentially a wide area and interspersed with neurons that carry out functions other than pitch analysis. Such a distributed arrangement would look messy to the investigator, but might bring advantages to the brain, such as improved fault tolerance (there are, for example, few cases of selective pitch deficits following strokes or small lesions to the brain) or improved interactions between pitch and nonpitch representations for auditory streaming or object recognition.

A number of studies have looked for putative pitch representations in the cortex of humans as well as other mammals, using either electrophysiological recordings or functional imaging methods. It is not uncommon for particular brain regions identified in these studies to be referred to as "pitch centers." However, we deliberately try to avoid this: To demonstrate that a cortical region is indeed a pitch center, showing that it responds selectively to sounds that evoke pitch is not enough. One would also need to demonstrate that it is playing an important role in shaping the listener's subjective pitch percept, and, to date, no study has fully achieved that, although some interesting pieces of the puzzle have been provided. We will first review the single neuron evidence.

In primary auditory cortex (A1), there appears to be no explicit and invariant representation of stimulus periodicity. There are now a fair number of studies that have failed to demonstrate pure sensitivity to periodicity in A1 neurons in a number of species, including cats and macaques (Qin et al., 2005; Schwarz & Tomlinson, 1990). But if A1 does not represent periodicity explicitly, higher-order cortical fields might.

The best evidence to date for neurons that might be specifically sensitive to periodicity is in a nonprimary area of the marmoset auditory cortex. This area, studied by Bendor and Wang (2005), lies adjacent to the low-frequency region of A1 but seems to be distinct from it. Some neurons in this area respond equally well to pure tones of some particular frequency and to harmonic complexes made up of multiples of that frequency but with a missing fundamental. Thus, these neurons appear to be specifically interested in stimulus periodicity, rather than responding merely to sound energy at F_0.

Figure 3.14 illustrates these responses. The neuron shown was tested with complexes consisting of three harmonics of 200 Hz up to high harmonic numbers (figure 3.14A). It responded to all of these complexes, although its responses decreased somewhat at very high harmonic numbers (figure 3.14B). The neuron also responded to pure tones around the same frequency (figure 3.14C), but its tuning was narrow enough that it didn't respond to any of the other harmonics of 200 Hz when presented by itself (figure 3.14E).

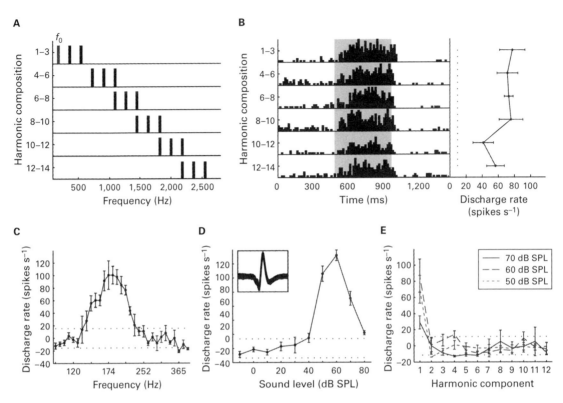

Figure 3.14

(A) Schematic representation of the stimuli used by Bendor and Wang, consisting of three successive harmonics with harmonic numbers from 1 to 14. (B) Peristimulus time histograms (left) and tuning curve (right) of a cortical neuron's response to these harmonic complexes. (C) Responses of the same neuron to pure tones, showing narrow tuning centered on 182 Hz. (D) Response of this neuron to its best sound frequency as a function of level. The inset shows superimposed action potentials recorded from the neuron. The neuron did not respond to a 182-Hz tone below the level of 40 dB SPL. (E) Responses to pure tones at the harmonic frequencies at three levels, showing that responses to pure sine waves occurred only to the first harmonic of the complexes in A.

From figure 1 in Bendor and Wang (2005) with permission from Macmillan Publishers Ltd.

While these data suggest that this neuron is, indeed, sensitive to the periodicity of the stimuli in figure 3.14A, such neurons have to pass two controls to be able to say with certainty that they qualify as bona fide periodicity-selective neurons. The first is to be able to generalize their responses to other periodic stimuli. The second, and possibly harder control to perform, is to exclude the possibility that the neuron might really respond to combination tones that are generated by nonlinearities in the cochlea. As we have seen in chapter 2, section 2.3, combination tones are cochlear responses at frequencies that are the sum and differences of the tone frequencies that compose the sound. The two main combination tones in the cochlea are f2–f1 (the difference between the frequency of the higher and lower tones) and 2f1–f2. It is therefore quite possible that the three-component harmonic complexes used by Bendor and Wang could generate combination tones at F_0. In other words, the cochlea might reinstate the missing fundamental, and the neurons, rather than being truly periodicity sensitive even in the absence of the fundamental, might simply be driven by the cochlear combination tone. Bendor and Wang tried to control for combination tones by using relatively low-level sounds, hoping that this would keep the amplitude of the combination tones too small to excite the neurons they investigated. How effective this was at keeping combination tones out of the picture is difficult to know. These controls are important since there is good evidence that pitch does not depend on combination tones. One example we encountered is the complex of 220, 320, and 420 Hz. This complex would create a cochlear combination tone at 100 Hz, but its pitch is 106 Hz, one semitone higher. So, while the neurons described by Bendor and Wang are the best candidates to date for encoding periodicity, they require a substantial amount of study to confirm them in this role.

Even if these neurons encode periodicity, their role as "pitch neurons" remains uncertain, chiefly because, so far, no evidence indicates that these neurons play a key role in generating or informing the animal's subjective pitch perception. If pitch neurons are really anatomically clustered in a small region, as Bendor and Wang suspect, investigating their role in perception would be relatively easier, because it would then be possible to combine behavioral studies to measure subjective pitch judgments with electrophysiological recording, microstimulation, or lesion studies.

The evidence from other animal experiments is conflicting. A number of studies tried to probe periodicity coding in cortex by imaging of intrinsic optical signals related to blood oxygenation and blood flow. In an influential study, Schulze and colleagues (2002) obtained data suggesting that a periodotopic map overlies the frequency map in A1 of gerbils, although with a different orientation. However, these experiments were carried out using sounds that do not evoke pitch in humans (when properly controlled for combination tones): high-frequency tones that were sinusoidally amplitude modulated with low-frequency envelopes (SAM tones). Other periodic sounds were not used, so we do not know whether the map identified is capable of representing the periodicity of different stimulus types in a similar, consistent manner. To investigate this, we have repeated these experiments in ferrets (Nelken et al., 2008), and though we did observe topographically organized periodicity sensitivity using the same SAM tones, these maps did not generalize to other periodic stimuli. Our experiments failed to find any consistent periodotopic representation either in A1 or the immediately adjacent secondary cortical fields, including areas that should correspond to the periodicity representation suggested by Bendor and Wang in marmosets.

It is possible, of course, perhaps even likely, that significant species differences may exist between marmosets, ferrets, and gerbils, so it is hard to be certain to what extent results obtained in any one of these species are indicative of mammalian auditory cortex in general. Furthermore, one may wonder whether optical imaging techniques, which, after all, rely on rather indirect measures of neural activity, are actually sensitive enough to reveal a true picture of the underlying functional organization of cortex. In the light of the experimental data available to date, however, many researchers remain sceptical about the existence of periodotopic maps in mammalian cortex that could represent pitch topographically.

Since we don't seem to be able to get a hold on periodotopic maps, can we at least identify a region of cortex that appears particularly responsive to stimulus periodicity, and might serve as the brain's "pitch processor," even if it does not represent stimulus periodicity topographically? A functional magnetic resonance imaging (fMRI) study by Patterson and colleagues (2002) suggests that, in humans, such a periodicity region may exist in the nonprimary regions surrounding A1, in particular the lateral portion of Heschl's gyrus (lHG, just lateral to A1, which in humans lies in the medial portion of Heschl's gyrus). In their experiments, Patterson and colleagues used IRN stimuli, because, as we mentioned earlier, these stimuli can be morphed from pitch-free rushing white noise into a pitch-evoking periodic sound. Thus, by comparing brain responses to white noise with those to pitch-evoking IRNs, we ought to be able to reveal brain regions with a particular interest in encoding periodicity.

Figure 3.15 shows the presumed location of A1 in humans (white regions in the lower panels). In the upper panels, the darker regions are those in which broadband noise gave rise to significant activation. They cover A1 but also regions posterior (commonly known as planum temporale) and lateral (closer to the skull, at the edge of the figure) to it. These lateral parts are mostly lighter, indicating that they were activated more strongly by pitch-evoking IRNs than by noise that does not evoke pitch.

Additional pieces of evidence support the notion that the lHG may play an important role in pitch processing. For example, the perception of pitch in sounds that lie at the borders of the existence regions for pitch varies among individuals—in some listeners

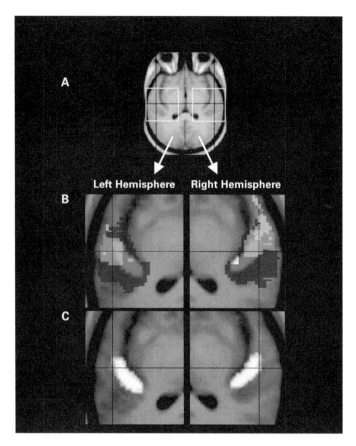

Figure 3.15

Imaging study of pitch encoding in human auditory cortex using fMRI. In the lower panels, the white regions indicate the location of human A1. In the upper panels, the darkest regions indicate the overall area activated as strongly by noise as by periodic stimuli (these regions include both A1 and nonprimary areas). The lighter regions, lying more laterally, were activated more strongly by periodic stimuli. The lightest regions were activated most strongly by stimuli that had additional structure in the sequence of pitches.

From figure 3 of Patterson, Uppenkamp, Johnsrude, and Griffiths (2002) with permission from Elsevier.

the existence regions are wider than in others. It turns out that such tendencies are cor-related, to a significant degree, with anatomical asymmetries in lHG, such that a larger lHG in the left hemisphere is related to larger existence regions (Schneider et al., 2005). Further support for the presence of a pitch center in lHG comes from local field potential recordings measuring neural activity in the auditory cortex of one human patient who was undergoing brain surgery (Schonwiesner & Zatorre, 2008). Electrodes had been positioned in this patient's auditory cortex to help localize an epileptic focus. While the patient was waiting for the onset of a seizure, he was asked to listen to noise-to-IRN transitions very similar to those used in the study by Krumbholz and her colleagues, discussed at the beginning of this section. The recorded responses agree with the findings of the fMRI study by Patterson and his collaborators illustrated in figure 3.15: Whereas noise evoked stronger responses in the medial part of the HG than in its lateral part, the transition from noise to IRN, and hence the onset of pitch, evoked stronger responses at electrodes positioned in lateral HG than in medial HG.

But despite these results, doubt remains about whether lHG really contains a center for encoding periodicity (and, a fortiori, pitch). One problem with these studies is that they have used essentially only one pitch-evoking stimulus—IRNs. Studies using addi-tional stimuli, and not just IRNs, have not necessarily come to the same conclusions. Thus, Hall and Plack (2009) found that, whereas IRNs indeed preferentially activated lHG, other pitch-evoking stimuli strongly activated other parts of auditory cortex, and not necessarily lHG. In fact, the area that was most consistently activated by different pitch-evoking stimuli in their study was the planum temporale, which lies posterior to HG, and may represent a higher processing stage for auditory information than lHG.

None of these studies has addressed the perceptual aspect of pitch perception. The first steps in this directions were performed in a series of recent studies in ferrets by Bizley and her coworkers. In an electrophysiological mapping study (Bizley et al., 2009), these authors recorded responses of hundreds of neurons from all over five different ferret auditory cortical fields. To address the properties of periodicity coding and its relationships with the coding of other sound attributes, they used artificial vowel sounds that varied systematically not just in F_0, but also in timbre and sound source direction. Not one of the neurons they recorded was sensitive to periodicity alone: They all also responded to changes in either timbre or source direction or both. And neurons that seemed particularly sensitive to periodicity were found more com-monly in low-frequency parts of auditory cortex, but were not confined to any one cortical area.

As we have already mentioned, ferrets are capable of categorizing F_0s as high or low, albeit with rather high thresholds (about 20%; Walker et al., 2009). To address the correspondence between neural activity and perception, Schnupp and colleagues (2010) recorded from another set of over 600 neurons in ferret auditory cortex, this time mapping out in much greater detail their periodicity tuning in response to artificial vowels. About half of these neurons were sensitive to changes in F_0, and, interestingly, about one third increased their firing rates monotonically with increasing F_0, while another third decreased their firing rate monotonically with increasing F_0. Such an arrangement of populations with opposite but monotonic dependence of firing rate on F_0 might well be able to provide a robust code for periodicity, one that would, for example, be independent of sound level, as increasing sound levels would not change the relative proportion of firing rates in the high-F_0 versus the low-F_0 preferring neurons. Indeed, Bizley and colleagues went on to show that relatively small ensembles of cortical neurons could be decoded to judge changes in F_0 with the same accuracy as that displayed by the animals in their behavioral tests. Such "F_0-coding neural ensembles" could be found all over the cortex.

However, we still do not know whether the ensemble codes identified by Bizley and colleagues really provide the neural basis for pitch perception. For example, we do not know whether these ensembles would be able to represent the pitch of a wide variety of periodic sounds, not just artificial vowels but also pure tones, missing fundamental harmonic complexes, or IRNs. Furthermore, if these ensembles do inform an animal's pitch judgments, then the ensembles and the animals should make the same occasional mistakes when asked to make a difficult discrimination. This expectation could be tested experimentally if responses of sufficiently large numbers of neurons were recorded from the ferrets while they performed the pitch discrimination task. For technical reasons, this is still difficult, and most of the data in the studies by Bizley and colleagues came from either anesthetized ferrets or awake, but nonbehaving animals. More work is therefore needed before we can be certain whether the ensemble codes proposed by Bizley and colleagues really do play an important role in informing an animal's pitch judgments, or whether the neural basis of pitch perception is of a different nature after all. What is certain is that a complete answer can emerge only from studies that successfully combine physiological and psychophysical approaches, and thereby monitor both the neural and the perceptual responses to sounds of varying pitch simultaneously.

3.9 Recapitulation: The Paradoxes of Pitch Perception

Pitch is a fundamental perceptual property of sounds—arguably the first that would come to mind when considering nonspeech sounds. It is perceived so effortlessly and automatically that we are mostly unaware of the large amount of processing required to extract it. Anyone who has tried to implement a pitch estimation algorithm for natural sounds is probably aware of the difficulties and ambiguities that arise with the use of any single measure of periodicity for pitch estimation.

We saw that pitch is strongly related to the periodicity of sounds, and learned how to estimate this periodicity either in the time domain or from frequency representations of sounds. We observed that the brain is ready to accept rather weak evidence for periodicity and transform it into the sensation of pitch. It is precisely because strict periodicity is not required for evoking pitch that pitch is difficult to compute but also useful as a perceptual cue in a noisy world.

This complexity is mirrored in the representation of pitch in the brain. We have a reasonably good understanding of how periodicity is expressed in the responses of auditory nerve fibers, and how to estimate pitch from the periodicity of auditory nerve fiber responses. However, it remains unclear where and how temporal patterns (which contain an implicit representation of F_0) are transformed into an explicit representation of F_0, and become the percept of pitch. To a considerable degree, we traced this difficulty to the fact that pitch requires generalization. We know that the early auditory system represents sounds in all their details. On the other hand, pitch represents a huge generalization—ignoring any feature of the sound except for its periodicity. Thus, an explicit representation of pitch is almost antithetical to the general rules of sound representation in the early auditory system, which seems to be optimized for keeping all details of the sounds, rather than ignoring those that may be irrelevant for a particular purpose. It makes sense for the auditory system (and presumably for any sensory system) to push generalizations far up in the processing hierarchy. It is therefore perhaps unsurprising that, whereas the information necessary to extract periodicity and possibly partial sensitivity to F_0 (as found by Bizley et al., 2009, in ferret auditory cortex) occurs throughout the auditory system, explicit, invariant representations of pitch (if they exist at all) apparently do not occur below the higher-order ("belt") areas of the auditory cortex, such as the lHG or planum temporale in humans. Similar phenomena may be observed in visual perception. For example, color is a salient perceptual attribute of a visual stimulus, yet neurons whose activity accurately represents the color of a stimulus are found only at rather high levels of the visual hierarchy, beyond both primary and second-order visual cortex. The fact that we perceive the higher-order, generalizing feature (pitch) much more easily than lower-level features (e.g., the sound level of a specific harmonic) suggests that perception follows the processing hierarchy in the reverse order—from the more abstract, generalized high-order representations to the more detailed, physically based ones. We will discuss this reverse relationship in greater depth in chapter 6, when we consider auditory scene analysis.

4 Hearing Speech

How our auditory system supports our ability to understand speech is without a doubt one of the most important questions in hearing research. Severe hearing loss often brings social isolation, particularly in those who were not born into deaf communities. For most of us, the spoken word remains the primary communication channel, particularly for the intimate, face-to-face exchanges and conversations that we value so much. Naturally, we hope that, in due course, a better understanding of the neurobiology of speech processing will improve our ability to repair problems if this system goes wrong, or may allow us to build artificial speech recognition systems that actually work, computers that we could actually talk to. But while the potential rewards of research into the auditory processing of speech are great, considerable technical and conceptual challenges also slow progress in this area.

One major challenge stems from the great complexity of speech. Essentially, a relatively modest number of speech sounds (sometimes called "phones") are recombined according to rules of morphology to form words, and the words are recombined according to the rules of grammar to form sentences. Our auditory brain can analyze the sound of any sentence in a language we have learned, and decipher its meaning, yet the number of correct, meaningful sentences in any language is so large as to be, for all practical intents and purposes, infinite. Thus, when we learn a language, we must not only acquire a sizeable lexicon of sound-to-meaning mappings, but also perfect our grasp of the rules of morphology and grammar, which allow us to manipulate and recombine the speech sounds to generate endless varieties of new meanings.

Many animal species use vocalizations to communicate with members of their own species, and sometimes these communication sounds can be quite elaborate—consider, for example, certain types of birdsong, or the song of humpback whales. Nevertheless, the complexity of human speech is thought to have no equal in the animal kingdom. Dogs and some other domestic animals can be trained to understand a variety of human vocal commands, and rhesus monkeys in the wild are thought to use between thirty and fifty types of vocalization sounds to convey different meanings. The number of different vocalizations used in these examples of inter- and intraspecies vocal communication is, however, fairly modest compared to the size of a typical human language vocabulary, which can comprise tens of thousand words.

Animals also seem to have only a limited capacity for recombining communication sounds to express new concepts or describe their relationships. Even the most mono-syllabic of human teenagers readily appreciates that the meaning of the sentence "*John eats and then flies*" is very different from that of "*And then John eats flies*," even though in both sentences the speech sounds are identical and only their order has changed a bit. Human children seem to learn such distinctions with little effort. But while you do not need to explain this difference to your child, you would have a terribly hard time trying to explain it to your dog. Indeed, many language researchers believe that humans must have an innate facility for learning and understanding grammar, which other animals seem to lack (Pinker, 1994).

Given this uniquely high level of development of speech and language in humans, some may argue that there is little point in studying the neural processing of speech and speechlike sounds in nonhuman animals. However, the tools available to study the neural processing of communication sounds in humans are very limited. Work with humans depends heavily either on lesion studies that attempt to correlate damage to particular brain areas with loss of function, on noninvasive functional imaging techniques, or on the rare opportunities where electrophysiological recording or stimulation experiments can be incorporated into open brain surgery for the treatment of epilepsy. Each of these methods has severe limitations, and the level of detail that is revealed by microelectrode recordings in animal brains is, as we shall see, still an invaluable source of complementary information.

But using animal experiments to shed light on the processing of vocalizations is not merely a case of "looking for the key where the light is." Human speech almost certainly evolved from the vocal communication system of our primate ancestors, and it evolved its great level of complexity in what is, in evolutionary terms, a rather short period of time. No one is quite certain when humans started to speak properly, but we diverged from the other surviving great ape species some 5 million years ago, and our brains reached their current size some 1 to 2 million years ago (no more than 100,000 generations). During this period, human speech circuits almost certainly arose as an adaptation and extension of a more or less generic, rudimentary mammalian vocal communication system, and animal experiments can teach us a great deal about these fundamental levels of vocalization processing.

Speech can be studied on many levels, from the auditory phonetic level, which considers the manner in which individual speech sounds are produced or received, to the syntactic, which considers the role of complex grammatical rules in interpreting speech, or the semantic, which asks how speech sounds are "mapped onto a particular meaning." As we have said, studies of animal brains are unlikely to offer deep parallels or insights into syntactic processing in the human auditory system, but neural representations of speech sounds or animal vocalizations on the auditory/phonetic level are likely to be very similar from one mammal to the next. Most mammals vocalize, and do so in much the same way as we do (Fitch, 2006). As we briefly described in section 1.6, mammals vocalize by pushing air through their larynx, causing their vocal folds to vibrate. The resulting sound is then filtered through resonant cavities in their vocal tracts, to impart on it a characteristic "formant" structure. (On the book's web site you can find short video clips showing the human vocal folds and vocal tract in action.) There are some differences in detail, for example, humans have a relatively deep-sitting larynx, which makes for a particularly long vocal tract, and may allow us to be a "particularly articulate mammal" (Ghazanfar & Rendall, 2008), but the basic layout is essentially the same in all mammals, and the sounds generated by the vocal tracts of different types of mammals consequently also have much in common. These similarities are more obvious in some cases than in others (few humans, for example, would be very flattered to hear that they sound like a donkey), but at times they can be very striking, as in the case of Hoover the talking harbor seal. Hoover was an orphaned seal pup, who had been adopted by a fisherman in Maine, and began to imitate the speech of his rescuer. Recordings of Hoover the talking seal can be found on the book's website, and even though it is hard to make out much meaning in them, they nevertheless sound uncannily like the slurred speech of an old sailor.

When vocalizing to communicate with each other, animals also face some of the same challenges we humans have to overcome to understand speech. For example, both human and animal vocalizations are subject to a fair amount of individual variability. No two humans pronounce the same word absolutely identically. Differences in gender, body size, emotional affect, as well as regional accents can all change the sound of a spoken word without necessarily changing its meaning. Similarly, dogs who differ in size or breed can produce rather different sounding barks, yet despite these differences they all remain unmistakably dog barks. Even songbirds appear to have pronounced "regional dialects" in their songs (Marler & Tamura, 1962). One common problem in the processing of human speech as well as in animal vocalizations is therefore how to correctly identify vocalizations, despite the often very considerable individual variability. The neural processes involved in recognizing communication sounds cannot be simple, low-level feature extractors, but must be sophisticated and flexible pattern classifiers. We still have only a very limited understanding of how animal and human brains solve this kind of problem, but in experimental animals, unlike in humans, these questions are at least in principle amenable to detailed experimental observation.

This chapter is subdivided into eight sections. In the first two sections, we examine the acoustic properties of speech in greater detail, consider how the acoustic features of speech evolve in time, and how they are categorized into distinct speech sounds. In the third section, we describe how speech sounds are thought to be encoded in subcortical structures. Our knowledge of these subcortical representations comes exclusively from animal experiments. In the fourth part, we briefly review the anatomy of the cortex, and in the fifth we summarize what clinical observations have taught us about the role played by various parts of the human cerebral cortex in speech processing. In the next two sections, we examine the roles of primary and higher-order cortical fields in greater detail, in the light of additional information from human brain imaging and animal experiments, before briefly considering the influence of vision on speech processing and perception.

4.1   Speech as a Dynamic Stimulus

When one considers speech as an auditory stimulus, one obvious question to ask is: Is speech radically different from other sounds, and if so, in what way? In section 1.6, we looked at the production of vocalization sounds, and we noted that the physics of vocal sound production is not particularly unusual, and contains nothing that might not have an equivalent in the inanimate world. (You may wish to glance through section 1.6, pages 34–39, quickly before you read on if this is not fresh in your mind.) The harmonics in voiced speech sounds produced by the oscillating vocal folds are not so different from harmonics that might be produced by vibrating taut strings or reeds. Unvoiced fricatives are caused by turbulent airflow through constrictions in the vocal tract, and they resemble the noises caused by rushing wind or water in both the way they are created and the way they sound. Resonant cavities in our vocal tract create the all-important formants by enhancing some frequencies and attenuating others, but they operate just like any other partly enclosed, air-filled resonant chamber. So if speech sounds are, in many respects, fundamentally similar to other environmental sounds and noises, we might also expect them to be encoded and processed in just the same way as any other sound would be by neurons of the auditory system.

Nevertheless, listeners only rarely mistake other environmental sounds for speech, so perhaps there is something about speech that makes it characteristically speechlike, even if it is not immediately obvious what this something is. Consider the sound of wind rushing through some trees. It may contain noisy hissing sounds that resemble fricative consonants (fffff-, sss-, shhh-like sounds), and it may also contain more harmonic, vaguely vowel-like "howling." But the pitch and amplitude contours of these sounds of howling wind usually change only slowly, much more slowly than they would in speech. Meanwhile, a small stream of water dropping into a pond might trickle, gurgle, and splash with an irregular rhythm rather faster than that of speech.

Thus, it seems that speech has its own characteristic rhythm. Speech sounds change constantly in a manner that is fast, but not too fast, and somewhat unpredictable yet not entirely irregular. But can we turn this intuition regarding possible characteristic rhythms of speech into something more tangible, more quantifiable?

One way to approach this question is to consider the mechanisms of speech production in a little more detail. A good example of this type of analysis can be found in a paper by Steven Greenberg (2006), in which he argues that the syllable may be the most appropriate unit of analysis for speech sounds. Based on a statistical analysis of a corpus of spoken American English, he concluded that syllables consist of an optional "onset" (containing between zero and three consonants), an obligatory "nucleus" (a vowel sound, which can be either a monophthong like the /a/ in "at," or a diphthong, like the /ay/ in "may"), and an optional "coda" (containing between zero and four consonants). A single English syllable can therefore be as simple as "a" or as elaborate as "straights." Greenberg would argue that more "atomic" speech sound units, such as the phoneme, or phone, are "unreal" in the sense that they have no independent existence outside the syllabic framework. Furthermore, he points out that the information content of consonants depends on the syllabic context. For example, onsets are more informative than codas, as can be seen by the fact that consonants in the coda can often be lost without any loss of intelligibility (consider the lost /d/ in "apples an' bananas"). Given the diversity of English syllables, it is unsurprising that they can also vary considerably in their temporal extent. English syllables are typically 100 to 500 ms long, and are characterized by an "energy arc," since the vowel nucleus is normally up to 40 dB more intense than the consonants of the onset or the coda. Note that not all languages exhibit as much phonetic diversity in their syllables as English. In spoken Japanese, for example, onsets very rarely comprise more than a single consonant, and the only commonly used coda to a syllable is an optional "n." Consequently, in Japanese there are only a few hundred possible syllables, while in English there are many thousands, but the onset-nucleus-coda syllabic structure is clearly a feature of both languages.

As mentioned in chapter 1, engineers like to refer to changes in a signal over time as "modulations", and they distinguish two fundamental types: amplitude modulation (AM, meaning the sound gets louder or quieter) and frequency modulation (FM, meaning the frequency content of the sound changes). Greenberg's observation of one energy arc in every spoken syllable, and one syllable every few hundreds of milliseconds or so would lead us to expect that speech sounds should exhibit marked AM at modulation rates of a few hertz. Is this expectation borne out? If you look at spectrograms of spoken sentences, like those shown in figure 2.13A (p. 81) or figure 4.1A, you do, of course, notice that speech contains plenty of both AM and FM. But it is not obvious, just from looking at the spectrograms, what the properties of these modulations really are, or whether speech exhibits characteristic modulations, which would be either

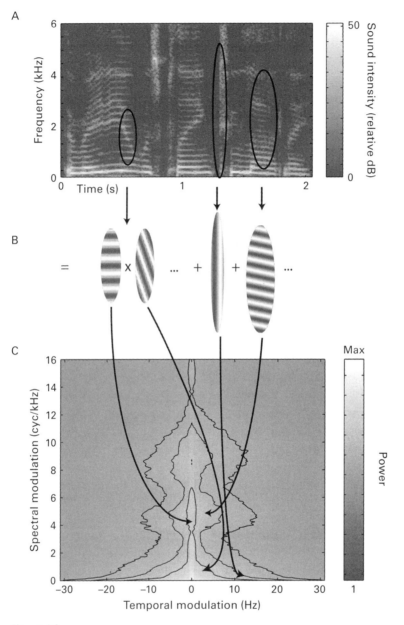

Figure 4.1

Modulation spectra of spoken English. Spectrograms of spoken sentences (example sentence "The radio was playing too loudly," shown in A) are subjected to a two-dimensional Fourier transform (2DFT) to calculate the sentence's modulation spectrum (C). Just as an ordinary Fourier transform particularly prominent in spoken sentences or particularly important in carrying the information encoded in the speech signal.

How best to identify and describe the modulations that are characteristic of speech is an old and important research question. One recent study by Elliott and Theunissen (2009) sheds new light on this by analyzing and manipulating the modulation spectra of speech. (At first glance, the concept of a modulation spectrum is perhaps a little technical and abstract, but it is useful, so hang in there for the next two pages or so.) Essentially, modulation spectra are the two-dimensional Fourier transforms (2DFTs) of the signal's spectrogram. This may appear terrifyingly complicated to the uninitiated, but it is not quite as bad as all that. The concept is illustrated in figure 4.1. Figure 4.1A shows the spectrogram of a spoken sentence. Recall from section 1.3 that ordinary Fourier transforms express a one-dimensional signal, like a sound, as a superposition (or sum) of a large number of suitably chosen sine waves. The 2DFT does a very similar thing, by expressing a two-dimensional "picture" as a superposition of sine wave gratings or "ripples." Think of these ripples as regular zebra stripes of periodically (sinusoidally) increasing and decreasing amplitude.

Figure 4.1B illustrates this by showing how regions within the spectrogram are well approximated by such ripples. Consider the region delineated by the leftmost black elliptic contour in the spectrogram. This patch contains a very obvious harmonic stack associated with one of the vowel sounds in the sentence, and the regularly spaced harmonics can be well approximated by a ripple with a matching spectral modulation rate, that is, stripes of an appropriate spacing along the vertical, frequency, or spectral dimension. In this conceptual framework, spectral modulations are therefore manifest as zebra stripes that run horizontally across the spectrogram, parallel to the time axis, and a set of harmonics with a fundamental frequency of 200 Hz would thus be captured to a large extent by a spectral modulation with a modulation rate of 5 cycles/kHz. Perhaps counterintuitively, a lower-pitched sound, with harmonics spaced, say, every 100 Hz, would correspond to a higher spectral modulation rate of 10 cycles/kHz, since low-pitched sounds with lower fundamental frequencies can squeeze a larger number of harmonics into the same frequency band.

But we cannot describe every aspect of a spectrogram solely in terms of horizontal stripes that correspond to particular spectral modulations. There is also variation in time. Particularly obvious examples are the short, sharp, broadband fricative and

represents a waveform as a superposition of sine waves, a 2DFT represents a spectrogram as a superposition of "spectrotemporal ripples." The spectrograms of the ripples themselves look like zebra stripes (B). Their temporal modulation captures the sound's AM, and their spectral modulation captures spectral features such as harmonics and formants.
Adapted from figure 1 of Elliott and Theunissen (2009).

plosive consonants which show up as vertical stripes in the spectrogram in figure 4.1A. In the modulation spectrum of a sound, these and other "vertical" features are captured by "temporal modulations," and this occurs in a relatively intuitive manner. Temporal modulations simply measure the amount of AM at some particular modulation rate, so high-frequency temporal modulations capture fast changes in amplitude, low temporal modulation frequencies capture slow changes in amplitude, and at 0 Hz temporal modulation we find the sound's grand average (constant) signal power.

Earlier, we mentioned that, according to Greenberg (2006), speech sounds are characterized by syllabic energy arcs, which are between 100 and 500 ms wide. These energy arcs should correspond to temporal modulation frequencies between 10 and 2 Hz. The fact that almost all the signal power in the speech modulation spectrum shown in figure 4.1C appears to be contained between + and –10 Hz temporal modulation is therefore compatible with Greenberg's observations.

Hang on a minute. Did we just say a temporal modulation of *minus* 10 Hz? It is relatively easy to imagine what a temporal modulation of 10 Hz might represent: Some property of the sound gets larger and then smaller and then larger again ten times a second. But what, you may ask, is a temporal modulation rate of *minus* 10 Hz supposed to mean? You would be right to think that, in our universe, where time never flows backward, a sound can hardly go through some cyclical changes once every minus 0.1 s. Indeed, these "negative" temporal modulation frequencies should simply be thought of as an expedient mathematical trick that allows us to represent acoustic features in which frequency changes over time, and which would show up as diagonal stripes in the spectrogram. The 2DFT captures such spectrotemporal modulations with diagonal ripples, and these diagonals come in two flavors: They either rise, or they fall. In the convention adopted here, a spectrotemporal ripple with a negative temporal modulation corresponds to rising frequency trajectories, while positive temporal frequencies correspond to falling frequencies. The fact that the modulation spectrum shown in figure 4.1C is fairly symmetrical around 0 Hz temporal modulation, thus, tells us that, in the sample of American English sentences analyzed here, features with rising frequency content are just as common as features with falling FM.

One very useful feature of the modulation spectrum is that it separates out low spectral frequency, that is, spectrally broad features such as the formants of speech, from high spectral frequency features, such as harmonic fine structure associated with pitch. The pitch of female speech tends to be noticeably higher than that of male speech, but the formants of female speech differ less from those of male speech, which presumably makes understanding speech, regardless of speaker gender, substantially easier. This is readily apparent in the modulation spectra shown in figure 4.2, which

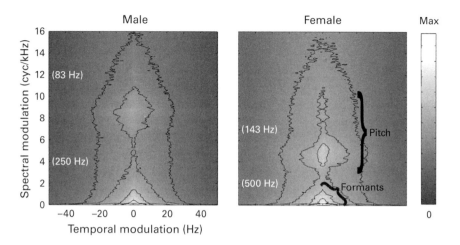

Figure 4.2

Modulation spectra of male and female English speech. Corresponding pitches are given in white.

From figure 2 of Elliott and Theunissen (2009).

are rather similar for the low spectral modulations (less than 3 cycles/kHz) associated with the broad formant filters, but much more dissimilar for the higher spectral modulations associated with pitch.

Given the crucial role of formants in speech, we might therefore expect the meaning of the spoken sentence to be carried mostly in the relatively low temporal and frequency modulations, and one rather nice feature of Elliott and Theunissen's (2009) use of the modulation spectrum is that they were able to demonstrate this directly. Modulation spectra, like ordinary Fourier transforms, are in principle "invertible," that is, you can use the spectrum to reconstruct the original signal. Of course, if you blank out or modify parts of the modulation spectrum before inversion, then you remove or modify the corresponding temporal or spectral modulations from the original speech.

By testing comprehension of sentences after filtering out various ranges of modulations, Elliott and Theunissen (2009) were able to demonstrate that spectral modulations of less than 4 cycles/kHz and temporal modulations between 1 and 7 Hz are critical for speech intelligibility. They refer to this as the core region of the human speech modulation spectrum, and it sits very much in those parts of modulation space where we would expect the formants of speech to reside. Filtering out modulations outside this core region has only a relatively small effect on speech intelligibility, but may make it much harder to distinguish male from female speakers, particularly if it affects spectral modulations between 4 and 12 cycles/kHz, which, as we have seen in figure 4.2, encapsulate much of the differences in male versus female voice pitch. Examples of such "modulation filtered" speech can be found in the online material accompanying Elliott and Theunissen's original (2009) paper, or on the Web site accompanying this book.

Many artificial speech recognition systems use a mathematical device that is conceptually closely related to the modulation spectrum, known as the "dynamic cepstrum." Like the modulation spectrum, the cepstrum is calculated as a Fourier transform along the frequency axis of the sound's spectrogram. The cepstrum can then be used to separate out the low spectral modulations that are associated with the relatively broadly tuned resonances of the vocal tract that mark the formants of speech, and discard the high spectral modulations associated with pitch.

Pitch, thus, seems to add little to speech comprehension, at least for English and most Indo-European languages. (You can find examples of speech samples with altered pitch contours that illustrate this on the book's Web site). But it is worth noting that many Asian languages are tonal, meaning that they may use pitch trajectories to distinguish the meanings of different words. To give one example: Translated into Mandarin Chinese, the sentence *"mother curses the horse"* becomes *"māma mà mă."* The symbols above the *"a"*s are Pinyin[1] tone markers, intended to indicate the required pitch. Thus, the *"ā"* is pronounced not unlike like the "a" in the English "bark," but with a pitch much higher than the speaker's normal, neutral speaking voice. The *"à,"* in contrast, must be pronounced with a rapidly falling pitch contour, and in the *"ă"*—particularly challenging for unaccustomed Western vocal tracts—the pitch must first dip down low, and then rise again sharply, by well over one octave, in a small fraction of a second. Remove these pitch cues, for example, by filtering out spectral modulations above 7 cycles/kHz, and the sentence becomes *"mamamama,"* which is gibberish in both Chinese and English. One consequence of this use of pitch to carry semantic meaning in tonal languages is that many current Western speech processing technologies, from speech recognition software for personal computers to speech processors for cochlear implants, are not well adapted to the needs of approximately one quarter of the world's population.

Nevertheless, even in tonal languages, the lion's share of the meaning of speech appears to be carried in the formants, and in particular in how formant patterns change (how they are modulated) over time. Relatively less meaning is encoded in pitch, but that does not mean that pitch is unimportant. Even in Western, nontonal languages, pitch may provide a valuable cue that helps separate a speech signal out from background noise, or to distinguish one speaker from another. (We shall return to the role of pitch as a cue in such auditory scene analysis problems in chapter 6.) In chapter 3, we looked in detail at how pitch information is thought to be represented in the auditory pathway, so let us now look in more detail at how the auditory system distinguishes different classes of speech sounds.

4.2 Categorical Perception of Speech Sounds

One crucial, but also poorly understood, part of the neural processing of speech is that sounds must be mapped onto categories. The physical properties of a sound can vary smoothly and continuously. Not only can we produce /a/ sounds and /i/ sounds, but also all manner of vowels that lie somewhere along the continuum between /a/ and /i/. However, perceiving a sound as "between /a/ and /i/" is unhelpful for the purpose of understanding speech. Our brains have to make categorical decisions. A person who is talking to us may be telling us about his "bun" or his "bin," but it has to be one or the other. There is no continuum of objects between "bun" and "bin." Once we use speech sounds to distinguish different, discrete objects, concepts, or grammatical constructs, we must subdivide the continuous space of possible speech sounds into discrete categories. Such categorical perception is therefore believed to be a key step in speech processing, and it has attracted much interest among researchers. What are the criteria that our brains use to distinguish sound categories? Are category boundaries arbitrary parcellations of the set of all possible speech sounds, and do different languages draw these boundaries differently? Or are there physical or physiological laws that dictate where the boundaries should fall? And does the human brain comprise specialized modules for recognizing such phoneme categories that other animals lack, or is categorical perception of speech sounds or vocalizations also seen in other animals?

Let us first consider the question of phoneme boundaries. One thing that is readily apparent to most students of foreign languages is that the phoneme boundaries are not the same in all languages. German, for example, has its Umlaute—"ä," "ü," and "ö"—effectively a set of additional vowels that are lacking in English. Some Scandinavian languages have even more vowels, such as the "å" and the "ø." Thus, English lacks certain phoneme categories that exist in other languages, but it also makes some distinctions other languages do not. Japanese people, for example, are famously unable to distinguish between "r" and "l" sounds. This inability is not innate, however, but emerges during the first year of life, as children are conditioned in their mother tongue (Kuhl et al., 2006). While these language-specific differences suggest that phonetic boundaries are largely determined by the environment we grow up in, they may nevertheless not be entirely arbitrary. In a recent review, Diehl (2008) discussed two theories, the quantal theory and the dispersion theory, which may help explain why phonetic category boundaries are where they are. Both theories emerge from considerations of the physical properties and limitations of the vocal tract.

To get a feeling for the ideas behind quantal theory, let us start with a simple experiment that you can try yourself. Make a long "ssssssss" sound, and then, while keeping the sound going, move the tip of your tongue very slowly backward in your mouth so as to gradually change the sound from /s/ to /sh/. When the tip of your tongue is near your teeth, you will make an /s/, and with the tip of your tongue further back against your palate you will make a /sh/. So far so good, but you may notice that placing your tongue halfway between the /s/ and /sh/ positions does not easily produce a sound halfway between /s/ and /sh/. As you move your tongue steadily forward or backward you may notice a very sudden transition (a "quantum leap") from /s/ to /sh/ or from /sh/ to /s/. Quantal theory posits that languages avoid using speech sounds that are very close to such quantal boundaries in the acoustics. We do not use speech sounds somewhere between /s/ and /sh/ because they would be too difficult to pronounce reliably. Near a quantal boundary, a small inaccuracy in the placement of the articulators will often lead to disproportionately large changes in the sound produced, and therefore any category of speech sounds that happened to live very close to a quantal boundary would be particularly easy to mispronounce and mishear. Making sure that speech sound categories keep a respectful distance from quantal boundaries would therefore make speech more robust.

Dispersion theory (Liljencrants & Lindblom, 1972) takes a different approach. It starts from the realization that there are limits to the range of speech sounds a normal human vocal tract can produce. The theory then makes the not unreasonable assumption that, to make speech sound categories easily distinguishable, they should be widely spread out (dispersed) across this space of all possible speech sounds. Figure 4.3 illustrates this for the case of vowel sounds. The coordinate axes of figure 4.3 show the first and second formant frequency of a particular vowel. The continuous contour shows the limits of the formant frequencies that a normal human vocal tract can easily produce, while the black dots show first and second formant frequencies for some of the major vowel categories of the world's languages. It, indeed, looks as if the vowels are not positioned randomly inside the space available within the contour, but instead are placed so as to maximize their distances, which should help make them easily distinguishable.

Thus, the quantal and dispersion theories establish some ground rules for where phonetic category boundary might fall, but there is nevertheless considerable scope for different languages to draw up these boundaries differently, as we have seen. And this means that at least some phoneme boundaries cannot be innate, but must be learned, typically early in life. Interestingly, the learning of some of these categorical boundaries appears to be subject to so-called critical or sensitive developmental periods (Kuhl et al., 2008), so that category distinctions that are learned in the early years of life are very hard or impossible to unlearn in adulthood. Thus, Japanese speakers who have not learned to differentiate between "r" and "l" early in life appear to find it very difficult even to hear a difference between these sounds in adulthood. (We will say more about sensitive periods in chapter 7.) However, that seems to be an extreme case, and most learned phoneme boundaries do not bring with them an inability to distinguish sounds that fall within a learned class. Thus, the English language has no

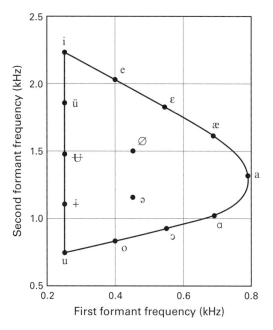

Figure 4.3

The contour shows the pairings of possible F1/F2 formant frequencies, which are as distinct as they could be, given the physical constraints of the human vocal tract. Symbols show approximately where vowels of the world's languages are located in this F1/F2 space.
Adapted from figure 7 of Diehl (2008) with permission from the Royal Society.

category boundary that distinguishes the vowels /ä/ or /å/, yet adult native English speakers can learn very quickly to distinguish and to recognize them.

So some phonetic category boundaries, such as those between /r/ and /l/ or between /a/, /ä/, and /å/, are therefore largely language specific and culturally determined, and children pick them up in early infancy. But other phoneme boundaries seem fixed across many languages, and may therefore be based on distinctions that are hard-wired into the auditory system of all humans, or perhaps all mammals. For example, you may recall that consonants differ either in their place or the manner of articulation. Thus, /p/ and /t/ are distinguished by place of articulation (one is made with the lips, the other with the tip of the tongue placed against the top row of teeth), but /b/ and /p/ both have the same "labial" place of articulation. What distinguishes /b/ from /p/ is that one is said to have a "voiced" manner of articulation while the other is "unvoiced," in other words the /p/ in "pad" and the /b/ in "bad" differ mostly in their "voice onset time" (VOT).[2] In "pad," there is a little gap of about 70 ms between the plosive /p/ sound and the onset of the vocal fold vibration that marks the vowel /a/, while in "bad," vocal fold vibration starts almost immediately after the /b/, with a gap typically no greater than 20 ms or so. Consequently, it is possible to morph a recording of the word "bad" to sound like "pad" simply by lengthening the gap between the /b/ and the /a/. What is curious about VOTs is that the length of VOTs does not seem to vary arbitrarily from one language to the next. Instead, VOTs occur in no more than three distinct classes, referred to as leading, short or long, which are conserved across the world's languages. In the leading category, voicing may start at about 100 ms before the consonant, while short VOTs imply that voicing starts 10 to 20 ms after the consonant, and long VOTs mean that voicing starts about 70 ms after the consonant (Lisker & Abramson, 1964). Leading voicing is not a typical feature of English, but it is common in other languages such as Spanish, where, for example, "v" is pronounced like a very soft /b/, so that the word "*victoria*" is pronounced "*mbictoria.*"

Several studies have shown that animals, such as chinchillas (Kuhl & Miller 1978) or quail (Kluender, Diehl, & Killeen, 1987), can be easily trained to discriminate stop consonants with short or long VOTs. Thus the three VOT categories may be "linguistic universals" because they are based on acoustic distinctions that are particularly salient for the auditory systems not just of humans but also of other animals.

4.3   Subcortical Representations of Speech Sounds and Vocalizations

You may recall from section 2.4, and in particular from figure 2.13, that the inner ear and auditory nerve (AN) are thought to operate like a filter bank, and firing rates along the tonotopic array of the auditory nerve fiber bundle create a sort of "neurogram," a rate-place code for the acoustic energy distribution in the incoming sound. The frequency resolution in that tonotopic rate-place code is not terribly sharp, but it is easily sharp enough to capture formant peaks. When we introduced the neurogram notion in figure 2.13, however, we did gloss over a small complication, which we now ought to come clean about. We mentioned only in passing in section 2.4 that the majority (roughly 80%) of AN fibers are high spontaneous rate fibers that saturate— that is, they cannot fire any faster, once the sound at their preferred frequency reaches a level of between 30 and 50 dB SPL. Over 30 years ago, Young and Sachs (1979) had already pointed out that this rate saturation can have awkward consequences for the place-rate representation of formants in the auditory nerve. Figure 4.4 illustrates some of their findings from a set of experiments in which they recorded AN responses to artificial vowel sounds presented at different sound levels.

Figure 4.4A shows the power spectrum of the stimulus Sachs and Young used: an artificial vowel with harmonics every 128 Hz, passed through a set of formant filters to impose formant peaks at about 400 Hz, as well as at about 2,000 and 2,800 Hz. The resultant sound is not too different from the human vowel /I/ (a bit like the "i" in

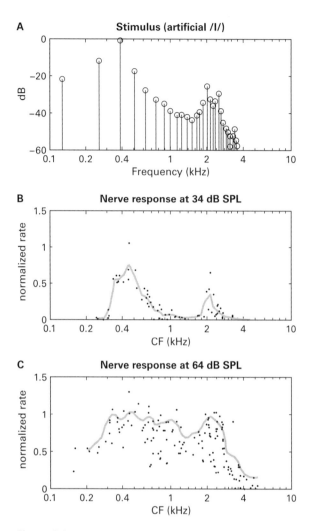

Figure 4.4

Responses in the auditory nerve of the cat to a steady-state artificial vowel /I/. (A) power spectrum of the vowel sound. It exhibits harmonics every 128 Hz, and formants at approximately 0.4, 2, and 2.8 kHz. (B) Nerve fiber responses when the vowel is presented at a relatively quiet 34 dB SPL. Each dot is the normalized evoked firing rate of a single nerve fiber, plotted against each fiber's CF. The continuous line is a moving average along the frequency axis. The observed nerve discharge rate distribution exhibits clear peaks near the stimulus formant frequencies. (C) Nerve fiber responses when the sound is presented at a moderately loud 64 dB SPL. Due to saturation of nerve fiber responses, the peaks in the firing distributions are no longer clear. Based on data published in Young and Sachs (1979).

"blitz"). Note that the figure uses a logarithmic frequency axis, which explains why the harmonics, spaced at regular 128-Hz intervals, appear to become more densely packed at higher frequencies. Sachs and Young recorded responses from many AN fibers in the anesthetized cat to presentations of this sound at various sound levels. Figure 4.4B summarizes their results for presentations of the artificial vowel at an intensity of 34 dB SPL. Each point in figure 4.4B shows the response for a single nerve fiber. The x-coordinate shows the nerve fiber's characteristic frequency (CF), and the y-coordinate shows the nerve fiber's firing rate, averaged over repeated presentations of the stimulus at 34 dB SPL, and normalized by subtracting the nerve fiber's spontaneous firing rate and dividing by the nerve fiber's maximal firing rate in response to loud pure tones at its CF. In other words, a normalized rate of 0 means the neuron fires no more strongly than it would in complete quiet, while a normalized rate of 1 means it fires almost as strongly as it ever will. The gray continuous line in figure 4.4B shows a moving average across the observed normalized firing rates for the AN fibers. This averaged normalized firing rate as a function of CF appears to capture the formant peaks in the stimulus quite nicely. So what's the problem?

The problem is that 34 dB SPL is really very quiet. Just the background hum generated by many air conditioning systems or distant traffic noise will have higher sound levels. Most people converse with speech sounds of an intensity closer to 65 to 70 dB SPL. But when Sachs and Young repeated their experiment with the artificial vowel presented at the more "natural" sound level of 64 dB SPL, the firing rate distribution in the auditory nerve was nothing like as pretty, as can be seen in figure 4.4C. The firing rate distribution has become a lot flatter, and the formant peaks are no longer readily apparent. The problem is not so much that the peaks in the firing rate distribution at the formants have disappeared, but rather that the valley between them has filled in. This is a classic example of the so-called dynamic range problem. Most AN fibers saturate at relatively modest sound intensities, and sounds don't have to become very loud before the AN fibers lose their ability to signal spectral contrasts like those between the formant peaks and troughs in a vowel.

The curious thing, of course, is that even though the representation of the formant peaks across the nerve fiber array appears to become degraded as sound levels increase, speech sounds do not become harder to understand with increasing loudness—if anything the opposite is true. So what is going on?

There are a number of possible solutions to the dynamic range problem. For example, you may recall from chapter 2 that AN fibers come in different classes: High spontaneous rate (HSR) fibers are very sensitive and therefore able to respond to very quiet sounds, but they also saturate quickly; low spontaneous rate (LSR) fibers are less sensitive, but they also saturate not nearly as easily. The plots in figure 4.4 do not distinguish between these classes of AN fibers. Perhaps the auditory pathway uses HSR fibers only for hearing in very quiet environments. HSR fibers outnumber LSR fibers about four to one, so the large majority of the nerve fibers sampled in figure 4.4 are likely to be HSR fibers, and using those to encode a vowel at 64 dB SPL might be a bit like trying to use night vision goggles to see in bright daylight.

Young and Sachs (1979) also proposed an alternative, perhaps better explanation when they noticed that, even though the nerve fibers with CFs between 300 and 3,000 Hz shown in figure 4.4C may all fire at similarly high discharge rates, they tend to phase lock to the formant frequencies close to their own CF. For example, you might find a 500-Hz fiber that is firing vigorously, but at an underlying 400-Hz rhythm. In that case you might conclude that the dominant frequency component in that frequency range is the frequency signaled by the temporal firing pattern (400 Hz) even if this is not the nerve fiber's preferred frequency (500 Hz). Such considerations led Young and Sachs (1979) to propose a response measure that takes both firing rate and phase locking into account. This response measure, the "average localized synchronized rate" (ALSR), quantifies the rate of spikes that are locked to the CF of the neuron. In the previous example, the ALSR would be rather low for the 500-Hz neuron, since most spikes are synchronized to the 400-Hz formant. The ALSR measure of auditory nerve discharges reflects formant frequencies much more stably than ordinary nonsynchronized rate-place codes could.

Whether your auditory brainstem solves the dynamic range problem by computing the ALSR, by listening selectively either to HSR or to LSR fibers depending on sound level, or by relying on some other as yet unidentified mechanism is not known. However, we can be pretty certain that the auditory brainstem does solve this problem, not only because your ability to understand speech tends to be robust over wide sound level ranges, but also because electrophysiological recordings have shown that so-called chopper neurons in the ventral cochlear nucleus can represent formants in a much more sound level invariant manner than the auditory nerve fibers do (Blackburn & Sachs, 1990).

At the level of the auditory brainstem, as well as in the inferior colliculus or the medial geniculate, and to some extent even in primary auditory cortex, this representation is thought to retain a somewhat spectrographic character. The pattern of neural discharges mostly reflects the waxing and waning of acoustic energy in the particular frequency bands to which these neurons happen to be tuned. But much experimental evidence suggests that this representation is not very isomorphic, in the sense that neural firing patterns in the brainstem and midbrain do not simply and directly reflect the rhythms of speech. Nor do the temporal response properties of neurons in the thalamus or cortex appear to be tuned to match the temporal properties of speech particularly well. Evidence for this comes from studies like those by Miller and colleagues (2002), who have analyzed response properties of thalamus and cortex neurons using synthetic dynamic ripple stimuli and reverse correlation. The dynamic ripple sounds they used are synthetic random chords that vary constantly and randomly in their frequency and amplitude. The rationale behind these experiments rests on the assumption that, at some periods, just by chance, this ever changing stimulus will contain features that excite a particular neuron, while at other times it will not. So, if one presents a sufficiently long random stimulus, and then asks what all those stimulus episodes that caused a particular neuron to fire had in common, one can characterize the neuron's response preferences. Often this is done by a (more or less) simple averaging of the spectrogram of the stimulus episodes that preceded a spike, and the resulting spike-triggered average of the stimulus serves as an estimate of the neuron's spectrotemporal receptive field (STRF).

You may recall from our discussions in chapter 2 that auditory neurons can be modeled, to a coarse approximation, as linear filters. For example, in figure 2.12, we illustrated similarities between auditory nerve fibers and so-called gamma-tone filters. Now, in principle, we can also try to approximate auditory neurons in the central nervous system with linear filter models (only the approximation risks becoming ever cruder and more approximate as each level of neural processing may contribute nonlinearities to the neural response properties). The way to think of a neuron's STRF is as a sort of spectrographic display of the linear filter that would best approximate the neuron's response properties. Consequently, we would expect a neuron to fire vigorously only if there is a good match between the features of the STRF and the spectrogram of the presented sound.

Figure 4.5A shows such an example of an STRF estimated for one neuron recorded in the auditory thalamus of the cat. The STRF shows that this particular neuron is excited by sound at about 9 kHz and the excitation kicks in with a latency of about 10 ms. There are inhibitory frequency regions both above and below the neuron's preferred frequency. But we also see that the excitatory region near 9 kHz is followed by "rebound inhibition," which should shut off this neuron's firing after about 10 ms or so of response. The STRF would thus predict that continuous, steady-state sounds are not particularly effective stimuli for this neuron.

In section 4.1, we discussed the dynamic properties of speech, and saw how its characteristic amplitude and frequency modulations can be captured by its modulation spectrum. We also saw how the modulation spectrum is generated from the sound's spectrogram by two-dimensional Fourier transformation. Now, if the STRF of a neuron is a sort of spectrographic display of the spectral and temporal features that that neuron prefers, we ought to be able to apply a similar thought process here, and transform the neuron's STRF with a 2DFT to reveal what sort of spectral and temporal modulations the neuron might respond to with particular vigor. To use the technical term, we can use the 2DFT of the STRF to obtain the neuron's "modulation transfer function" (MTF). Figure 4.5B shows the MTF obtained in this manner from the STRF shown in figure 4.5A.

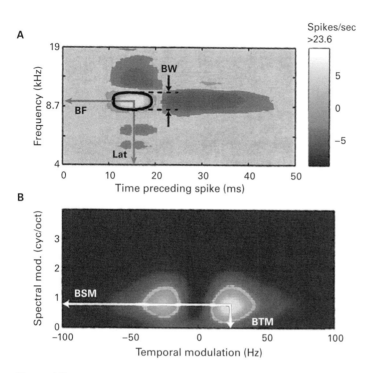

Figure 4.5

(A) Spectrotemporal receptive field of a neuron recorded in the auditory thalamus of the cat. BW: spectral bandwidth, BF: best frequency, Lat: response latency. (B) Modulation transfer function for the same neuron. BSM, best spectral modulation, BTM, best temporal modulation. Reproduced from figure 1 of Miller et al. (2002) with permission from the American Physiological Society.

When many neurons are characterized in this manner, it is possible to investigate what range of temporal and spectral modulations the population of neurons, on average, might be able to represent effectively through equivalent modulations of their own firing rates. We can then ask, is this population MTF well matched to the modulations encountered in speech? Figure 4.6 shows population MTFs determined in this manner for the main auditory thalamic relay station to the cortex, the ventral part of the medial geniculate (MGv), and for the primary auditory cortex of the cat.

Comparing the population MTFs of auditory thalamus and cortex shown in figure 4.6 to the speech modulation spectra shown in figures 4.1C and 4.2, we notice that the neural MTFs at these, still relatively early, auditory processing stations are not obviously well matched to the temporal modulations characteristic of speech. However, it would probably have been surprising if they were. For starters, the MTFs shown in figure 4.6

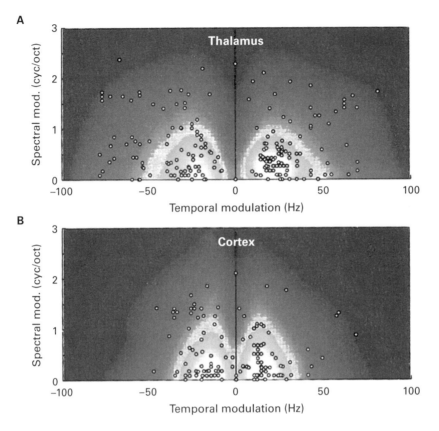

Figure 4.6
(A) Population MTF of the auditory thalamus in the cat. The dots show best temporal and spectral modulation values for individual neurons. The gray values show the averaged MTF. (B) Population MTF for cat A1.
Reproduced from figure 8 of Miller et al. (2002) with permission from the American Physiological Society.

were recorded in cats, and the cat auditory system is hardly likely to be optimized for the processing of human speech. However, we have no reason to assume that the population MTFs of human thalamus or primary auditory cortex would look much different. The shape of the population MTF can provide some insights into the nature of the neural code for sounds in the brain that are likely to be true for most mammals. The best temporal modulation frequencies for these neurons are often higher than they would need to be for the purposes of speech encoding (extending out to 50 Hz and above while speech modulations rarely exceed 30 Hz). In contrast, the best frequency modulations are not nearly high enough to capture the pitch part of the speech modulation spectrum, but they do appear quite well matched to the frequency modulation spectra of formants. We saw in chapters 2 and 3 that, already at the level of the auditory nerve, frequency tuning of individual nerve fibers is not usually sharp enough to resolve the harmonics that would reveal the pitch of a periodic sound, and the low-pass nature of the population MTF suggests that neurons at higher levels of the pathway cannot resolve harmonics in the sound's spectrum either.

Another striking mismatch between the speech modulation spectrum and the neural population MTF can be seen at temporal modulation frequencies near zero. Speech modulation spectra have a lot of energy near 0-Hz temporal modulation, which reflects the fact that, on average, there is some sound almost all the time during speech. However, as one ascends the auditory pathway toward cortex, auditory neurons appear increasingly unwilling to respond to sustained sound with sustained firing. Instead, they prefer to mark sound onsets and offsets with transient bursts of firing, and then fall silent. Slow temporal modulations of their firing rates are consequently rare. With this emphasis on change in the spectrum, rather than sustained sound energy levels, the representation of sounds in the thalamus and cortex resembles the derivative of the spectrogram with respect to time, but since speech sounds are rarely sustained for long periods of time, this emphasis on time-varying features does not change the representation dramatically. In fact, as we shall see later, even at the level of the primary auditory cortex, speech sounds appear to be represented in a manner that is perhaps more spectrographic (or neurographic) than one might expect. Consequently, much interesting processing of speech remains to be done when the sounds arrive at higher-order cortical fields. Where and how this processing is thought to take place will occupy us for much of the rest of this chapter.

4.4 Cortical Areas Involved in Speech Processing: An Overview

Before we start our discussion of the cortical processing of speech sounds in earnest, let us quickly revise some of the key anatomical terms, so we know which bit is which. Figure 4.7 shows anatomical drawings of the human cerebral cortex. Figure 4.7A shows the left side of the cortex, reminding you that the cortex on each hemisphere is subdivided into four lobes: The occipital lobe at the back deals mostly with visual processing; the parietal lobe deals with touch, but also integrates information across sensory modalities to keep track of the body's position relative to objects and events around us; the frontal lobe is involved in planning and coordinating movements, short-term working memory, and other cognitive functions; and, finally, the temporal lobe is involved in hearing, but also in high-level vision, general object recognition, and the formation of long-term memories.

In the human brain, many of the auditory structures of the temporal lobe are not visible on the surface, but are tucked away into the sylvian fissure, which forms the

A 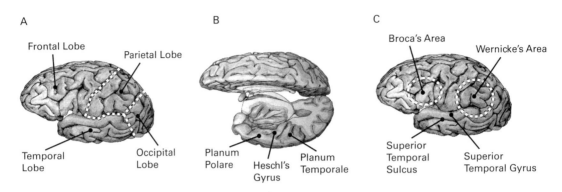 B   C

Figure 4.7

(A) Drawing of a lateral view of the human brain, showing the four principal lobes. (B) Human cortex seen from above, with the frontal and parietal lobe cut away to expose the superior bank of the temporal lobe, where the primary auditory cortex (Heschl's gyrus) and auditory belt areas (planum temporale and polare) are situated. (C) Lateral view showing higher-order cortical areas commonly associated with higher-order auditory processing and speech.
Original artwork kindly provided by Jo Emmons (www.joemmons.com).

boundary between the temporal, frontal and parietal lobes. Figure 4.7B therefore shows a view of the human brain from above, with the left frontal and parietal lobes cut away to show the upper bank of the temporal lobe. Most of the auditory afferents from the thalamus terminate in Heschl's gyrus, where primary auditory cortex is found in humans. To the front and back of Heschl's gyrus lie the planum polare and the planum temporale, where second-order auditory belt areas are situated.

But the processing of speech certainly also involves cortical areas well beyond the auditory areas on the upper bank of the temporal lobe. A few of the other key areas are shown in figure 4.7C, including the superior temporal gyrus (STG) and sulcus (STS), and Broca's and Wernicke's areas. The latter two are both named after nineteenth-century neurologists who associated damage to these areas with disturbances of either speech production (Broca's aphasia) or speech comprehension (Wernicke's aphasia. See the book's Web site for short video clips showing patients with Broca's and Wernicke's aphasia.) Note that the definitions of Broca's and Wernicke's areas are not based on anatomical landmarks, but instead derived from case studies of patients with injuries to these parts of the brain. Since the damage caused by such injuries is rarely confined to precisely circumscribed regions, the exact boundaries of Broca's and Wernicke's areas are somewhat uncertain, although a consensus seems to be emerging among neuroanatomists that Broca's area should be considered equivalent to the cytoarchitectonically defined and well-circumscribed Brodmann areas 44 and 45. In any case, both Wernicke's and Broca's areas clearly lie either largely or entirely outside the temporal lobe, which is traditionally associated with auditory processing. Note also that, while both hemispheres of the cortex have frontal, parietal, occipital, and temporal lobes, as well as Heschl's gyri and superior temporal sulci, much clinical evidence points to the left hemisphere playing a special role in speech processing, and Broca's and Wernicke's areas appear normally to be confined largely or wholly to the left hemisphere.

4.5   The Role of Auditory Cortex: Insights from Clinical Observations

Paul Broca, who lived from 1824 to 1880, and in whose honor one of the brain areas we just encountered is named, was one of the first to observe that speech processing may be asymmetrically distributed in cortex. He stated that the left hemisphere was "dominant" for language. Broca chose his words carefully. The left hemisphere's dominance is not meant to imply that the right hemisphere contributes nothing to speech comprehension or production. Rather, the left hemisphere, in most but not all individuals, is capable of carrying out certain key speech processing functions even if the right hemisphere is not available to help, but the right hemisphere on its own would not succeed. We might envisage the situation as similar to that of a lumberjack who, if forced to work with one hand only, would be able to wield his axe with his right hand, but not with his left. This "righthand-dominant lumberjack" would nevertheless work at his best if allowed to use both hands to guide his axe, and his left hand would normally be neither idle nor useless.

Since Broca's time, a wealth of additional clinical and brain imaging evidence has much refined our knowledge of the functional roles of the two brain hemispheres and their various areas in both the production and the comprehension of speech. Much of that work was nicely summarized in a review by Dana Boatman (2004), from which we present some of the highlights.

Much of the research into human speech areas has been driven forward by clinical necessity, but perhaps surprisingly not as much from the need to understand and diagnose speech processing deficits as from the desire to cure otherwise intractable epilepsy by surgical means. In these epilepsy surgeries, neurosurgeons must try to identify the "epileptic focus," a hopefully small piece of diseased brain tissue that causes seizures by triggering waves of uncontrollable hyperexcitation which spread through much of the patient's brain. Successful identification and removal of the epileptic focus can cure the patient of a debilitating disease, but there are risks. For example, if the operation were to remove or damage one of the brain's crucial speech modules, the patient would be left dumb or unable to understand speech. That would be a crippling side effect of the operation one would like to avoid at all cost. So, the more we know about the location of such crucial brain regions, the better the surgeon's chances are to keep the scalpel well away from them.

One complicating factor which neurosurgeons have appreciated for a long time is that the layout of cortex is not absolutely identical from one person to the next, and it is therefore desirable to test each individual patient. One such test that has been administered frequently since the 1960s is the so-called Wada procedure (Wada & Rasmussen, 1960), during which a short-acting anesthetic (usually sodium amytal) is injected into the carotid artery, one of the main blood supply routes for the cerebral hemispheres of the brain. After injecting the anesthetic on either the left or right side only, one can then try to have a conversation with a patient who is literally half asleep, because one of his brain hemispheres is wide awake, while the other is deeply anesthetized. Records of such Wada tests have revealed that approximately 90% of all right-handed patients and about 75% of all left-handed patients display Broca's classic "left hemisphere dominance" for speech. The remaining patients are either "mixed dominant" (i.e., they need both hemispheres to process speech) or have a "bilateral speech representation" (i.e., either hemisphere can support speech without necessarily requiring the other). Right hemisphere dominance is comparatively rare, and seen in no more than 1 to 2% of the population.

The Wada procedure has its usefulness—for example, if we needed to perform surgery on the right brain hemisphere, it would be reassuring to know that the patient can speak and comprehend speech with the spared left hemisphere alone. However, often one would like more detailed information about the precise localization of certain functions than the Wada test can provide. To obtain more detailed information, neurosurgeons sometimes carry out electrocortical mapping studies on their patients. Such mappings require preparing a large part of one of the patient's brain hemispheres for focal electrical stimulation either by removing a large section of the skull to make the brain accessible for handheld electrodes, or by implanting a large electrode array over one of the hemispheres. During the actual mapping, the patient receives only local anesthetic and analgesics, and is therefore awake and can engage in conversation or follow simple instructions.

The patients are then tested on simple speech tasks of varying level of complexity. The simplest, so called acoustic-phonetic tasks, require only very simple auditory discriminations; for example, the patient is asked whether two syllables presented in fairly quick succession are the same or different. The next level, so called phonological tasks, require a slightly deeper level of analysis of the presented speech sounds. For example, the patient might be asked whether two words rhyme, or whether they start with the same phoneme. Note that neither acoustic-phonetic nor phonological tasks require that the tested speech sounds be understood. For example, we can easily repeat the syllable "shmorf," we can tell that it rhymes with "torf," and that "shmorf" and "torf" do not start with the same phoneme. We can do all this even though both "shmorf" and "torf" are completely meaningless. The ability to use speech sounds for meaningful exchanges requires a further so-called lexical-semantic level of analysis, which is typically tested by asking a patient to carry out simple instructions (such as "please wiggle the ring finger on your left hand") or to answer questions of varying level of grammatical complexity.

While the patients are grappling with these acoustic, phonological, or semantic tasks, the surgeon will sneakily send small bursts of electric current to a particular spot on their brain. The current is just large enough to disrupt the normal activity of the neurons in the immediate vicinity of the stimulating electrodes, and the purpose of this is to test whether the highly localized disruption makes any obvious difference to the patient's ability to perform the task.

In such electrocortical mapping studies, one does observe a fair degree of variation from one patient to another, as no two brains are exactly alike. But one can neverthe-less observe clear trends, and Dana Boatman (2004) has summarized which parts of cortex appear to be essential for acoustic, phonological, or semantic tasks across a large numbers of patients. The results of her analysis are shown in figure 4.8.

The data in figure 4.8 suggest a hierarchical arrangement. The more complex the task, the larger the number of cortical sites that seem to make a critical contribution because disruptive stimulation at these sites impairs performance. Acoustic-phonetic tasks (figure 4.8A) are not easily disrupted. Only at a single spot on the superior tem-poral gyrus (STG) could electrical stimulation reliably interfere with phonetic process-ing in all patients. Phonological processing (figure 4.8B) requires a greater degree of analysis of the speech sounds, and it seems to involve large parts of STG, as well as some points on Broca's area in the frontal lobe, since focal stimulation of any of these areas impairs performance. Lexical-semantic tasks (figure 4.8C) are yet more complex, and seem to involve yet more cortical territory because they are even more vulnerable

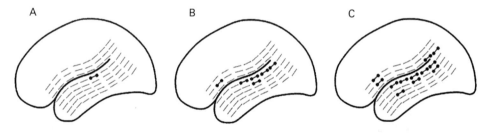

Figure 4.8
Sites where acoustic (A), phonological (B), or lexical-semantic (C) deficits can be induced by disruptive electrical stimulation. The light gray symbols show locations on perisylvian cortex that were tested by applying disruptive electrical stimulation. The black symbols show sites where such stimulation interfered with the patient's ability to perform the respective task.
Reproduced from figures 1 through 3 of Boatman (2004), with permission from Elsevier, copy-right (2004).

to disruption. Focal stimulation not just of the superior temporal sulcus (STS), STG, and Broca's area, but also of Wernicke's area in the parietal lobe can disrupt the performance of this type of task.

In figure 4.8 we also notice that the sites where one can disrupt processing on the next higher level of complexity always appear to include the sites that were involved in the lower processing levels. That is perhaps unsurprising. If some focal electrical stimulation perturbs our perception of speech sounds to the point where we can no longer tell whether two words spoken in sequence were the same or different, then it would be odd if we could nevertheless tell whether those words rhymed, or what they meant.

The clinical data thus suggests a cortical processing hierarchy, which begins with acoustic-phonetic processing in or near primary auditory cortex, and engages ever-increasing amounts of cortical territory as the brain subjects vocalizations to phonological and semantic analysis. But the clinical data cannot provide much detail on what exactly each particular cortical area contributes to the process. For example, the fact that semantic processing of sounds can be disrupted by electrical stimulation of parts of Wernicke's area does not mean that important steps toward this semantic processing may not have already begun at much earlier levels in the cortical hierarchy. In fact, some results from animal research might be interpreted as evidence for "semantic preprocessing" from the earliest levels.

4.6   The Representation of Speech and Vocalizations in Primary Auditory Cortex

Since semantic processing involves finding the "meaning" of a particular speech sound or animal vocalization, one can try to investigate semantic processing by comparing neural responses to "meaningful" sounds with responses to sounds that are "meaningless" but otherwise very similar. One simple trick to make speech sounds incomprehensible, and hence meaningless, is to play them backward. Time reversing a sound does not change its overall frequency content. It will flip its modulation spectrum along the time axis, but since speech modulation spectra are fairly symmetrical around $t = 0$ (see figure 4.1C), this does not seem to matter much. Indeed, if you have ever heard time-reversed speech, you may know that it sounds distinctly speechlike, not unlike someone talking in a foreign language (you can find examples of such time reversed speech in the book's Web site). Of course, one can also time reverse the vocalizations of other animals, and indeed, in certain songbird species, brain areas have been identified in which neurons respond vigorously to normal conspecific songs, but not to time-reversed songs (Doupe and Konishi, 1991). Typically, the songbird brain areas showing such sensitivity to time reversal seem to play an important role in relating auditory input to motor output, for example, when a bird learns to sing or monitors its own song.

Interestingly, Xiaoqin Wang and colleagues (1995) have used the same trick in marmosets, a species of new world monkey, and found that already in primary auditory cortex, many neurons respond much more vigorously to natural marmoset twitter calls than to time-reversed copies of the same call. Could it be that marmoset A1 neurons fire more vigorously to the natural calls because they are "meaningful," while the time-reversed ones are not? If the same natural and time-reversed marmoset calls are presented to cats, one observes no preferential responses in their A1 for the natural marmoset calls (Wang & Kadia, 2001), perhaps because neither the natural nor the reversed marmoset calls are particularly meaningful for cats.

However, the interpretation of these intriguing data is problematic. One complicating factor, for example, is the fact that the relationship between the number of spikes fired by a neuron during some relatively long time interval and the amount of information or meaning that can be extracted from the neuron's firing pattern is not straightforward. A more vigorous response does not necessarily convey proportionally more information. This was clearly illustrated in a study by Schnupp and colleagues (2006), who used the same marmoset calls as those used by Wang et al. (1995), but this time played them either to naïve ferrets, or to ferrets who had been trained to recognize marmoset twitter calls as an acoustic signal that helped them find drinking water. For the trained ferrets, the marmoset calls had thus presumably become "meaningful," while for the naïve ferrets they were not. However, neither in the naïve nor the trained ferrets did primary auditory cortex neurons respond more strongly to the natural marmoset calls than to the time-reversed ones. Instead, these neurons responded vigorously to either stimuli, but many of the neurons exhibited characteristic temporal firing patterns, which differed systematically for different stimuli. These temporal discharge patterns were highly informative about the stimuli, and could be used to distinguish individual calls, or to tell normal from time-reversed ones. However, these neural discharge patterns had to be "read out" at a temporal resolution of 20 ms or finer; otherwise this information was lost. Figure 4.9 illustrates this. Schnupp and colleagues (2006) also showed that training ferrets to recognize these marmoset vocalizations did not change the nature of this temporal pattern code, but did make it more reliable and hence more informative.

These results indicate that the representation of complex stimuli like vocalizations or speech at early stages of the cortical processing hierarchy is still very much organized around "acoustic features" of the stimulus, and while this feature-based representation does not directly mirror the temporal fine structure of the sound with submillisecond precision, it does nevertheless reflect the time course of the stimulus at coarser time resolutions of approximately 10 to 20 ms. It may or may not be a coincidence that the average phoneme rate in human speech is also approximately one every 20 ms, and that, if speech is cut into 20-ms-wide strips, and each strip is time-reversed and their order is maintained, speech remains completely

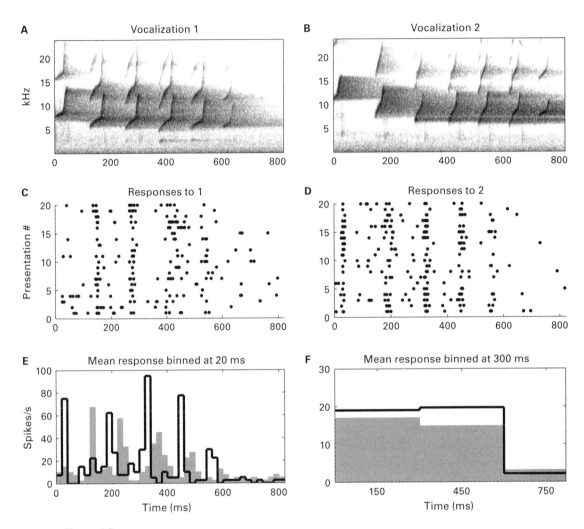

Figure 4.9
(A, B) Spectrograms of two marmoset "twitter calls." (C, D) Dot rasters showing responses of a neuron in ferret primary auditory cortex to these sounds. Each dot represents one nerve impulse, each row of dots an impulse train fired in response to a single presentation of the corresponding stimulus. The neuron fires similar mean spike counts but with different temporal discharge patterns in response to each stimulus. (E, F) Responses shown in C and D are plotted as histograms, showing the mean firing rate poststimulus onset, with the responses to stimulus 1 shown in gray, those to stimulus 2 in black. At fine temporal resolutions (small histogram bin width, e.g., 20 ms shown in E) the differences in the response patterns are very clear and, as shown by Schnupp et al. (2006), contain much information about stimulus identity. However, at coarser temporal resolutions (300 ms bin width, shown in F), the responses look very similar, and information about stimulus identity is lost.

comprehensible (Saberi & Perrott, 1999) (A sound example demonstrating this can be found on the book's Web site.)

Further evidence for such a feature-based representation of vocalizations and speech sounds in mammalian A1 comes from a recent study by Engineer and colleagues (2008), who trained rats to recognize consonants of American English. The rats were trained to distinguish nonsense syllables that differed only in their onset consonant: "pad" from "bad," "zad" from "shad," "mad" from "nad," and so on. Some of these distinctions the rats learned very easily, while they found others more difficult. Engineer and colleagues then proceeded to record responses to these same syllables from hundreds of neurons in the auditory cortex of these animals. These responses are reproduced here in figure 4.10 as neurogram-dot raster displays. Each panel shows the responses of a large number of A1 neurons, arranged by each neuron's characteristic frequency along the y-axis. The x-axis shows time after stimulus onset. The panels zoom in on the first 40 ms only to show the response to the onset consonant.

Figure 4.10 shows that the A1 neurons normally respond to the onset syllable with one or occasionally with two bursts of activity, but the bursts do not all start at the same time, nor are they all equally strong. Instead, they vary systematically, depending on the sound stimulus and the neuron's frequency tuning. In fact, the firing pattern is still very much like the neurogram responses we saw in figure 2.13 for auditory nerve fiber responses. When presented with an /m/ or an /n/, which contain little acoustic energy at high frequencies, the high-frequency A1 neurons fail to fire. Conversely, in response to an /s/, which contains little energy at low frequencies, only the high-frequency neurons respond. This interplay between frequency sensitivity and the acoustic properties of the stimulus leads to each consonant having its own response pattern across the population of cortical neurons. Interestingly, when Engineer and colleagues (2008) used pattern classifier algorithms similar to those used by Schnupp et al. (2006) to quantify the differences between the cortical activity patterns evoked by the different speech sounds, they noticed that these differences predicted how easily a rat would learn to distinguish the sounds. Thus, /m/ and /n/ evoked rather similar response patterns, and rats found it very hard to distinguish them, but /p/ and /b/ evoked rather different response patterns, and rats learned to distinguish the sounds easily.

The responses to /p/ and /b/ shown in figure 4.10 are, in fact, particularly interesting, because they exhibit a phenomenon that had previously been described by Steinschneider, Fishman, and Arezzo (2003) in the primary auditory cortex of rhesus monkeys and by Eggermont (1995) in cortex of cats. In response to /p/, the low- to mid-frequency neurons produce two bursts of impulses, while in response to /b/ they produce just one. In fact, the second burst of action potentials in the response to /p/ is not strictly a response to /p/, but a response to the onset of voicing, to the /a/ in

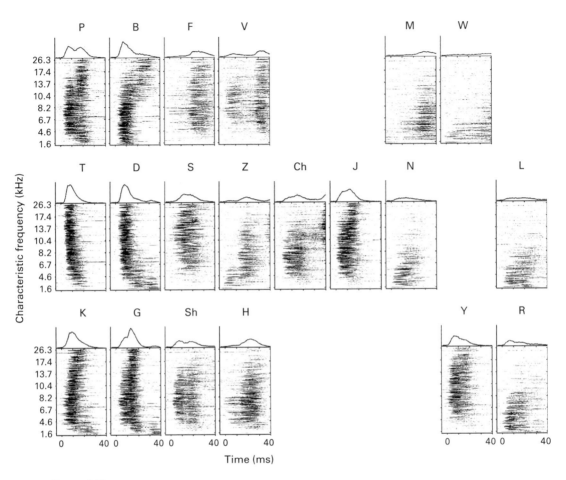

Figure 4.10
Responses of rat A1 neurons to 20 different consonants.
Adapted from figures 1 and 2 of Engineer et al. (2008) with permission from Macmillan Publishers, Ltd., copyright (2008).

the syllables "pad" and "bad" that were presented to the animals. There is, of course, an /a/ in "bad" as well, yet the response to it is suppressed in the low- and mid-frequency neurons, probably due to the phenomenon of "forward masking." You may recall from section 4.2 that the key distinguishing feature between /p/ and /b/ is that the former has a longer VOT; that is, in "pad" the gap between the consonant and the vowel may be some 60 to 70 ms long, while in "bad" it may be no longer than 20 ms. The longer gap in "pad" gives the neurons time to recover from forward masking and to respond vigorously to both the /p/ and the /a/, whereas in "bad," forward masking much reduces the response to the /a/. Neural response patterns tend to transition fairly abruptly from single-peaked to double-peaked responses when a "ba" sound is morphed to a "pa" by lengthening the VOT. Forward masking is thus one aspect of neural processing that leads to a deviation in the neural firing patterns from what might be expected on the basis of a purely spectrographic representation, and it may be responsible for the categorical perceptual boundaries associated with VOTs that we discussed in section 4.2. Thus, although responses at the earliest cortical processing levels appear to represent purely acoustic-phonetic aspects of vocalizations, the neuronal response properties found there may nevertheless account for at least some aspects of categorical perception.

4.7 Processing of Speech and Vocalizations in Higher-Order Cortical Fields

As we have just seen, the representation of animal vocalizations or speech sounds in early stages of auditory cortex still appears to be fairly "raw," and rather directly related to physical stimulus attributes. A somewhat categorical distinction between /p/ and /b/ based on a relative suppression of the response to the voice onset seems to be as good as it gets. One might reasonably assume that neural responses would become fairly specific if they reflected the result of lexical-semantic processing, yet most studies indicate that neurons in early cortical processing stages are not very selective but respond more or less vigorously to all manner of vocalizations as well as to other sounds from inanimate objects. It therefore looks as if many of the most interesting aspects of speech and vocalization processing occur "beyond" the primary auditory fields.

Unfortunately, when it comes to the study of speech and vocalization processing in higher-order cortical areas, obtaining the very detailed data against which to test particular theories is very difficult. One of the main experimental approaches for this type of work is noninvasive functional imaging in normal human volunteers, using techniques like positron emission tomography (PET) or functional magnetic resonance imaging (fMRI). These approaches can yield interesting results. For example, a study by Scott and colleagues (2000) provided intriguing evidence that parts of the left anterior STG may be activated selectively by intelligible speech. This conclusion was based on a comparison of cortical activation patterns obtained either with normal speech sounds or with speech rendered unintelligible by inverting sound along the frequency axis. (You can find an example of such spectrally rotated speech on the book's Web site).

However, as Scott herself points out in a comprehensive review (Scott & Wise, 2004), word deafness (i.e., the inability to recognize the meaning of words) only rarely results from damage to the left STG alone, and usually occurs only in patients who

suffered injury to the STG on both sides. This highlights one methodological limitation inherent in functional brain imaging studies. When a particular area of the brain
appears to "light up" under the scanner, what we really see is a marginally greater
blood supply to this area during some particular stimulus regime than during another.
As a measure of brain activity, this is very indirect. One problem is that it reveals only
the tip of the iceberg; it shows which brain area blushed significantly more under the
effort of the neural processing it carried out than some neighboring area. And here
"significantly more" is to be understood in the statistical sense, meaning that the difference can be measured with a fair degree of confidence, not that it is very large.
Neighboring areas may have made crucial contributions to the processing, but these
fail to show up in the functional scan because they were performed "relatively
effortlessly."

Another limitation of fMRI and PET stems from their inherently poor temporal
resolution, as they effectively measure responses of the brain's vasculature that reflect
the relatively slowly changing metabolic demands of the neural tissue. Consequently,
fMRI and PET cannot resolve any brain processes that occur on timescales faster than
a few seconds. As we saw in the previous section, deciphering the cortical code is likely
to require a temporal resolution approximately 1,000-fold faster. Consequently, a
number of elegant theories that have recently emerged remain largely untestable with
functional imaging techniques. For example, it has been suggested that certain brain
areas may be specialized for processing slow aspects of speech, such as "prosody"—that
is, the overall melody and rhythm of a speech, which convey emotional undertones
or label sentences as questions or statements—while other brain areas may specialize
in processing fast features, such as formant transitions that identify individual speech
sounds (Poeppel & Hickok, 2004). Whether, or to what extent, this is really true we
will know only when techniques that provide more direct observations of neural activity on a millisecond timescale become widely available.

Detailed and direct observations are, of course, possible in animal experiments,
where microelectrodes can be implanted directly in the areas of interest. However, the
layout of higher-order cortical fields may not be identical from one species of mammal
to the next, and humans not only have a uniquely rich, complex vocal communication system, they also have substantially larger cortices than almost any other mammal.
Studies carried out on some of our primate cousins, such as rhesus macaques, may
nevertheless provide interesting insights that are likely to be representative of the
processes we would expect to take place in human brains.

Based on anatomical observations, it has been suggested that auditory cortical areas
in primate brain may be organized into two more or less discrete processing streams
(Romanski et al., 1999): a dorsal stream, which may be concerned mostly with identifying sound source locations, and a ventral stream, which is thought to play the lead
role in identifying sounds. Anatomical evidence from tracer studies (figure 4.11) indi-

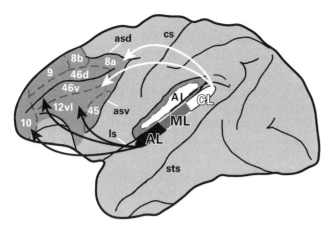

Figure 4.11
Putative dorsal and ventral processing streams in macaque auditory cortex, as suggested from anatomical tracer studies.
Adapted from figure 3D of Romanski et al. (1999) with permission from the author and from Macmillan Publishers Ltd., copyright (1999).

cates that this ventral stream should run from primary auditory cortex via medial belt (secondary) areas to anterior STG and inferotemporal cortex, and from there finally to areas in the ventral prefrontal cortex (vPFC). Recognizing and distinguishing different types of vocalizations or spoken words should most certainly be a "ventral stream task," and the notion that the ventral stream may form the "sound-meaning interface" in human speech processing is often discussed in the literature (Hickok & Poeppel, 2004; Scott & Wise, 2004).

Against this background, a recent set of experiments by Russ and colleagues (2008) is therefore of particular interest, as these investigators were able to record activity from individual neurons in the STG and the vPFC of awake rhesus macaques, who were listening to ten very different types of rhesus vocalization calls. These calls are acoustically very distinct, the animals make different calls in different social situations, and there is little doubt that each of these calls therefore has a different meaning for the animals. If neurons in the ventral stream indeed represent the meaning of a vocalization, then one might expect these neurons to be rather selective in their response to these calls; that is, each neuron might respond to only a small subset of calls with similar meanings. We might also expect that this specificity would increase as one ascends along the ventral path from STG to vPFC. Finally, we would not expect neurons in the vPFC to be very interested in minute acoustic details, such as the temporal fine structure of the sound, or to represent much information in the temporal fine structure of their discharges. After all, if we pronounce a particular word the meaning of this utterance does not depend on whether we speak fast or slowly or introduce small gaps between the syllables, and even speaking very rapidly we would find it difficult to convey more than two or three concepts per second on average. Meaning therefore unfolds relatively slowly, and the temporal fine structure of sounds becomes irrelevant once their meaning has been identified. Consequently, if neurons in vPFC, at the end of the ventral stream, really represent the abstracted, lexical meaning of a vocalization rather than the sound itself, we would not expect their temporal firing patterns to convey much stimulus-related information on a millisecond timescale.

What makes the experiments by Russ and colleagues (2008) so interesting and surprising is that they produced a wealth of data that clearly runs counter to all these expectations. Neurons in the STG and vPFC are not very selective in their responses. The large majority of neurons respond vigorously (with >50% of their maximal firing rate) to more than half of the vocalizations tested. Nor do responses become more specific as one ascends from STG to vPFC—if anything, the reverse is true. But both STG and vPFC neurons convey a great deal of information about which of the vocalizations was presented in the temporal fine structure of their discharges. Using spike pattern classification techniques identical to those used by Schnupp and colleagues (2006) to analyze neural discharge patterns recorded in ferret A1, Russ et al. (2008) were able to show that responses of neurons in macaque STG and vPFC also need to be decoded at a resolution of a few milliseconds if the individual vocalizations are to be correctly identified. Furthermore, the reliance on precise temporal patterning of the discharges is, if anything, larger in vPFC than in STG.

Do the results of Russ and colleagues (2008) mean that our intuitions about how our brain "ought to" represent the meaning of sounds are simply wrong, and that the meaning of a sound is never represented explicitly through invariant, sparse, and categorical responses? Perhaps, but alternatively it could be that, to see such meaning-specific responses, one needs to look outside the auditory pathway. After all, meaning is abstracted somewhat beyond the level of any particular sensory modality, and it is not uncommon that the same meaning can be conveyed with both sounds and pictures. Interestingly, recent work by Quian Quiroga and colleagues (2009) found neurons in structures buried inside the temporal lobe, such as the hippocampus, the amygdala, and the entorhinal cortex, that may respond to pictures of some specific familiar object, say a landmark or a person or a pet, and these same neurons may also respond to that object's name, either spoken or written. These object-specific neurons are highly selective for stimulus category, responding typically to only one or two stimulus objects out of over a hundred tested. At the same time, they are unselective for the sensory modality, as they frequently respond as vigorously to a spoken name or a characteristic sound as to a visual image. They have long response latencies (300 ms or so for images, 500 ms or more for sounds), and their discharges appear not to reflect acoustic features of the auditory waveform in any way.

It is curious that such "semantic" responses to the meaning of sound have so far been observed only in structures such as the amygdala (which is thought to process the emotional significance of stimuli, e.g., "are they scary or not") or the hippocampus (which seems to serve as the gateway to long-term episodic memory). As we have seen, even at the highest levels of the auditory "what stream," neural responses appear overwhelmingly tuned to acoustic stimulus properties, not their semantics. Perhaps we simply haven't yet looked hard enough for semantically tuned responses in higher-order auditory cortex. It is worth bearing in mind, however, that such semantic responses may also be rare in the hippocampus, the amygdala, and entorhinal cortex. Quian Quiroga and colleagues (2009) tested 750 neurons, and found that fewer than 4% of neurons (25 in total) seemed to be object specific and responsive to sound. If semantically tuned neurons formed a small subset of the neural population in higher-order auditory cortex, and if their responses were very highly selective and "sparse," then they could have slipped through the net in previous investigations.

4.8 Visual Influences

The brain does, of course, rely mostly on acoustic information to process speech and vocalizations, but it will also happily incorporate visual information if this is useful. Listeners who suffer from hearing impairments or who have to operate under difficult conditions with large amounts of background noise often find it much easier to understand a speaker if they can also observe the movement of his or her mouth, and "lip read." At a very basic level, lip reading can be helpful simply because of the temporal cueing it provides: Sounds you hear when the speaker's mouth is not moving are bound to be purely background noise. But since the lips (together with the tongue and the soft palate) are among the chief articulators used to shape speech sound, visual observation of the lips provides information that can help distinguish different phonemes and influence their perception.

This is vividly illustrated by a visual-auditory illusion known as the McGurk effect (McGurk & MacDonald, 1976). To create the McGurk effect, a video is made showing a person articulating the syllables "gaga" over and over again. The video is then synchronized with a soundtrack of the person speaking the syllables "baba." If you watch a McGurk video, your ears will hear the syllables "baba," but you can also see that the lips are not closed at the onset of the syllables, so your eyes tell you that the syllables you heard could not have started with a labial plosive. You will therefore not perceive the /ba/ that was actually delivered to your ears, but instead hear a /da/ or a /tha/, as these are acoustically similar to the actual sound, but are articulated by the tip of the tongue, which is not visible, so the eyes do not provide evidence against them. The /da/ or /tha/ you perceive is, in effect, the most plausible compromise between the /ga/ that is shown and the /ba/ that is played. You can find a McGurk effect video on the book's Web site. Try watching it, and then just listening to it with your eyes closed. The difference in the sound you hear depending on whether your eyes are open or not is quite compelling. With your eyes closed you will clearly hear that the movie's sound track consists entirely of the syllables "baba," but when you open your eyes the sound appears to change instantly to "dada" or "thatha."

The McGurk effect nicely illustrates how visual information can directly and powerfully influence and enrich our auditory perception of speech sounds, and it probably exercises this influence through visual inputs that feed directly into the auditory cortex. A number of electrophysiological studies have reported responses in auditory cortex to visual stimuli (Bizley et al., 2007; Brosch, Selezneva, & Scheich, 2005). Also, imaging experiments have shown that auditory cortex can be activated by silent lip reading (Calvert et al., 1997), and activity in auditory cortex can be enhanced when speech is presented along with a movie showing the face of a speaker (Callan et al., 2003). Selective enhancement of responses to vocalization stimuli that are seen as well as heard has also been described in monkeys (Ghazanfar et al., 2005).

Thus, visual information can contribute significantly to the neural processing of vocalization stimuli, but it is important to remember that the role of the visual modality is nevertheless a minor one. Telecommunications technology has advanced to the point where video telephony is becoming widely available, yet most of us do not feel the need for it. Nobody would think it a practical idea to rely on the video only and switch the sound off. Educational policies that discourage profoundly deaf children from learning sign language and instead try to teach them to understand normal speech through lip reading alone are well intended, but nevertheless badly flawed. They ignore the important fact that the most of the articulatory gestures we use to encode our thoughts in speech, such as voicing and all the subtle movements of the tongue and the soft palate, simply cannot be observed by looking at a speaker's face. They are accessible to us only through their acoustic fingerprints, which a healthy auditory system can decipher with surprising ease.

4.9 Summary

As we have seen, speech most likely evolved from initially rather simple vocal communication systems, comprising perhaps less than a dozen or so distinct messages, such as mating calls, alarm calls, pup calls, threats, and a few others. From these humble beginnings, speech evolved into a staggeringly sophisticated communication system, in which humans can combine and recombine a relatively modest number of speech sounds to communicate a seemingly limitless variety of ideas. These ideas reach the ear of the listener encoded as a more or less continuous stream of amplitude- and frequency-modulated sound. But not all spectral and temporal modulations in the speech signal are equally important. Relatively coarse levels of detail (temporal modulations between 1 and 7 Hz and spectral modulations of less than 4 cycles/kHz) are usually sufficient for a successful decoding of the message.

The auditory system is thought to decipher speech sounds through a hierarchy of successive analyses, which operate on different timescales. Acoustic-phonetic analysis examines amplitude and frequency modulations in the incoming sound in order to detect and characterize speech sounds within the signal, phonological processing aims to reconstruct how speech sounds are arranged to form syllables and words, while lexical-semantic analysis aims to decipher the meaning of the sounds. Most of these processing steps are thought to involve areas of cortex, particularly those on the upper part of the temporal lobe, but also some frontal and parietal areas, especially in the left cerebral hemisphere. Many important details of how these cortical areas operate remain obscure.

5 Neural Basis of Sound Localization

Most of our senses can provide information about where things are located in the surrounding environment. But the auditory system shares with vision and, to some extent, olfaction the capacity to register the presence of objects and events that can be found some distance away from the individual. Accurate localization of such stimuli can be of great importance to survival. For example, the ability to determine the location of a particular sound source is often used to find potential mates or prey or to avoid and escape from approaching predators. Audition is particularly useful for this because it can convey information from any direction relative to the head, whereas vision operates over a more limited spatial range. While these applications may seem less relevant for humans than for many other species, the capacity to localize sounds both accurately and rapidly can still have clear survival value by indicating, for example, the presence of an oncoming vehicle when crossing the street. More generally, auditory localization plays an important role in redirecting attention toward different sources. Furthermore, the neural processing that underlies spatial hearing helps us pick out sounds—such as a particular individual's voice—from a background of other sounds emanating from different spatial locations, and therefore aids source detection and identification (more about that in chapter 6). Thus, it is not surprising that some quite sophisticated mechanisms have evolved to enable many species, including ourselves, to localize sounds with considerable accuracy.

If you ask someone where a sound they just heard came from, they are most likely to point in a particular direction. Of course, pinpointing the location of the sound source also involves estimating its distance relative to the listener. But because humans, along with most other species, are much better at judging sound source direction, we will focus primarily on this dimension of auditory space. A few species, though, notably echolocating bats, possess specialized neural mechanisms that make them highly adept at determining target distance, so we will return to this later.

5.1   Determining the Direction of a Sound Source

Registering the location of an object that we can see or touch is a relatively straight-forward task. There are two reasons for this. First, the receptor cells in those sensory systems respond only to stimuli that fall within restricted regions of the visual field or on the body surface. These regions, which can be extremely small, are known as the spatial receptive fields of the cells. For example, each of the mechanoreceptors found within the skin has a receptive field on a particular part of the body surface, within which it will respond to the presence of an appropriate mechanical stimulus. Second, the receptive fields of neighboring receptor cells occupy adjacent locations in visual space or on the body surface. In the visual system, this is possible because an image of the world is projected onto the photoreceptors that are distributed around the retina at the back of the eye, enabling each to sample a slightly different part of the field of view. As we have seen in earlier chapters, the stimulus selectivity of the hair cells also changes systematically along the length of the cochlea. But, in contrast to the receptor cells for vision and touch, the hair cells are tuned to different sound frequencies rather than to different spatial locations. Thus, while the cochlea provides the first steps in identifying what the sound is, it appears to reveal little about where that sound originated.

Stimulus localization in the auditory system is possible because of the geometry of the head and external ears. Key to this is the physical separation of the ears on either side of the head. For sounds coming from the left or the right, the difference in path length to each ear results in an interaural difference in the time of sound arrival, the magnitude of which depends on the distance between the ears as well as the angle subtended by the source relative to the head (figure 5.1). Depending on their wave-length, incident sounds may be reflected by the head and torso and diffracted to the ear on the opposite side, which lies within an "acoustic shadow" cast by the head. They may also interact with the folds of the external ears in a complex manner that depends on the direction of sound incidence. Together, these filtering effects produce monaural localization cues as well as a second binaural cue in the form of a difference in sound level between the two ears (figure 5.1).

Figure 5.2 shows how the different localization cues vary with sound direction. These measurements were obtained by placing a very small microphone in each ear canal of a human subject (King, Schnupp, & Doubell, 2001). The ears are usually pretty symmetrical, so locations along the midsagittal plane (which bisects the head down the middle, at right angles to the interaural axis) will generate interaural level differences (ILDs; figure 5.2A and B) and interaural time differences (ITDs; figure 5.2C) that are equal or very close in value to zero. If the sound source shifts from directly in front (represented by 0° along the horizontal axis of these plots) to one side, both ILDs and ITDs build up and then decline back toward zero as the source moves behind the

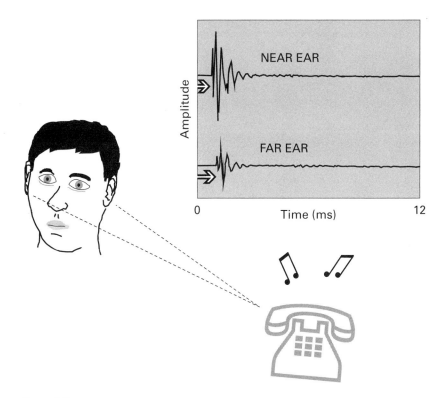

Figure 5.1
Binaural cues for sound localization. Sounds originating from one side of the head will arrive first at the ear closer to the source, giving rise to an interaural difference in time of arrival. In addition, the directional filtering properties of the external ears and the shadowing effect of the head produce an interaural difference in sound pressure levels. These cues are illustrated by the waveform of the sound, which is both delayed and reduced in amplitude at the listener's far ear.

subject. A color version of this figure can be found in the "spatial hearing" section of the book's Web site).

ITDs show some variation with sound frequency, becoming smaller at higher frequencies due to the frequency dispersion of the diffracted waves. Consequently, the spectral content of the sound must be known in order to derive its location from the value of the ITD. However, the ITDs measured for different frequencies vary consistently across space, with the maximum value occurring on the interaural axis where the relative distance from the sound source to each ear is at its greatest (figure 5.2C). By contrast, the magnitude of the ILDs changes considerably with the wavelength and therefore the frequency of the sound. Low-frequency (long wavelength) sounds propagate around the head with little interference, and so the resulting ILDs are very

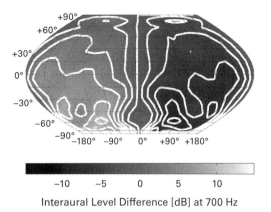

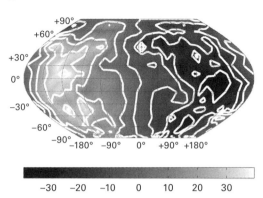

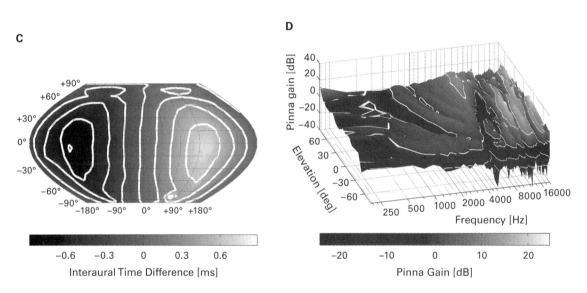

Figure 5.2
Acoustic cues underlying the localization of sounds in space. (A, B) Interaural level differences (ILDs) measured as a function of sound azimuth (horizontal axis) and elevation (vertical axis) in a human subject for 700-Hz tones (A) and 11-kHz tones (B). (C) Spatial pattern of interaural time differences (ITDs). In each of these plots, sound source direction is plotted in spherical coordinates, with 0° indicating a source straight in front of the subject, while negative numbers represent angles to the left and below the interaural axis. Regions in space generating the same ILDs or ITDs are indicated by the white lines, which represent iso-ILD and iso-ITD contours. (D) Monaural spectral cues for sound location. The direction-dependent filtering effects produced by the external ears, head, and torso filter are shown by plotting the change in amplitude or gain measured in the ear canal after broadband sounds are presented in front of the subject at different elevations. The gain is plotted as a function of sound frequency at each of these locations.

small if present at all. This is illustrated in figure 5.2A for the spatial pattern of ILDs measured for 700-Hz tone pips; for most locations, the ILDs are around 5 to 10 dB and therefore provide little indication as to the origin of the sound source. But at higher frequencies, ILDs are larger and, above 3 kHz, become reliable and informative cues to sound source location. For example, at 11 kHz (figure 5.2B), the ILDs peak at about 40 dB, and show much more variation with sound source direction. This is partly due to the growing influence of the direction-dependent filtering of the incoming sound by the external ears on frequencies above about 6 kHz. This filtering imposes a complex, direction–dependent pattern of peaks and notches on the sound spectrum reaching the eardrum (figure 5.2D).

In adult humans, the maximum ITD that can be generated is around 700 µs. Animals with smaller heads have access to a correspondingly smaller range of ITDs and need to possess good high-frequency hearing to be able to use ILDs at all. This creates a problem for species that rely on low frequencies, which are less likely to be degraded by the environment, for communicating with potential mates over long distances. One solution is to position the ears as far apart as possible, as in crickets, where they are found on the front legs. Another solution, which is seen in many insects, amphibians, and reptiles as well as some birds, is to introduce an internal sound path between the ears, so that pressure and phase differences are established across each eardrum (figure 5.3). These ears are known as pressure-gradient or pressure-difference receivers, and give rise to larger ILDs and ITDs than would be expected from the size of the head (Christensen-Dalsgaard, 2005; Robert, 2005). For species that use pressure gradients to localize sound, a small head is a positive advantage as this minimizes the sound loss between the ears.

Mammalian ears are not pressure-gradient receivers; in contrast to species such as frogs that do use pressure gradients, mammals have eustachian tubes that are narrow and often closed, preventing sound from traveling through the head between the two ears. Directional hearing in mammals therefore relies solely on the spatial cues generated by the way sounds from the outside interact with the head and external ears. Fortunately, mammals have evolved the ability to hear much higher frequencies than other vertebrates, enabling them to detect ILDs and monaural spectral cues, or have relatively large heads, which provide them with a larger range of ITDs.

Because several physical cues convey information about the spatial origin of sound sources, does this mean some of that information is redundant? The answer is no, because the usefulness of each cue varies with the spectral composition of the sound and the region of space from which it originates. We have already seen that low frequencies do not generate large ILDs or spectral cues. In contrast, humans, and indeed most mammals, use ITDs only for relatively low frequencies. For simple periodic stimuli, such as pure tones, an interaural difference in sound arrival time is equivalent to a difference in the phase of the wave at the two ears (figure 5.4), which can be

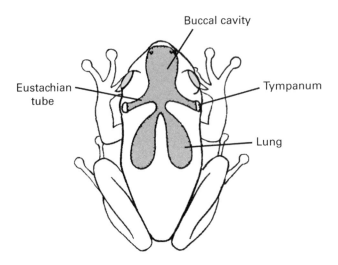

Figure 5.3
In species with pressure-gradient receiver ears, sound can reach both sides of the eardrum. In frogs, as shown here, sound is thought to arrive at the internal surface via the eustachian tubes and mouth cavity and also via an acoustic pathway from the lungs. The eardrums, which are positioned just behind the eyes flush with the surrounding skin, are inherently directional, because the pressure (or phase) on either side depends on the relative lengths of the different sound paths and the attenuation across the body. This depends, in turn, on the angle of the sound source. Artwork by Peter Navins, reproduced by kind permission.

registered in the brain by the phase-locked responses of auditory nerve fibers. However, these cues are inherently ambiguous. Note that in figure 5.4, the ITD corresponds to the distance between the crests of the sound wave received in the left and right ears, respectively, but it is not a priori obvious whether the real ITD of the sound source is the time from crest in the right ear signal to crest in the left (as shown by the little double-headed black arrow), or whether it is the time from a left ear crest to the nearest right ear crest (gray arrow). The situation illustrated in figure 5.4 could thus represent either a small, right ear–leading ITD or a large left ear–leading one. Of course, if the larger of the two possible ITDs is "implausibly large," larger than any ITD one would naturally expect given the subject's ear separation, then only the smaller of the possible ITDs need be considered. This "phase ambiguity" inherent in ITDs is therefore easily resolved if the temporal separation between subsequent crests of the sound wave is at least twice as long as the time it takes for the sound wave to reach the far ear, imposing an upper frequency limit on the use of interaural phase differences for sound localization. In humans, that limit is 1.5 to 1.6 kHz, which is where the period of the sound wave is comparable to the maximum ITD available. Consequently, it may still

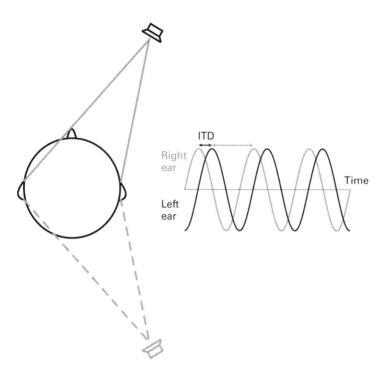

Figure 5.4

The interaural time delay for a sinusoidal stimulus results in a phase shift between the signals at each ear. For ongoing pure-tone stimuli, the auditory system does not know at which ear the sound is leading and which it is lagging. There are therefore two potential ITDs associated with each interaural phase difference, as shown by the black and gray arrows. This is known as a phase ambiguity. However, the shorter ITD normally dominates our percept of where the sound is located. Even so, the same ITD will be generated by a sound source positioned at an equivalent angle on the other side of the interaural axis (gray loudspeaker). This cue is therefore spatially ambiguous and cannot distinguish between sounds located in front of and behind the head.

be difficult to tell whether the sound is located on the left or the right unless it has a frequency of less than half that value (Blauert, 1997).

We can demonstrate the frequency dependence of the binaural cues by presenting carefully calibrated sounds over headphones. When identical stimuli are delivered directly to the ears in this fashion, the sound will be perceived in the middle of the head. If, however, an ITD or ILD is introduced, the stimulus will still sound as though it originates inside the head, but will now be "lateralized" toward the ear through which the earlier or more intense stimulus was presented. If one tone is presented to the left ear and a second tone with a slightly different frequency is delivered at the same time to the right ear, the tone with the higher frequency will begin to lead because it has a shorter period (figure 5.5). This causes the sound to be heard as if it is moving from the middle of the head toward that ear. But once the tones are 180° out of phase, the signal leads in the other ear, and so the sound will shift to that side and then move back to the center of the head as the phase difference returns to zero. This oscillation is known as a "binaural beat," and occurs only for frequencies up to about 1.6 kHz (Sound Example "Binaural Beats" on the book's Web site).

The fact that the binaural cues available with pure-tone stimuli operate over different frequency ranges was actually recognized as long ago as the beginning of the twentieth century, when the Nobel Prize–winning physicist Lord Rayleigh generated binaural beats by mistuning one of a pair of otherwise identical tuning forks. In an early form of closed-field presentation, Rayleigh used long tubes to deliver the tones from each tuning fork separately to the two ears of his subjects. He concluded that

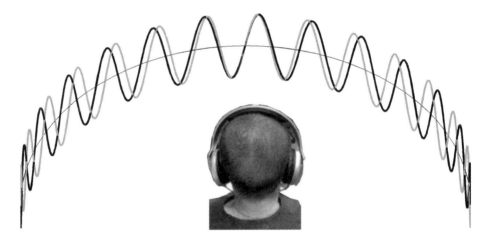

Figure 5.5
Schematic showing what the interaural phase relationship would be for sound source directions in the horizontal plane in front of the listener. For source directions to the left, the sound in the left ear (black trace) leads in time before the sound in the right ear (gray trace), while for source directions to the right, the right ear leads. Consequently, tones of slightly different frequencies presented over headphones to each ear, so that their interaural phase difference constantly shifts (so-called binaural beat stimuli), may create the sensation of a sound moving from one side to the other, then "jumping back" to the far side, only to resume a steady movement. Note that the perceived moving sound images usually sound as if they move inside the head, between the ears. The rate at which the sound loops around inside the head is determined by the difference between the two tone frequencies.

ITDs are used to determine the lateral locations of low-frequency tones, whereas ILDs provide the primary cue at higher frequencies. This finding has since become known as the "duplex theory" of sound localization. Studies in which sounds are presented over headphones have provided considerable support for the duplex theory. Indeed, the sensitivity of human listeners to ITDs or ILDs (Mills, 1960; Zwislocki & Feldman, 1956) can account for their ability to detect a change in the angle of the sound source away from the midline by as little as 1° (Mills, 1958). This is the region of greatest spatial acuity and, depending on the frequency of the tone, corresponds to an ITD of just 10 to 15 μs or an ILD of 0.5 to 0.8 dB.

Although listeners can determine the lateral angle of narrowband stimuli with great accuracy, they struggle to distinguish between sounds originating in front from those coming from behind the head (Butler, 1986). These front-back confusions are easily explained if we look at the spatial distribution of ITDs and ILDs. For a given sound frequency, each binaural cue value will occur at a range of stimulus locations, which are indicated by the white contours in figures 5.2A–C. These iso-ILD or iso-ITD contours are aptly referred to as "cones of confusion," because, in the absence of any other information, listeners (or neurons) will be unable to distinguish between the sound directions that lie on each contour. In the case of ITDs, the cones of confusion are centered on the interaural axis (figure 5.2C), giving rise to the type of front-back confusion illustrated in figure 5.4. The situation is once again more complex for ILDs, where cones of confusion take a different shape for each sound frequency (figure 5.2A and B).

We must not forget, however, that natural sounds tend to be rich in their spectral composition and vary in amplitude over time. (The reasons for this we discussed in chapter 1.) This means that, when we try to localize natural sounds, we will often be able to extract and combine both ITD and ILD information independently from a number of different frequency bands. Moreover, additional cues become available with more complex sounds. Thus, timing information is not restricted to ongoing phase differences at low frequencies, but can also be obtained from the envelopes of high-frequency sounds (Henning, 1974). Broadband sound sources also provide the auditory system with direction-dependent spectral cues (figure 5.2D), which are used to resolve front-back confusions, as illustrated by the dramatic increase in these localization errors when the cavities of the external ears are filled with molds (Oldfield & Parker, 1984).

The spectral cues are critical for other aspects of sound localization, too. In particular, they allow us to distinguish whether a sound comes from above or below. It is often thought that this is a purely monaural ability, but psychophysical studies have shown that both ears are used to determine the vertical angle of a sound source, with the relative contribution of each ear varying with the horizontal location of the source (Hofman & Van Opstal, 2003; Morimoto, 2001). Nevertheless, some individuals who are deaf in one ear can localize pretty accurately in both azimuth and elevation (Slattery & Middlebrooks, 1994; Van Wanrooij & Van Opstal, 2004). To some extent, this can be attributed to judgments based on the variations in intensity that arise from the shadowing effect of the head, but there is no doubt that monaural spectral cues are also used under these conditions. The fact that marked individual variations are seen in the accuracy of monaural localization points to a role for learning in this process, an issue we shall return to in chapter 7.

Because front-back discrimination and vertical localization rely on the recognition of specific spectral features that are imposed by the way the external ears and head filter the incoming stimulus, the auditory system is faced with the difficulty of dissociating those features from the spectrum of the sound that was actually emitted by the source. Indeed, if narrowband sounds are played from a fixed loudspeaker position, the perceived location changes with the center frequency of the sound, indicating that specific spectral features are associated with different directions in space (Musicant & Butler, 1984). But even if the sounds to be localized are broadband, pronounced variations in the source spectrum will prevent the extraction of monaural spectral cues (Wightman & Kistler, 1997). Consequently, these cues provide reliable spatial information only if the source spectrum is relatively flat, familiar to the listener, or can be compared between the two ears.

It should be clear by now that to pinpoint the location of a sound source both accurately and consistently, the auditory system has to rely on a combination of spatial cues. It is possible to measure their relative contributions to spatial hearing by setting the available cues to different values. The classic way of doing this is known as time-intensity trading (Sound Example "Binaural Cues and Cue Trading" on the book's Web site) (Blauert, 1997). This involves presenting an ITD favoring one ear together with an ILD in which the more intense stimulus is in the other ear. The two cues will therefore point to opposite directions. But we usually do not hear such sounds as coming from two different directions at the same time. Instead, we typically perceive a sort of compromise sound source direction, somewhere in the middle. By determining the magnitude of the ILD required to pull a stimulus back to the middle of the head in the presence of an opposing ITD, it is possible to assess the relative importance of each cue. Not surprisingly, this depends on the type of sound presented, with ILDs dominating when high frequencies are present.

Although presenting sounds over headphones is essential for measuring the sensitivity of human listeners or auditory neurons to binaural cues, this approach typically overlooks the contribution of the spectral cues in sound localization (as unfortunately do many textbooks). Indeed, the very fact that sounds are perceived to originate within the head or at a position very close to one or the other ear indicates that localization per se is not really being studied. If the filter properties of the head and external ears—

the so-called head-related transfer function—are measured and then incorporated in the signals played over headphones, however, the resulting stimuli will be externalized, that is, they will sound as though they come from outside rather than inside the head (Hartmann & Wittenberg, 1996; Wightman & Kistler, 1989). The steps involved in generating "virtual acoustic space" (VAS) stimuli, which can be localized just as accurately as real sound sources in the external world (Wightman & Kistler, 1989), are summarized in figure 5.6 (Sound Example "Virtual Acoustic Space" on the book's Web site).

You might ask why we would want to go to so much trouble to simulate real sound locations over headphones when we could just present stimuli from loudspeakers in the free field. This comes down to a question of stimulus control. For example, one of the great advantages of VAS techniques is that ITDs, ILDs, and spectral cues can be manipulated largely independently. Using this approach, Wightman and Kistler (1992) measured localization accuracy for stimuli in which ITDs signaled one direction and ILDs and spectral cues signaled another. They found that ITDs dominate the localization of broadband sounds that contain low-frequency components, which is in general

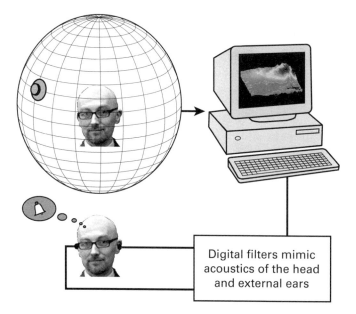

Figure 5.6

Construction of virtual acoustic space. Probe tube microphones are inserted into the ear canal of the subject, and used to measure the directional filtering properties of each ear. Digital filters that replicate the acoustical properties of the external ears are then constructed. With these digital filters, headphone signals can be produced that sound as though they were presented out in the real external world.

agreement with the duplex theory mentioned previously. Nevertheless, you may be aware that many manufacturers of audio equipment have begun to produce "surround-sound" systems, which typically consist of an array of perhaps five mid- to high-frequency loudspeakers, but only a single "subwoofer" to deliver the low frequencies. These surround-sound systems can achieve fairly convincing spatialized sound if the high-frequency speaker array is correctly set up. But since there is only one subwoofer (the positioning of which is fairly unimportant), these systems cannot provide the range of low-frequency ITDs corresponding to the ILDs and spectral cues available from the array of high-frequency speakers. Thus, ITDs do not dominate our percept of sound source location for the wide gamut of sounds that we would typically listen to over devices such as surround-sound home theater systems. Indeed, it is becoming clear that the relative weighting the brain gives different localization cues can change according to how reliable or informative they are (Kumpik, Kacelnik, & King, 2010; Van Wanrooij & Van Opstal 2007). Many hours of listening to stereophonic music over headphones, for example, which normally contains no ITDs and only somewhat unnatural ILDs, may thus train our brains to become less sensitive to ITDs. We will revisit the neural basis for this type of reweighting of spatial cues in chapter 7, when we consider the plasticity of spatial processing.

5.2 Determining Sound Source Distance

The cues we have described so far are useful primarily for determining sound source direction. But being able to estimate target distance is also important, particularly if, as is usually the case, either the listener or the target is moving. One obvious, although not very accurate, cue to distance is loudness. As we previously mentioned in section 1.7, if the sound source is in an open environment with no walls or other obstacles nearby, then the sound energy radiating from the source will decline with the inverse square of the distance. In practice, this means that the sound level declines by 6 dB for each doubling of distance. Louder sounds are therefore more likely to be from nearby sources, much as the size of the image of an object on the retina provides a clue as to its distance from the observer. But this is reliable only if the object to be localized is familiar, that is, the intensity of the sound at the source or the actual size of the visual object is known. It therefore works reasonably well for stimuli such as speech at normal conversational sound levels, but distance perception in free field conditions for unfamiliar sounds is not very good.

And things become more complicated either in close proximity to the sound source or in reverberant environments, such as rooms with walls that reflect sound. In the "near field," that is, at distances close enough to the sound source that the source cannot be approximated as a simple point source, the sound field can be rather complex, affecting both spectral cues and ILDs in idiosyncratic ways (Coleman, 1963).

As a consequence, ILDs and spectral cues in the near field could, in theory, provide potential cues for sound distance as well as direction. More important, within enclosed rooms, the human auditory system is able to use reverberation cues to base absolute distance judgments on the proportion of sound energy reaching the ears directly from the sound source compared to that reflected by the walls of the room. Bronkhorst and Houtgast (1999) used VAS stimuli to confirm this by showing that listeners' sound distance perception is impaired if either the number or level of the "reflected" parts of the sound are changed.

While many comparative studies of directional hearing have been carried out, revealing a range of abilities (Heffner & Heffner, 1992), very little is known about acoustic distance perception in most other species. It is clearly important for hunting animals, such as barn owls, to be able to estimate target distance as they close in on their prey, but how they do this is not understood. An exception is animals that navigate and hunt by echolocation. Certain species of bat, for example, emit trains of high-frequency pulses, which are reflected off objects in the animal's flight path. By registering the delay between the emitted pulse and its returning echo, these animals can very reliably catch insects or avoid flying into obstacles in the dark.

5.3   Processing of Spatial Cues in the Brainstem

In order to localize sound, binaural and monaural spatial cues must be detected by neurons in the central auditory system. The first step is, of course, to transmit this information in the activity of auditory nerve fibers. As we have seen in chapter 2, the firing rates of auditory nerve fibers increase with increasing sound levels, so ILDs will reach the brain as a difference in firing rates of auditory afferents between the left and right ears. Similarly, the peaks and notches that constitute spectral localization cues are encoded as uneven firing rate distributions across the tonotopic array of auditory nerve fibers. Although most of those fibers have a limited dynamic range, varying in their discharge rates over a 30- to 40-dB range, it seems that differences in thresholds among the fibers, together with those fibers whose firing rates do not fully saturate with increasing level, can provide this information with sufficient fidelity. ITDs, in turn, need to be inferred from differences in the temporal firing patterns coming from the left versus the right ear. This depends critically on an accurate representation of the temporal fine structure of the sounds through phase locking, which we described in chapter 2.

Information about the direction of a sound source thus arrives in the brain in a variety of formats, and needs to be extracted by correspondingly different mechanisms. For ITDs, the timing of individual discharges in low-frequency neurons plays a crucial role, whereas ILD processing requires comparisons of mean firing rates of high-frequency nerve fibers from the left and right ears, and monaural spectral cue detection involves making comparisons across different frequency bands in a single ear. It is therefore not surprising that these steps are, at least initially, carried out by separate brainstem areas.

You may recall from chapter 2 that auditory nerve fibers divide into ascending and descending branches on entering the cochlear nucleus, where they form morphologically and physiologically distinct synaptic connections with different cell types in different regions of the nucleus. The ascending branch forms strong connections with spherical and globular bushy cells in the anteroventral cochlear nucleus (AVCN). As we shall see later, these bushy cells are the gateway to brainstem nuclei specialized for extracting binaural cues. As far as spatial processing is concerned, the important property of the descending branch is that it carries information to the dorsal cochlear nucleus (DCN), which may be particularly suited to extracting spectral cues. We will look at each of these in turn, beginning with spectral cue processing in the DCN.

5.3.1 Brainstem Encoding of Spectral Cues

The principal neurons of the DCN, including the fusiform cells, often fire spontaneously at high rates, and they tend to receive a variety of inhibitory inputs. Consequently, these cells can signal the presence of sound features of interest either by increasing or reducing their ongoing firing rate. When stimulated with tones, the responses of some of these cells are dominated by inhibition. Such predominantly inhibitory response patterns to pure tones are known as "type IV" responses, for historical reasons. In addition to this inhibition in response to pure tones, type IV neurons respond to broadband noises with a mixture of excitation as well as inhibition from a different source (the "wideband inhibitor," which we shall discuss further in chapter 6). The interplay of this variety of inhibitory and excitatory inputs seems to make type IV neurons exquisitely sensitive to the spectral shape of a sound stimulus. Thus, they may be overall excited by a broadband noise, but when there is a "notch" in the spectrum of the sound near the neuron's characteristic frequency, the noise may strongly inhibit the neuron rather than excite it. This inhibitory response to spectral notches can be tuned to remarkably narrow frequency ranges, so that the principal neurons of the DCN can be used not just to detect spectral notches, but also to determine notch frequencies with great precision (Nelken & Young, 1994). That makes them potentially very useful for processing spectral localization cues.

Spectral notches are particularly prominent features of the HRTF in the cat, the species most used to study this aspect of sound localization. Figure 5.7A shows HRTF measurements made by Rice and colleagues (1992) for three different sound source directions. In the examples shown, the sound came from the same azimuthal angle but from three different elevations. Moving from 15° below to 30° above the horizon

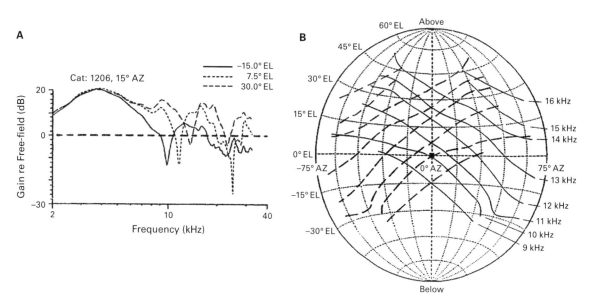

Figure 5.7

(A) Head-related transfer functions of the cat for three sound source directions. Note the prominent "first notch" at frequencies near 10 kHz. (B) Map of the frontal hemifield of space, showing
sound source directions associated with particular first-notch frequencies. With the cat facing
the coordinate system just as you are, the solid diagonals connect all source directions associated
with the first-notch frequencies in the right ear (as indicated along the right margin). Dashed
lines show equivalent data for the left ear. Together, the first-notch frequencies for the left
and right ears form a grid of sound source direction in the frontal hemifield. AZ, azimuth;
EL, elevation.
From Rice et al. (1992) with permission from Elsevier.

made very little difference to the HRTF at low frequencies, whereas at frequencies
above 7 kHz or so, complex peaks and notches can be seen, which vary in their frequency and amplitude with sound source direction. The first obvious notch (also
referred to as the "mid-frequency notch") occurs at frequencies near 10 kHz and shifts
to higher frequencies as the sound source moves upward in space. In fact, Rice et al.
(1992) found that such mid-frequency notches can be observed in the cat's HRTF
through much of the frontal hemifield of space, and the notch frequency changes
with both the horizontal and vertical angles of the sound source.

This systematic dependency of notch frequency on sound source direction is shown
in figure 5.7B. The solid diagonal lines show data from the right ear, while the dashed
lines show data from the left. The lowest diagonal connects all the source directions
in the frontal hemisphere that have a first notch at 9 kHz, the second diagonal

connects those with a first notch at 10 kHz, and so on, all the way up to source directions that are associated with first notches at 16 kHz. What figure 5.7B illustrates very nicely is that these first notch cues form a grid pattern across the frontal hemisphere. If the cat hears a broadband sound and detects a first notch at 10 kHz in both the left and the right ears, then this gives a strong hint that the sound must have come from straight ahead (0° azimuth and 0° elevation), as that is the only location where the 10-kHz notch diagonals for the left and right ears cross. On the other hand, if the right ear introduces a first notch at 12 kHz and the left ear at 15 kHz, this should indicate that the sound came from 35° above the horizon and 30° to the left, as you can see if you follow the fourth solid diagonal and seventh dashed diagonal from the bottom in figure 5.7B to the point where they cross.

This grid of first-notch frequencies thus provides a very neatly organized system for representing spectral cues within the tonotopic organization of the DCN. Type IV neurons in each DCN with inhibitory best frequencies between 9 and 15 kHz are "spatially tuned" to broadband sound sources positioned along the diagonals shown in figure 5.7B, in the sense that these locations would maximally suppress their high spontaneous firing. Combining this information from the two nuclei on each side of the brainstem should then be sufficient to localize broadband sources unambiguously in this region of space. There is certainly evidence to support this. Bradford May and colleagues have shown that localization accuracy by cats in the frontal sound field is disrupted if the frequency range where the first notch occurs is omitted from the stimulus (Huang & May, 1996), while cutting the fiber bundle known as the dorsal acoustic stria, which connects the DCN to the inferior colliculus (IC), impairs their ability to localize in elevation without affecting hearing sensitivity (May, 2000).

It may have occurred to you that cats and some other species can move their ears. This has the effect of shifting the locations at which the spectral notches occur relative to the head. Such movements are extremely useful for aligning sounds of interest with the highly directional ears, so that they can be detected more easily. However, ITDs are little affected by pinna movements, so it would appear that these animals effectively perform their own cue trading experiments whenever the ears move. Consequently, a continuously updated knowledge of pinna position is required to maintain accurate sound localization. This is provided in the form of somatosensory input to the DCN, which mostly originates from the muscle receptors found in the pinna of the external ear (Kanold & Young, 2001).

Although spectral notches are undoubtedly important localization cues, psychophysical studies in humans indicate that multiple spectral features contribute to sound localization (Hofman & Van Opstal, 2002; Langendijk & Bronkhorst, 2002). Moreover, nobody has documented an arrangement of HRTF notches or peaks in other mammalian species that is as neat and orderly as that of the cat. This implies that it is necessary to learn through experience to associate particular spectral cues with a specific source direction. But even in the absence of a systematic pattern, notch-sensitive type IV neurons in the DCN would still be useful for detecting spectral cues and sending that information on to the midbrain, and they are thought to serve this role not just in cats but in many mammalian species.

5.3.2 Brainstem Encoding of Interaural-Level Differences

As we have seen, binaural cues provide the most important information for localization in the horizontal plane. ILDs are perhaps the most familiar spatial cue to most of us because we exploit them for stereophonic music. To measure these differences, the brain must essentially subtract the signal received at one side from that received at the other and see how much is left. Performing that subtraction appears to be the job of a nucleus within the superior olivary complex known as the lateral superior olive (LSO). The neural pathways leading to the LSO are shown schematically in figure 5.8.

Since ILDs are high-frequency sound localization cues, it is not surprising that neurons in the LSO, although tonotopically organized, are biased toward high frequencies. These neurons are inhibited by sound from the contralateral ear and excited by sound from the ipsilateral ear; they are therefore often referred to as "IE" neurons. The excitation arrives directly via connections from primary-like bushy cells in the AVCN, while the inhibition comes from glycinergic projection neurons in the medial nucleus of the trapezoid body (MNTB), which, in turn, receive their input from globular bushy cells in the contralateral AVCN.

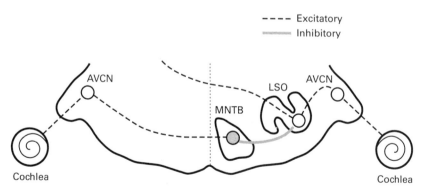

Figure 5.8
Schematic of the ILD processing pathway in the auditory brainstem. AN, auditory nerve; AVCN, anteroventral cochlear nucleus; MNTB, medial nucleus of the trapezoid body; LSO, lateral superior olive.
Artwork by Prof. Tom Yin, reproduced with kind permission.

Given this balance of excitatory and inhibitory inputs, an IE neuron in the LSO will not respond very strongly to a sound coming from straight ahead, which would be of equal intensity in both ears. But if the sound source moves to the ipsilateral side, the sound intensity in the contralateral ear will decline due to the head shadowing effects described earlier. This leads to lower firing rates in contralateral AVCN neurons, and hence a reduction in inhibitory inputs to the LSO, so that the responses of the LSO neurons become stronger. Conversely, if the sound moves to the contralateral side, the LSO receives less excitation but stronger inhibition, and LSO neuron firing is suppressed. A typical example of this type of ILD tuning in LSO neurons is shown in figure 5.9. In this manner, LSO neurons establish a sort of rate coding for sound source location. The closer the sound source is to the ipsilateral ear, the more strongly the neurons fire. Note that this rate code is relatively insensitive to overall changes in sound intensity. If the sound source does not move, but simply grows louder, then both the excitatory and the inhibitory drives will increase, and their net effect is canceled out.

IE neurons in the LSO are unusual in that they prefer stimuli presented to the ipsilateral side. However, sensory neurons in most brain areas tend to prefer stimulus locations on the opposite side of the body. To make ILD-derived spatial sensitivity of LSO neurons conform to the contralateral sensory representations found elsewhere, those neurons send excitatory projections to the contralateral IC. Consequently, from the midbrain onwards, central auditory neurons, just like those processing touch or

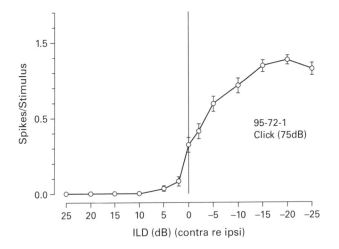

Figure 5.9
Firing rate as a function of ILD for a neuron in the LSO of the rat.
Adapted from Irvine, Park, and McCormick (2001) with permission from the American Physiological Society.

vision, will typically prefer stimuli presented in the contralateral hemifield. The output from the LSO to the midbrain is not entirely crossed, however, as a combination of excitatory and inhibitory projections also terminate on the ipsilateral side (Glendenning et al., 1992). The presence of ipsilateral inhibition from the LSO also contributes to the contralateral bias in the spatial preferences of IC neurons.

5.3.3 Brainstem Encoding of Interaural Time Differences

Although creating ILD sensitivity in the LSO is quite straightforward, the processing of ITDs is rather more involved and, to many researchers, still a matter of some controversy. Clearly, to measure ITDs, the neural circuitry has to somehow measure and compare the arrival time of the sound at each ear. That is not a trivial task. Bear in mind that ITDs can be on the order of a few tens of microseconds, so the arrival time measurements have to be very accurate. But arrival times can be hard to pin down. Sounds may have gently ramped onsets, which can make it hard to determine, with submillisecond precision, exactly when they started. Even in the case of a sound with a very sharp onset, such as an idealized click, arrival time measurements are less straightforward than you might think. Recall from chapter 2 that the mechanical filters of the cochlea will respond to click inputs by ringing with a characteristic impulse response function, which is well approximated by a gamma tone. Thus, a click will cause a brief sinusoidal oscillation in the basilar membrane (BM), where each segment of the membrane vibrates at its own characteristic frequency. Hair cells sitting on the BM will pick up these vibrations and stimulate auditory nerve fibers, causing them to fire not one action potential, but several, and those action potentials will tend to phase lock to the crest of the oscillations (compare figures 2.4 and 2.12 in chapter 2).

Figure 5.10 illustrates this for BM segments tuned to 1 kHz in both the left (shown in black) and right (shown in gray) ear, when a click arrives in the left ear shortly before it arrives in the right. The continuous lines show the BM vibrations, and the dots above the lines symbolize the evoked action potentials that could, in principle, be produced in the auditory nerve. Clearly, if the brain wants to determine the ITD of the click stimulus that triggered these responses, it needs to measure the time difference between the black and the gray dots. Thus, even if the sound stimuli themselves are not sinusoidal, ITDs give rise to interaural phase differences.

To make ITD determination possible, temporal features of the sound are first encoded as the phase-locked discharges of auditory nerve fibers, which are tuned to relatively narrow frequency bands. To a sharply tuned auditory nerve fiber, every sound looks more or less like a sinusoid. In the example shown in figure 5.10, this phase encoding of the click stimulus brings both advantages and disadvantages. An advantage is that we get "multiple looks" at the stimulus because a single click produces regular trains of action potentials in each auditory nerve. But there is also a

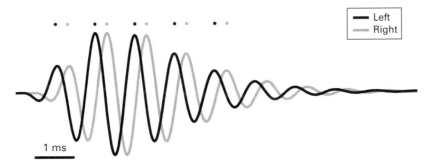

Figure 5.10
Basilar membrane impulse responses in the cochlea of each ear to a click delivered with a small interaural time difference.

potential downside. As we pointed out in section 5.1, it may not be possible to determine from an interaural phase difference which ear was stimulated first. Similarly, in the case of figure 5.10, it is not necessarily obvious to the brain whether the stimulus ITD corresponds to the distance from a black dot to the next gray dot, or from a gray dot to the next black dot. To you this may seem unambiguous if you look at the BM impulse functions in figure 5.10, but bear in mind that your auditory brainstem sees only the dots, not the lines, and the firing of real auditory nerve fibers is noisy, contains spontaneous as well as evoked spikes, and may not register some of the basilar membrane oscillations because of the refractory period of the action potential. Hence, some of the dots shown in the figure might be missing, and additional, spurious points may be added. Under these, more realistic circumstances, which interaural spike interval gives a correct estimate of the ITD is not obvious. Thus, the system has to pool information from several fibers, and is potentially vulnerable to phase ambiguities even when the sounds to be localized are brief transients.

The task of comparing the phases in the left and right ear falls on neurons in the medial superior olive (MSO), which, appropriately and in contrast to those found in the LSO, are biased toward low frequencies. As shown schematically in figure 5.11, the MSO receives excitatory inputs from both ears (MSO neurons are therefore termed "EE" cells) via monosynaptic connections from spherical bushy cells in the AVCN. The wiring diagram in the figure is strikingly simple, and there seem to be very good reasons for keeping this pathway as short and direct as possible.

Neurons in the central nervous system usually communicate with each other through the release of chemical neurotransmitters. This allows information to be combined and modulated as it passes from one neuron to the next. But this method of processing comes at a price: Synaptic potentials have time courses that are usually significantly slower and more spread out in time than neural spikes, and the process of transforming presynaptic spikes into postsynaptic potentials, only to convert them

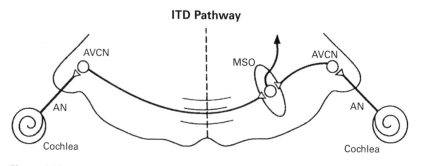

Figure 5.11

Connections of the medial superior olive.

Artwork by Prof. Tom Yin, reproduced with kind permission.

back into postsynaptic spikes, can introduce noise, uncertainty, and temporal jitter into the spike trains. Because ITDs are often extremely small, the introduction of temporal jitter in the phase-locked spike trains that travel along the ITD-processing pathway would be very bad news. To prevent this, the projection from auditory nerve fibers to AVCN bushy cells operates via unusually large and temporally precise synapses known as endbulbs of Held. Although many convergent synaptic inputs in the central nervous system are normally required to make a postsynaptic cell fire, a single presynaptic spike at an endbulb of Held synapse is sufficient to trigger a spike in the postsynaptic bushy cell. This guarantees that no spikes are lost from the firing pattern of the auditory nerve afferents, and that phase-locked time structure information is preserved. In fact, as figure 5.12 shows, bushy cells respond to the sound stimulus with a temporal precision that is greater than that of the auditory nerve fibers from which they derive their inputs.

AVCN bushy cells therefore supply MSO neurons with inputs that are precisely locked to the temporal fine structure of the sound in each ear. All the MSO neurons need to do to determine the sound's ITD is compare these patterns from the left and right ears. For a long time, it has been thought that MSO neurons carry out this interaural comparison by means of a delay line and coincidence detector arrangement, also known as the Jeffress model (Jeffress, 1948). The idea behind the Jeffress model is quite ingenious. Imagine a number of neurons lined up in a row, as shown schematically in figure 5.13. The lines coming from each side indicate that all five neurons shown receive inputs, via the AVCN, from each ear. Now let us assume that the neurons fire only if the action potentials from each side arrive at the same time, that is, the MSO neurons act as "coincidence detectors." However, the axons from the AVCN are arranged on each side to form opposing "delay lines," which results in the action potentials arriving at each MSO neuron at slightly different times from the left and right ears. Thus, for our hypothetical neuron A in figure 5.13, the delay from the left ear is only 0.1 ms, while that from the right ear is 0.5 ms. For neuron B,

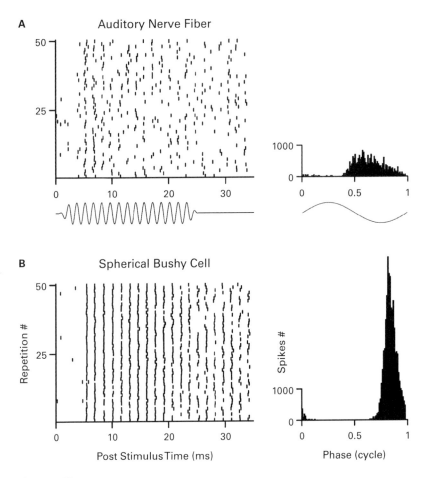

Figure 5.12

Phase-locked discharges of an auditory nerve fiber (A) and a spherical bushy cell of the AVCN (B). The plots to the left show individual responses in dot raster format. Each dot represents the firing of an action potential, with successive rows showing action potential trains to several hundred repeat presentations of a pure-tone stimulus. The stimulus waveform is shown below the upper raster plot. The histograms on the right summarize the proportion of spikes that occurred at each phase of the stimulus. The bushy cell responses are more reliable and more tightly clustered around a particular stimulus phase than those of the auditory nerve fiber. From Joris, Smith, and Yin (1998) with permission from Elsevier.

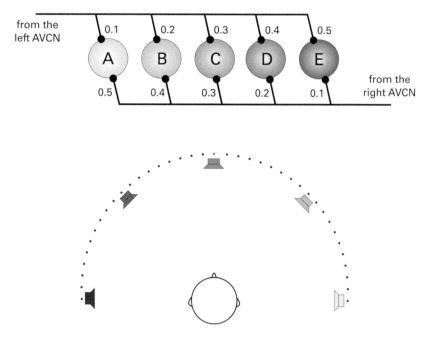

Figure 5.13

The Jeffress delay-line and coincidence detector model. A–E represent MSO neurons that receive inputs from the AVCN on both sides of the brain. The numbers next to each neuron indicate the conduction delay (in milliseconds) from each side. Because the model neurons act as coincidence detectors, they will respond best to ITDs that offset the difference in conduction delay from each ear. The pattern of delay lines therefore means that each neuron is tuned to a different ITD, and therefore location in space, as indicated by the corresponding grayscale of the loudspeaker icons in the lower part of the figure.

the left ear delay has become a little longer (0.2 ms) while that from the right ear is a little shorter (0.4 ms), and so on. These varying delays could be introduced simply by varying the relative length of the axonal connections from each side. But other factors may also contribute, such as changes in myelination, which can slow down or speed up action potentials, or even a slight "mistuning" of inputs from one ear relative to the other. Such mistuning would cause small interaural differences in cochlear filter delays, as we discussed in chapter 2 in the context of figures 2.4 and 2.5.

Now let us imagine that a sound comes from directly ahead. Its ITD is therefore zero, which will result in synchronous patterns of discharge in bushy cells in the left and right AVCN. The action potentials would then leave each AVCN at the same time, and would coincide at neuron C, since the delay lines for that neuron are the same on each side. None of the other neurons in figure 5.13 would be excited, because their inputs would arrive from each ear at slightly different times. Consequently, only neuron C would respond vigorously to a sound with zero ITD. On the other hand, if the sound source is positioned slightly to the right, so that sound waves now arrive at the right ear 0.2 ms earlier than those at the left, action potentials leaving from the right AVCN will have a head start of 0.2 ms relative to those from left. The only way these action potentials can arrive simultaneously at any of the neurons in figure 5.13 is if those coming from the right side are delayed so as to cancel out that head start. This will happen at neuron B, because its axonal delay is 0.2 ms longer from the right than from the left. Consequently, this neuron will respond vigorously to a sound with a right ear–leading ITD of 0.2 ms, whereas the others will not. It perhaps at first seems a little counterintuitive that neurons in the left MSO prefer sounds from the right, but it does make sense if you think about it for a moment. If the sound arrives at the right ear first, the only way of getting the action potentials to arrive at the MSO neurons at the same time is to have a correspondingly shorter neural transmission time from the left side, which will occur in the MSO on the left side of the brain. An animation of the Jeffress model can be found on the book's Web site.

A consequence of this arrangement is that each MSO neuron would have a preferred or best ITD, which varies systematically to form a neural map or "place code" corresponding to the different loudspeaker positions shown in the lower part of figure 5.13. All of our hypothetical neurons in this figure would be tuned to the same sound frequency, so that each responds to the same sound, but does so only when that sound is associated with a particular ITD. This means that the full range of ITDs would have to be represented in the form of the Jeffress model within each frequency channel of the tonotopic map.

The Jeffress model is certainly an attractive idea, but showing whether this is really how the MSO works has turned out to be tricky. The MSO is a rather small nucleus buried deep in the brainstem, which makes it difficult to study its physiology. However, early recordings were in strikingly good agreement with the Jeffress model. For example, Carr and Konishi (1988) managed to record from the axons from each cochlear nucleus as they pass through the nucleus laminaris, the avian homolog of the MSO, of the barn owl. They found good anatomical and physiological evidence that the afferent fibers act as delay lines in the predicted fashion, thereby providing the basis for the topographic mapping of ITDs. Shortly thereafter, Yin and Chan (1990) published recordings of cat MSO neurons, which showed them to behave much like "cross-correlators," implying that they may also function as coincidence detectors.

So what does it mean to say that MSO neurons act like cross-correlators? Well, first of all let us make clear that the schematic wiring diagrams in figures 5.11 and 5.13 are highly simplified, and may give the misleading impression that each MSO neuron receives inputs from only one bushy cell axon from each AVCN. That is not the case. MSO neurons have a distinctive bipolar morphology, with a dendrite sticking out from either side of the cell body. Each dendrite receives synapses from numerous bushy cell axons from either the left or right AVCN. Consequently, on every cycle of the sound, the dendrites receive not one presynaptic action potential, but a volley of many action potentials, and these volleys will be phase locked, with a distribution over the cycle of the stimulus much like the histogram shown at the bottom right of figure 5.12. These volleys will cause fluctuations in the membrane potential of the MSO dendrites that look a lot like a sine wave, even if the peak may be somewhat sharper, and the valley rather broader, than those of an exact sine wave (Ashida et al., 2007). Clearly, these quasi-sinusoidal membrane potential fluctuations in each of the dendrites will summate maximally, and generate the highest spike rates in the MSO neuron, if the inputs to each side are in phase.

Thus, an MSO neuron fires most strongly if, after compensation for stimulus ITD through the delay lines mentioned above, the phase delay between the inputs to the dendrites is zero, plus or minus an integer number of periods of the stimulus. Thus, as you can verify in figure 5.14, an MSO neuron that responds strongly to a 250-Hz tone (i.e., a tone with a 4,000 µs long period) with an ITD of 600 µs will also respond strongly at ITDs of 4,600 µs, or at –3,400 µs, although these "alternative best ITDs" are too large to occur in nature. The output spike rates of MSO neurons as a function of stimulus ITD bear more than a passing resemblance to the function you would obtain

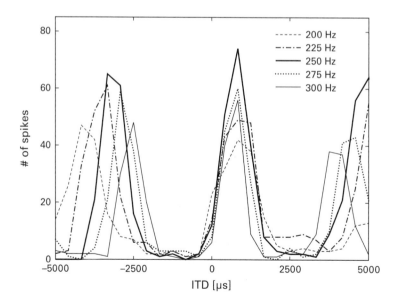

Figure 5.14
Spike rate of a neuron in the MSO of a gerbil as a function of stimulus ITD. The stimuli were pure-tone bursts with the frequencies shown.
Adapted from Pecka and colleagues (2008).

if you used a computer to mimic cochlear filtering with a bandpass filter and then calculated the cross-correlation of the filtered signals from the left and right ears. (Bandpass filtering will make the stimuli look approximately sinusoidal to the cross-correlator, and the cross-correlation of two sinusoids that are matched in frequency is itself a sinusoid.)

A cross-correlator can be thought of as a kind of coincidence detector, albeit not a very sharply tuned one. The cross-correlation is large if the left and right ear inputs are well matched, that is, if there are many temporally coincident spikes. But MSO neurons may fire even if the synchrony of inputs from each ear is not very precise (in fact, MSO neurons can sometimes even be driven by inputs from one ear alone). Nevertheless, they do have a preferred interaural phase difference, and assuming that phase ambiguities can be discounted, the preferred value should correspond to a single preferred sound source direction relative to the interaural axis, much as Jeffress envisaged.

The early experimental results, particularly those from the barn owl, made many researchers in the field comfortable with the idea that the Jeffress model was essentially correct, and chances are you have read an account of this in a neuroscience textbook. However, more recently, some researchers started having doubts that this strategy operates universally. For example, McAlpine, Jiang, and Palmer (2001) noticed that certain properties of the ITD tuning functions they recorded in the IC of the guinea pig appeared to be inconsistent with the Jeffress model. Now the output from the MSO to the midbrain is predominantly excitatory and ipsilateral. This contrasts with the mainly contralateral excitatory projection from the LSO, but still contributes to the contralateral representation of space in the midbrain, because, as we noted earlier, neurons in each MSO are sensitive to ITDs favoring the opposite ear and therefore respond best to sounds on that side. In view of this, McAlpine and colleagues assumed that ITD tuning in the IC should largely reflect the output of MSO neurons. They found that, for many neurons, the best ITDs had values so large that a guinea pig, with its relatively small head, would never experience them in nature (figure 5.15). If we assume that a neuron's best ITD is meant to signal a preferred sound source direction, then it must follow that the neurons are effectively tuned to sound source directions that do not exist.

These authors also observed that the peaks of the ITD tuning curves depend on each neuron's preferred sound frequency: The lower the characteristic frequency, the larger the best ITD. That observation, too, seems hard to reconcile with the idea that ITDs are represented as a place code, because it means that ITDs should vary across rather than within the tonotopic axis. The dependence of ITD tuning on the frequency tuning of the neurons is easy to explain. As we have already said, these neurons are actually tuned to interaural phase differences, so the longer period of lower frequency sounds will result in binaural cross-correlation at larger ITDs. You can see this in figure 5.14, where successive peaks in the ITD tuning curve are spaced further apart at lower

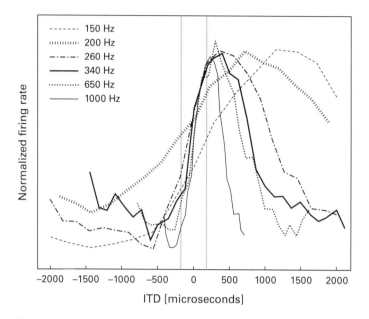

Figure 5.15

ITD tuning varies with neural frequency sensitivity. Each function represents the ITD tuning of a different neuron recorded in the guinea pig inferior colliculus. Each neuron had a different characteristic frequency, as indicated by the values in the inset. Neurons with high characteristic frequencies have the sharpest ITD tuning functions, which peak close to the physiological range (±180 μs, indicated by the vertical lines), whereas neurons with lower characteristic frequencies have wider ITD functions, which peak at longer ITDs that are often well outside the range that the animal would encounter naturally.

Adapted from McAlpine (2005) with permission from John Wiley and Sons.

frequencies, with their spacing corresponding to one stimulus period. This also means that the ITD tuning curves become broader at lower frequencies (figure 5.15), which does not seem particularly useful for mammals that depend on ITDs for localizing low-frequency sounds.

There is, however, another way of looking at this. You can see in figure 5.15 that the steepest region of each of the ITD tuning curves is found around the midline, and therefore within the range of naturally encountered ITDs. This is the case irrespective of best frequency. These neurons therefore fire at roughly half their maximal rate for sounds coming from straight ahead, and respond more or less strongly depending on whether the sound moves toward the contra- or ipsilateral side, respectively. Such a rate code would represent source locations near the midline with great accuracy, since small changes in ITD would cause relatively large changes in firing rate. Indeed, this is the region of space where, for many species, sound localization accuracy is at its best.

Studies of ITD coding in mammals have also called another aspect of the Jeffress model into question. We have so far assumed that coincidence detection in the MSO arises through simple summation of excitatory inputs. However, in addition to the excitatory connections shown in figure 5.11, the MSO, just like the LSO, receives significant glycinergic inhibitory inputs from the MNTB and the lateral nucleus of the trapezoid body. Furthermore, the synaptic connections to the MNTB that drive this inhibitory input are formed by a further set of unusually large and strong synapses, the so-called calyces of Held. It is thought that these calyces, just like the endbulbs of Held that provide synaptic input from auditory nerve fibers to the spherical bushy cells, ensure high temporal precision in the transmission of signals from globular bushy cells to MNTB neurons. As a result, inhibitory inputs to the MSO will also be accurately phase locked to the temporal fine structure of the sound stimulus.

The Jeffress model has no apparent need for precisely timed inhibition, and these inhibitory inputs to the MSO have therefore often been ignored. But Brand and colleagues (2002) showed that blocking these inhibitory inputs, by injecting tiny amounts of the glycinergic antagonist strychnine into the MSO, can alter the ITD tuning curves of MSO neurons, shifting their peaks from outside the physiological range to values close to 0µs. This implies that, without these inhibitory inputs, there may be no interaural conduction delay. How exactly these glycinergic inhibitory inputs influence ITD tuning in the MSO remains a topic of active research, but their role can no longer be ignored.

Based on the ITD functions they observed, McAlpine and colleagues proposed that it should be possible to pinpoint the direction of the sound source by comparing the activity of the two broadly tuned populations of neurons on either side of the brain. Thus, a change in azimuthal position would be associated with an increase in the activity of ITD-sensitive neurons in one MSO and a decrease in activity in the other. This notion that sound source location could be extracted by comparing the activity of neurons in different channels was actually first put forward by von Békésy, whose better known observations of the mechanical tuning of the cochlea are described in chapter 2. There is a problem with this, though. According to that scheme, the specification of sound source direction is based on the activity of neurons on both sides of the brain. It is, however, well established that unilateral lesions from the midbrain upward result in localization deficits that are restricted to the opposite side of space (Jenkins & Masterton, 1982), implying that all the information needed to localize a sound source is contained within each hemisphere.

In view of these findings, do we have to rewrite the textbook descriptions of ITD coding, at least as far as mammals are concerned? Well, not completely. In the barn owl, a bird of prey that is studied intensively because its sound localization abilities are exceptionally highly developed, the evidence for Jeffress-like ITD processing is strong. This is in part due to the fact that barn owl auditory neurons are able to phase lock, and thus to use ITDs, for frequencies as high as 9 kHz. Interaural cross-correlation of sounds of high frequency, and therefore short periods, will lead to steep ITD functions with sharp peaks that lie within the range of values that these birds will encounter naturally. Consequently, a place code arrangement as envisaged by Jeffress becomes an efficient way of representing auditory space.

By contrast, in mammals, where the phase locking limit is a more modest 3 to 4 kHz, the correspondingly shallower and blunter ITD tuning curves will encode sound source direction most efficiently if arranged to set up a *rate* code (Harper & McAlpine, 2004). However, the chicken seems to have a Jeffress-like, topographic arrangement of ITD tuning curves in its nucleus laminaris (Köppl & Carr, 2008). This is perhaps surprising since its neurons cannot phase lock, or even respond, at the high frequencies used by barn owls, suggesting that a rate-coding scheme ought to be more efficient given the natural range of ITDs and audible sound frequencies in this species. Thus, there may be genuine and important species differences in how ITDs are processed by birds and mammals, perhaps reflecting constraints from evolutionary history as much as or more than considerations of which arrangement would yield the most efficient neural representation (Schnupp & Carr, 2009).

5.4 The Midbrain and Maps of Space

A number of brainstem pathways, including those from the LSO, MSO, and DCN, converge in the IC and particularly the central nucleus (ICC), which is its main subdivision. To a large extent, the spatial sensitivity of IC neurons reflects the processing of sound localization cues that already took place earlier in the auditory pathway. But brainstem nuclei also project to the nuclei of the lateral lemniscus, which, in turn, send axons to the IC. Convergence of these various pathways therefore provides a basis for further processing of auditory spatial information in the IC. Anatomical studies carried out by Douglas Oliver and colleagues (Loftus et al., 2004; Oliver et al., 1997) have shown that some of these inputs remain segregated, whereas others overlap in the IC. In particular, the excitatory projections from the LSO and MSO seem to be kept apart even for neurons in these nuclei with overlapping frequency ranges. On the other hand, inputs from the LSO and DCN converge, providing a basis for the merging of ILDs and spectral cues, while the ipsilateral inhibitory projection from the LSO overlaps with the excitatory MSO connections.

In keeping with the anatomy, recording studies have shown that IC neurons are generally sensitive to more than one localization cue. Steven Chase and Eric Young (2008) used virtual space stimuli to estimate how "informative" the responses of individual neurons in the cat IC are about different cues. You might think that it would be much easier to combine estimates of sound source direction based on different spatial cues if the cues are already encoded in the same manner. And as we saw in the previous section, it looks as though the mammalian superior olivary complex employs a rate code for both ITDs and ILDs. Chase and Young found, however, that slightly different neural coding strategies are employed for ITDs, ILDs, and spectral cues. ITDs are represented mainly by the firing rate of the neurons, whereas the onset latencies and temporal discharge patterns of the action potentials make a larger contribution to the coding of ILDs and spectral notches. This suggests a way of combining different sources of information about the direction of a sound source, while at the same time preserving independent representations of those cues. The significance of this remains to be seen, but it is not hard to imagine that such a strategy could provide the foundations for maintaining a stable spatial percept under conditions where one of the cues becomes less reliable.

Another way of probing the relevance of spatial processing in the IC is to determine how well the sensitivity of the neurons found there can account for perceptual abilities. Skottun and colleagues (2001) showed that the smallest detectable change in ITD by neurons in the guinea pig IC matched the performance of human listeners. There is also some evidence that the sensitivity of IC neurons to interaural phase differences can change according to the values to which they have recently been exposed in ways that could give rise to sensitivity to stimulus motion (Spitzer & Semple, 1998). This is not a property of MSO neurons and therefore seems to represent a newly emergent feature of processing in the IC.

Earlier on in this chapter, we drew parallels between the way sound source direction has to be computed within the auditory system and the much more straightforward task of localizing stimuli in the visual and somatosensory systems. Most of the brain areas responsible for these senses contain maps of visual space or of the body surface, allowing stimulus location to be specified by which neurons are active. As we saw in the previous section, a place code for sound localization is a key element of the Jeffress model of ITD processing, which does seem to operate in the nucleus laminaris of birds, and barn owls in particular, even if the evidence in mammals is somewhat weaker.

The neural pathways responsible for sound localization in barn owls have been worked out in considerable detail by Masakazu Konishi, Eric Knudsen, and their colleagues. Barn owls are unusual in that they use ITDs and ILDs for sound localization over the same range of sound frequencies. Thus, the duplex theory does not apply. They also use these binaural localization cues in different spatial dimensions. Localization in the horizontal plane is achieved using ITDs alone, whereas ILDs provide the basis for vertical localization. This is possible because barn owls have asymmetric ears: The left ear opening within the ruff of feathers that surrounds the face is positioned higher up on the head than the right ear opening. Together with other differences between the left and right halves of the facial ruff, this leads to the left ear being more sensitive to sounds originating from below the head, while the right ear is more sensitive to sounds coming from above. The resulting ILDs are processed in the posterior part of the dorsal lateral lemniscal nucleus, where, like ITDs in the nucleus laminaris, they are represented topographically (Manley, Koppl, & Konishi, 1988).

The ITD and ILD processing pathways are brought together in the lateral shell of the central nucleus of the IC. Because they use ITDs at unusually high frequencies, barn owls have a particularly acute need to overcome potential phase ambiguities, which we discussed in the context of figures 5.4 and 5.10 (Saberi et al., 1999). The merging of information from different frequency channels is therefore required to represent sound source location unambiguously. This happens in the external nucleus of the IC, where the tonotopic organization that characterizes earlier levels of the auditory pathway is replaced by a map of auditory space (Knudsen & Konishi, 1978). In other words, neurons in this part of the IC respond to restricted regions of space that vary in azimuth and elevation with their location within the nucleus (figure 5.16). This is possible because the neurons are tuned to particular combinations of ITDs and ILDs (Peña & Konishi, 2002).

Constructing a map of the auditory world may, on the face of it, seem like an effective way of representing the whereabouts of sound sources within the brain, but it leaves open the question of how that information is read out to control behavior. The key to this lies in the next stage in the pathway. The external nucleus of the IC projects topographically to the optic tectum, which also receives substantial visual inputs. Knudsen (1982) demonstrated that auditory and visual inputs carrying signals from the same regions in space converge onto single neurons in the optic tectum. Thus, the tectum represents stimulus location independent of whether that stimulus was heard or seen, and uses this information to guide head-orienting behavior.

The discovery of a topographic representation of auditory space in the midbrain of the barn owl led to invigorated efforts to determine whether space maps are also present in the mammalian auditory system. Palmer and King (1982) showed that this is the case in the guinea pig superior colliculus (SC), the mammalian equivalent of the barn owl's optic tectum, and this has since been confirmed in other species. Given the need to combine information across different frequencies to establish a spatial topography, it should come as no surprise to learn that the mammalian SC is not tonotopically organized. The acoustical basis for the space map in mammals differs from that in owls, however, since this seems to rely exclusively on ILDs and spectral cues (figure 5.17) (Campbell et al., 2008; Palmer & King, 1985).

Like the optic tectum in the barn owl, the mammalian SC is a multisensory structure, and the auditory representation is superimposed on maps of visual space and of the body surface that are also present there. Indeed, one of the more striking features of the auditory topography in different species is that the range of preferred sound directions covaries with the extent of the visual map, as shown in figure 5.17C for the auditory and visual azimuth representations in the ferret SC. These different sensory inputs are transformed by the SC into motor commands for controlling orienting movements of the eyes, head, and, in species where they are mobile, the external ears. Besides providing a common framework for sensorimotor integration, aligning the

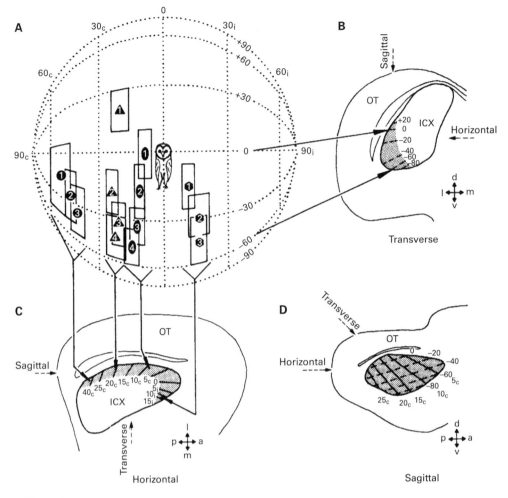

Figure 5.16

Topographic representation of auditory space in the external nucleus of the inferior colliculus (ICX) of the barn owl. (A) The coordinates of the auditory "best areas" of fourteen different neurons are plotted on an imaginary globe surrounding the animal's head. (B) As each electrode penetration was advanced dorsoventrally, the receptive fields of successively recorded neurons gradually shifted downwards, as indicated on a transverse section of the midbrain, in which isoelevation contours are depicted by the numbered dashed lines within the ICX. (C) These neurons were recorded in four separate electrode penetrations, whose locations are indicated on a horizontal section of the midbrain. Note that the receptive fields shifted from in front of the animal round to the contralateral side as the location of the recording electrode was moved from the anterior to the posterior end of the ICX. This is indicated by the solid lines within the ICX, which represent isoazimuth contours. (D) The full map of auditory space can be visualized in a sagittal section of the midbrain. The location of the optic tectum is indicated on each section: a, anterior; p, posterior; d, dorsal; v, ventral; m, medial; l, lateral.

Adapted from Knudsen and Konishi (1978) with permission from AAAS.

different sensory inputs allows interactions to take place between them, which give rise to enhanced responses to stimuli that are presented in close temporal and spatial proximity (Stein, Meredith, & Wallace, 1993).

Attractive though this arrangement is, transforming auditory inputs into a format that is dictated by other sensory modalities presents a new challenge. We have already seen that estimates of current pinna position are required in cats to ensure that movements of the ears do not result in conflicting information being provided by different acoustic localization cues. But merging auditory and visual inputs makes sense only if current eye position is also taken into account, so that the accuracy of a gaze shift toward an auditory target will be preserved irrespective of the initial position of the eyes. This is indeed the case in the SC, where recordings in awake animals (Hartline et al., 1995; Jay & Sparks, 1984), and even in anesthetized animals in which the eyes are displaced passively (Zella et al., 2001), have shown that auditory responses can be modulated by eye position; this indicates that, at least to some degree, auditory space is represented there in eye-centered coordinates, rather than the purely head-centered reference frame in which the localization cues are thought to be initially encoded. What is more surprising, though, is that the activity of neurons in tonotopically organized areas, including the IC (Groh et al., 2001) and the auditory cortex (Werner-Reiss et al., 2003), can also change with gaze direction.

5.5   What Does the Auditory Cortex Add?

Because many aspects of auditory spatial perception can apparently be accounted for by the substantial processing that takes place subcortically, it is tempting to conclude that the process of sound localization is largely complete at the level of the midbrain. This is not the end of the story, however, since we know the auditory cortex also plays an essential part in supporting spatial perception and behavior.

The clearest evidence for this comes from the prominent localization deficits that result from ablating or reversibly deactivating particular auditory cortical areas (Heffner & Heffner, 1990; Jenkins & Masterton, 1982; Lomber & Malhotra, 2008). In these studies, the ability of animals to discriminate between or pick out the location of sound sources on the opposite side of space is disrupted if the cortex is silenced on one side. If both the left and right sides of the cortex are affected, then the animals perform poorly on each side while retaining some ability to distinguish between sound sources positioned on either side of the midline. The deficits are most pronounced in species such as primates and carnivores with a well-developed cortex, and are also seen in humans with temporal lobe damage. In contrast to other species, however, humans appear to show a right-hemisphere dominance for sound localization. Thus, Zatorre and Penhune (2001) found that damage to the right auditory cortex can impair spatial perception on both sides, whereas left-sided lesions may have little effect on sound localization.

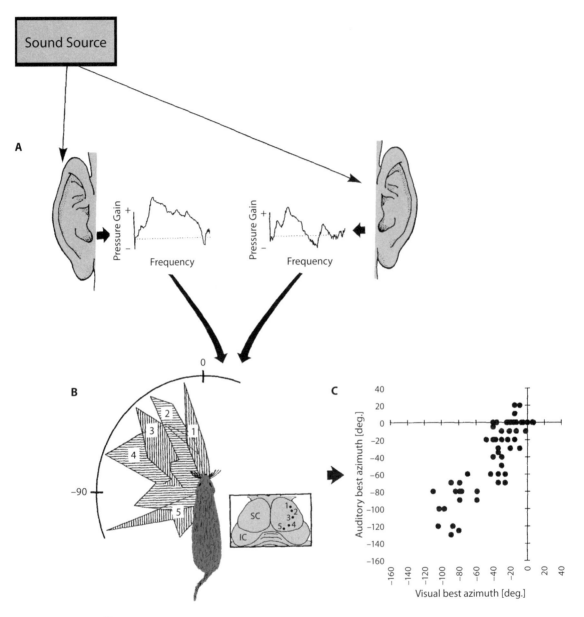

Figure 5.17
Representation of auditory space in the mammalian superior colliculus (SC). (A) The spectral localization cues generated by each external ear are shown for a sound source in the anterior hemifield. Both ILDs and spectral cues are used in the synthesis of the neural map of auditory space. (B) Spatial response profiles, plotted in polar coordinates centered on the head, for different neurons recorded in the right SC at the positions indicated by the corresponding numbers

As with other aspects of auditory perception, an important question in these studies is the relative involvement of different cortical areas. Jenkins and Merzenich (1984) addressed this issue by attempting to lesion the representation of a restricted band of frequencies in A1 of the cat, leaving the rest of the cortex intact, or, conversely, by destroying the whole of auditory cortex with the exception of a region of A1 that represented a narrow band of frequencies. In this ambitious experiment, they found that the small lesions resulted in localization deficits that were specific to the sound frequencies represented within the damaged area, whereas the larger lesions impaired the localization of brief sounds at all frequencies except those spared by the lesion.

While many other studies support the conclusion that A1 is necessary for normal sound localization, it is no longer possible to claim that this cortical area is sufficient. For one thing, larger deficits are observed if aspiration lesions include surrounding areas as well as A1 than if they are restricted to it. But more convincing are studies in which specific cortical fields are temporarily deactivated. Using this approach, Stephen Lomber and colleagues (Malhotra, Hall, & Lomber, 2004) have shown that certain cortical areas are involved in sound localization, whereas others are not. In one of these experiments, Lomber and Malhotra (2008) found that cooling the posterior auditory field produced a localization deficit in cats, but had no effect on their ability to carry out an auditory pattern discrimination task, whereas deactivation of the anterior auditory field produced the opposite result (figure 5.18). This suggests that a division of labor exists within the auditory cortex, with different areas being responsible for the processing of spatial and nonspatial information. But as we saw in chapters 3 and 4, this may have more to do with where those areas project than with fundamental differences in the way they process different types of sound.

These experiments clearly establish that the auditory cortex plays an essential role in spatial hearing. But how is sound source location represented there? As in other brain regions, the spatial receptive fields of cortical neurons have been mapped out

on the surface view of the midbrain. Each response profile indicates how the action potential firing rate varies with the azimuthal angle of the loudspeaker. Neurons in rostral SC (recording site 1) respond best to sounds located in front of the animal, whereas the preferred sound directions of neurons located at progressively more caudal sites (1→5) shift systematically into the contralateral hemifield. IC, inferior colliculus. (C) Relationship between the visual and auditory space maps in the ferret SC. For each vertical electrode penetration, the auditory best azimuths (loudspeaker direction at which the maximal response was recorded) of neurons recorded in the intermediate and deep layers of the SC are plotted against the corresponding visual coordinates of neurons recorded in the overlying superficial layers. 0° refers to the anterior midline, and negative numbers denote positions in the hemifield contralateral to the recording site. A similar correspondence between the visual and auditory maps is also found for stimulus elevation, which is mapped mediolaterally across the surface of the SC.
Adapted from King (1999).

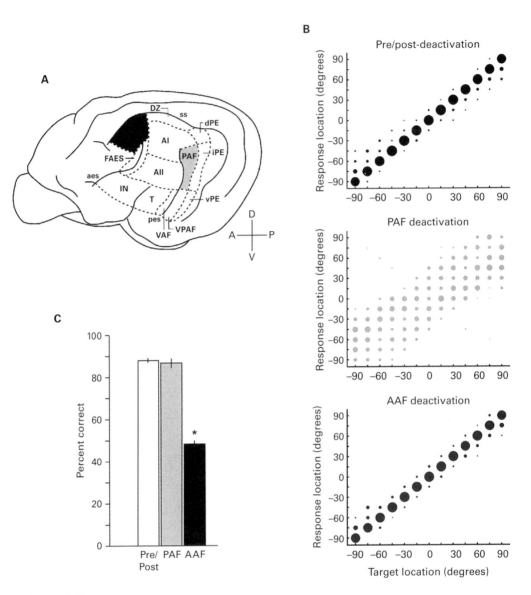

Figure 5.18

Behavioral evidence for the involvement of separate cortical areas in spatial and nonspatial auditory tasks. (A) Lateral view of the left cerebral hemisphere of the cat showing the auditory areas.
AAF, anterior auditory field (dark gray); AI, primary auditory cortex; AII, secondary auditory cortex;
dPE, dorsal posterior ectosylvian area; DZ, dorsal zone of auditory cortex; FAES, auditory field of
the anterior ectosylvian sulcus; IN, insular region; iPE, intermediate posterior ectosylvian area;
PAF, posterior auditory field (light gray); T, temporal region; VAF, ventral auditory field; VPAF,
ventral posterior auditory field; vPE, ventral posterior ectosylvian area. Sulci (lowercase): aes,

by recording the spiking activity of neurons in response to sounds delivered from free-field loudspeakers positioned around the head. These studies showed that cortical receptive fields vary in size both from one neuron to another and with the type of stimulus used, and they generally expand as the sound level is increased (Middlebrooks & Pettigrew, 1981; Rajan et al., 1990; Woods et al., 2006). In keeping with the behavioral deficits produced by ablation or deactivation of the auditory cortex in one hemisphere, the receptive fields of most cortical neurons are found on the contralateral side of the animal, although some neurons prefer sound sources near the frontal midline or on the ipsilateral side (figure 5.19).

We have already seen that different localization cues can be combined by individual neurons in the IC. Insofar as those neurons contribute to the ascending pathways, this must be the case for the cortex, too. As in subcortical nuclei, low-frequency cortical neurons are sensitive to ITDs, whereas high-frequency neurons rely more on ILDs. But spectral cues generated by the filter properties of the external ear are also important. Thus, at near-threshold sound levels, high-frequency A1 neurons have "axial" receptive fields that are centered on the acoustical axis of the contralateral ear. This is the region where the acoustical gain is at its maximum, indicating that the receptive fields of the neurons are shaped by pinna directionality.

As for the study of subcortical stations, the use of VAS techniques to change stimulus location digitally over headphones has also proved very valuable, making it possible to map out the spatial receptive field properties of cortical neurons in great detail (Brugge et al., 2001; Mrsic-Flogel, King, & Schnupp, 2005) and even to chart their spatiotemporal receptive fields (Jenison et al., 2001). Furthermore, using this technique to substitute spectral cues so that one animal is made to listen through the "virtual ears" of another changes cortical spatial receptive field properties, implying that individuals probably have to learn to localize using the particular cues provided by their own ears (Mrsic-Flogel et al., 2001). We will show in chapter 7 that this is indeed the case. Schnupp and colleagues (2001) extended this study to demonstrate that, in many cases, the location and shape of the spatial receptive fields of neurons in ferret A1 can be explained by a linear combination of their frequency sensitivity to stimulation of each ear and the directional properties of the auditory periphery

anterior ectosylvian; pes, posterior ectosylvian; ss, suprasylvian. Other abbreviations: A, anterior; D, dorsal; P, posterior; V, ventral. (B) Localization performance for one cat before and following cooling deactivation (top panel), during bilateral cooling of PAF cortex (middle panel) and during bilateral cooling of AAF cortex (bottom panel). Target location is indicated on the x-axis and response location on the y-axis. Area of the circle at each position indicates the percentage of responses made to that location. (C) Mean temporal pattern discrimination performance (mean ± s.e.m.) for the same cat before and following cooling deactivation (pre/post, white), during bilateral cooling of PAF cortex (light gray), and during bilateral cooling of AAF cortex (dark gray). Adapted from Lomber and Malhotra (2008) with permission from Macmillan Publishers Ltd.

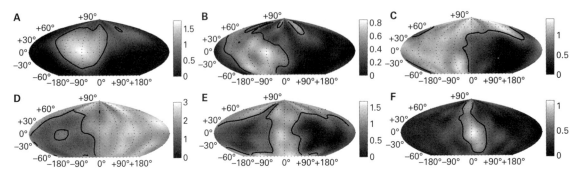

Figure 5.19
Six examples of spatial receptive fields recorded from different neurons in the primary auditory cortex (A1) of the ferret using virtual acoustic space stimuli derived from acoustical measurements of the animals' own ears. The grayscale indicates the numbers of spikes per stimulus presentation at each location.
Adapted from Mrsic-Flogel, King, and Schnupp (2005).

(figure 5.20). This linear estimation model can also account for the way receptive fields change with increasing sound level, although it works better for neurons that receive predominantly excitatory inputs from the contralateral ear and inhibitory inputs from the ipsilateral ear, and are therefore sensitive to ILDs, than for those receiving excitatory binaural inputs and likely to be sensitive to ITDs (Mrsic-Flogel et al., 2005). Intriguingly, it also predicts changes in the spatial receptive field caused by "listening through foreign virtual ears," and it can predict the observed improvement in spatial sensitivity seen with age as the head and ears grow (Mrsic-Flogel, Schnupp, & King, 2003), a finding that we shall also return to in chapter 7.

Early studies of the binaural sensitivity of A1 neurons suggested that EI and EE neurons are arranged in a series of bands that run orthogonal to the tonotopic axis, giving rise to the notion that A1 may possess a series of intertwined maps of different sound features, not unlike the regular organization of stimulus preferences in the visual cortex. As binaural response properties have been classified in greater detail, however, it has become clear that there is nothing more than a local clustering of neurons with similar response properties (Nakamoto, Zhang, & Kitzes, 2004; Rutkowski et al., 2000). This is also the case for the spatial receptive fields (Middlebrooks & Pettigrew, 1981; Rajan et al., 1990). As we saw in figure 5.19, the spatial sensitivity of cortical neurons can vary from one side of the midline to the other, indicating marked differences in their sensitivity to different localization cues, but there is no evidence for a map of auditory space in the cortex equivalent to that seen in the SC or to the maps of stimulus location that characterize the visual and somatosensory cortices.

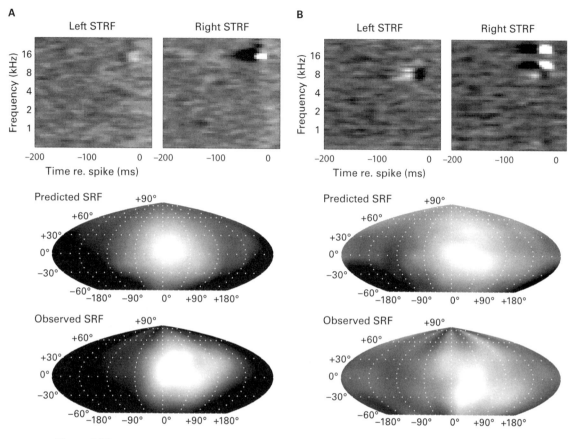

Figure 5.20

Predicting spatial sensitivity from the frequency tuning of two different neurons (A, B) recorded in the primary auditory cortex of the ferret. The upper plots show the spectrotemporal receptive fields (STRFs) measured by reverse correlation to random chord stimuli for each ear. The STRFs define the spectrotemporal structure of the sounds that elicit a response from the neurons. Each STRF was convolved with the energy spectrum vectors of virtual space stimuli presented to that ear for different virtual sound directions, and used to predict the spatial receptive field (SRF) of the neuron (middle row). Comparison with the observed SRF (bottom row) reveals a close fit between the two.

Adapted from Schnupp, Mrsic-Flogel, and King (2001).

Given the importance of the auditory cortex in sound localization, you might find this surprising. It is clearly possible to construct a map of auditory space in the brain, as studies of the SC and parts of the IC have shown, but we have to be clear about how that information is used. In the SC, auditory, visual, and somatosensory inputs combine to guide reflexive orienting movements. That is clearly a key function of the ability to determine the whereabouts of objects of interest in the world, but processing in the auditory cortex is responsible for much more, underlying our perception of what the sound source is in addition to where it is located.

We saw in the previous section that IC neurons can carry spatial information not just in their firing rates, but also in the timing of their action potentials. The potential importance of spike timing has been investigated extensively in the cortex. As the example in figure 5.21 shows, first-spike latencies tend to vary inversely with spike counts, with sounds at the more effective stimulus locations evoking more spikes with shorter latencies. However, temporal discharge patterns can be modulated across the receptive field independently of changes in firing rate, and a number of studies have shown that spike timing can carry as much or even more information about sound-source location than firing rate (Brugge, Reale, & Hind, 1996; Middlebrooks et al., 1998; Nelken et al., 2005). Indeed, Jenison (1998) showed that temporal response gradients across a population of cat A1 neurons can account for localization performance in both cats and humans.

As we have already stated, the impact of cortical deactivation on sound localization depends on which areas are silenced. There is also evidence in human imaging studies that the areas that show the greatest changes in blood oxygenation when subjects are asked to perform localization tasks are different from those engaged during sound recognition tasks (Alain et al., 2001; Barrett & Hall, 2006; Maeder et al., 2001). But recording studies have failed to reveal the clear division of labor that these imaging results might imply, since some sensitivity to sound source location is a property of all areas that have been investigated. Of course, that is not particularly surprising in view of the extensive subcortical processing of spatial information. Nevertheless, differences in spatial sensitivity have been observed. Thus, in monkeys, neurons in caudal auditory cortical areas are more sharply tuned for sound source location, and show a closer match to the ability of the animals to detect a change in sound direction, than those in core or rostral fields (Woods et al., 2006) (figure 5.22).

Regional differences are also found in cats. We saw in figure 5.18 that localization responses are impaired if the posterior auditory field (PAF) is silenced, whereas this is not the case if the anterior auditory field (AAF) is deactivated instead. Consistent with this, both the spike counts and first-spike latencies of neurons in PAF are more strongly modulated by changes in stimulus location and less affected by changes in sound level than those in AAF. On the other hand, it is likely that most cortical neurons are sensitive to both spatial and nonspatial sound attributes (Bizley et al., 2009), so these

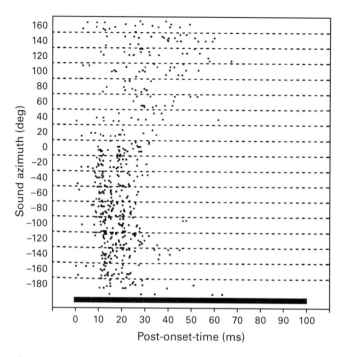

Figure 5.21
Auditory spatial information carried by temporal spike patterns. Responses of a neuron in the cat cortical anterior ectosylvian area to 100-ms noise bursts presented from various azimuthal positions, as indicated along the y-axis. The dots indicate the timing of action potential discharges. Each row of dots shows the temporal discharge pattern evoked by one stimulus presentation. Repeated presentations are shown in consecutive rows. Although individual responses are highly variable, one can nevertheless observe a systematic change in the temporal firing pattern as the sound source azimuth moves from the ipsilateral to the contralateral side.
Adapted from Middlebrooks et al. (1998) with permission from the American Physiological Society.

represent quantitative rather than qualitative differences in the preferences of the cortical neurons.

Although the spatial receptive fields of cortical neurons tend to be very large in relation to behavioral measures of spatial acuity, this does provide a means by which individual neurons can convey spatial information in their spike discharge patterns across a large range of stimulus locations. Based on responses like the one illustrated in figure 5.21, Middlebrooks and colleagues (1998) showed that computer-based classifiers can estimate sound source location from the firing patterns of individual neurons. However, the accuracy with which they do so is insufficient to account for sound localization behavior. Consequently, attention has switched to the role of population

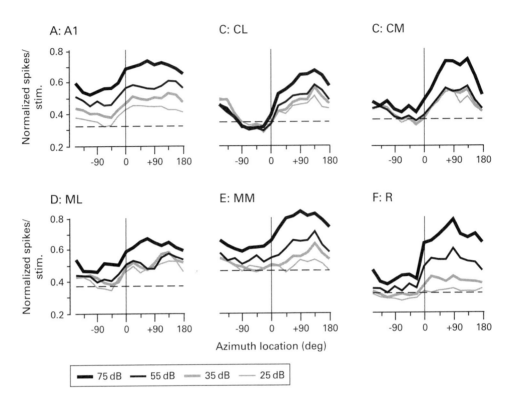

Figure 5.22
Normalized distribution of activity as a function of stimulus level and azimuth recorded in different areas of the monkey auditory cortex. Line thickness and shading corresponds to the different levels (see inset). The horizontal dashed line is the normalized spontaneous activity. Overall, the pooled responses increased in strength with increasing stimulus levels and were more sharply tuned for sound azimuth in the caudal belt fields (CM and CL) than in other areas of the auditory cortex.
From Woods et al. (2006) with permission from the American Physiological Society.

coding schemes, based on either the full spike discharge patterns (Stecker & Middlebrooks, 2003) or just the spike firing rates (Miller & Recanzone, 2009) or spike latencies (Reale, Jenison, & Brugge, 2003). These population codes tend to match behavioral performance more closely than those based on the responses of individual neurons.

We saw in section 5.3 that one school of thought is that sound direction based on ITDs might be extracted by comparing activity in the left and right MSOs. We also pointed out that this scheme is not readily compatible with the localization deficits incurred when auditory cortical areas are lesioned or deactivated on one side of the brain only. But while most cortical neurons respond preferentially to sounds located in the contralateral hemifield, others have ipsilateral receptive fields. This led Stecker and colleagues (2005) to propose that sound localization might be based on a comparison between the activity of populations of contralateral and ipsilateral neurons *within* each hemisphere. Although this has the attraction of embracing several of the ideas we have described in this chapter, how auditory space is represented in the cortex has yet to be fully established.

5.6 Localization in More Complex Environments: Echoes, Cocktail Parties, and Visual Cues

We have so far considered sound localization in the simple and rather artificial situation in which there is only one source. The reason for this is straightforward— the vast majority of studies have been done that way. Moreover, in order to exclude reflected sounds, psychophysical and recording experiments tend to be carried out in anechoic chambers. A more natural situation would be one where multiple sound sources are present at the same time in an environment with lots of room reflections and echoes. Instead of having a single source, the reflected sound waves will reach the listener from multiple directions, thereby distorting the spatial cues associated with the direct sound. In fact, in many modern environments, such as a typical office or bedroom, the portion of the sound energy that we receive indirectly as echoes from the walls and ceiling can be substantially greater than the direct sound.

In spite of this, human listeners are normally entirely unaware of the "reflected sound images" that each echoic surface creates, nor do these images confuse or impair localization accuracy of the true source as much as might be expected. The critical factor here seems to be that the reflected sound waves arrive at the ears slightly later than the direct sound. The simplest way of demonstrating the importance of the order in which sounds arrive is to present a pair of brief sounds from different directions in space. For short interstimulus delays of up to about 1 ms, the two sounds are fused by the auditory system, and their perceived location lies between the two source locations. This is known as "summing localization." At slightly longer delays, a single sound is still heard, but the second, or lagging, sound is suppressed and the perceived location is dominated by the actual location of the first sound. This is known as the "precedence effect" (Wallach, Newman, & Rosenzweig, 1949). But if the lagging sound arrives more than about 10 ms after the leading sound, the precedence effect breaks down, and two separate sounds are heard, each close to its true location. Neural correlates of the precedence effect have been described at various stages of the central auditory pathway (Fitzpatrick et al., 1999; Litovsky, 1998; Mickey & Middlebrooks, 2005). However, neural responses to the lagging sound tend to be suppressed in the cortex to longer delays than the precedence effect persists for in humans, and modeling studies suggest that part of this phenomenon can be accounted for by peripheral filtering together with compression and adaptation in the responses of the cochlear hair cells (Hartung & Trahiotis, 2001).

While the precedence effect describes what happens when a single echo is simulated, this is still a far cry from the more realistic situation in which sound waves traveling from a source are reflected many times by objects in the environment, and therefore arrive at the listener's ears over a protracted period of time. (See the book's web site, for a demonstration of a reverberant acoustic environment.) Devore and colleagues (2009) showed that reverberation affects the ITD sensitivity of IC neurons and lateralization judgments by human listeners in a similar fashion. They found that the spatial sensitivity of the neurons is better near the start of a reverberant stimulus and degrades over time, which is consistent with the gradual build up of reverberant energy as more and more reflections are generated.

Binaural processing is important not only for localizing sounds, but also for improving the detection of signals against a background of interfering noise (Blauert, 1997). Imagine that you are in a busy restaurant and trying to keep up with a particularly interesting conversation while other people are speaking at the same time. If you block one ear, this task becomes much harder. This is because binaural stimulation results in less masking of the sound source of interest by the "noise" emanating from other directions. Consequently, this important phenomenon is often referred to as the "cocktail party effect." It can be studied in the free field and over headphones, but the classical paradigm involves the presentation of a signal, usually a low-frequency tone, together with an interfering noise to both ears. Inverting the phase of either the signal or the noise can result in a 12- to 15-dB improvement in signal detection, a measure known as the binaural masking level difference (BMLD) (Licklider, 1948). More ecologically valid free-field studies, in which signal detection thresholds are measured when the signal and masker are spatially separated, have obtained similar levels of unmasking in both humans (Saberi et al., 1991) and ferrets (Hine, Martin, & Moore, 1994). Although concerned more with stimulus detection than localization, the responses of IC neurons to BMLD stimuli (Jiang, McAlpine, & Palmer, 1997) are consistent with their ITD sensitivity to tones and noise and with the results of human psychophysical studies.

In addition to considering how spatial hearing is affected in the presence of multiple sound sources, we also need to bear in mind that real objects very often stimulate more than one of the senses. Just as we saw in chapter 4 in the context of speech perception, visual cues can have a profound effect on sound localization. Thus, localization accuracy can improve if the source is also visible to the subject (Shelton & Searle, 1980; Stein, Huneycutt, & Meredith, 1988). On the other hand, the presence of a synchronous visual stimulus that is displaced slightly to one side of the auditory target can "capture" the perceived location of the sound source, causing it to be mislocalized (Bertelson & Radeau, 1981). This interaction between the senses provides the basis for the ventriloquist's illusion, and also explains why we readily link sounds with their corresponding visual events on a television or movie theater screen, rather than with the loudspeakers to one side. How vision exerts these effects at the neuronal level is not understood, but we now know that some neurons in the auditory cortex, as well as certain subcortical areas, are also sensitive to visual or tactile stimulation. Indeed, Bizley and King (2009) showed that visual inputs can sharpen the spatial sensitivity of auditory cortical neurons, highlighting the importance of nonacoustic factors in the neural representation of sound source location.

6 Auditory Scene Analysis

6.1 What Is Auditory Scene Analysis?

I'm sitting at the doors leading from the kitchen out into a small back garden. I hear the traffic in the nearby main road, and the few cars that turn from the main road into the little alley where the house stands. I hear birds—I can recognize the song of a blackbird. I hear the rustling of the leaves and branches of the bushes surrounding the garden. A light rain starts, increasing in intensity. The raindrops beat on the roofs of the nearby houses and on the windows of the kitchen.

Sounds help us to know our environment. We have already discussed, in some detail, the physical cues we use for that purpose. In previous chapters we discussed the complex processing required to extract the pitch, the phonemic identity (in case of speech), or the spatial location of sounds. However, so far we implicitly assumed that the sounds that need to be processed arise from a single source at any one time. In real life, we frequently encounter multiple sound sources, which are active simultaneously or nearly simultaneously. Although the sound waves from these different sources will arrive at our ears all mixed together, we nevertheless somehow hear them separately—the birds from the cars from the wind in the leaves. This, in a nutshell, is auditory scene analysis.

The term "auditory scene analysis" was coined by the psychologist Albert Bregman, and popularized through his highly influential book with that title. In parallel with the by now classic studies of auditory scene analysis as a psychoacoustic phenomenon, the field of computational auditory scene analysis has emerged in recent years, which seeks to create practical, computer-based implementations of sound source separation algorithms, and feeds back experience and new insights into the field.

Auditory scene analysis today is not yet a single, well-defined discipline, but rather a collection of questions that have to do with hearing in the presence of multiple sound sources. The basic concept that unifies these questions is the idea that the sounds emitted by each source reflect its distinct properties, and that it is possible to *group* those elements of the sounds in time and frequency that belong to the same source, while *segregating* those bits that belong to different sources. Sound elements that have been grouped in this manner are sometimes referred to as an "auditory stream," or even as an "auditory object." If auditory scene analysis works as it should, one such stream or object would typically correspond to the sound from a single source. However, "grouping," "segregation," "streams," and "auditory objects" are not rigorously defined terms, and often tested only indirectly, so be aware that different researchers in the field may use these terms to describe a variety of phenomena, and some may even reject the idea that such things exist at all.

In our survey of auditory scene analysis, we will therefore reexamine the idea that we group or segregate sounds, or construct auditory objects under different experimental conditions. We will start with a very simple situation—a pure tone in a background noise—in which different descriptions of auditory scene analysis can be discussed in very concrete settings. Then we will discuss simultaneous segregation—the ability to "hear out" multiple sounds that occur at the same time, and we will consider the way information about the composition of the auditory scene accumulates with time. Finally, with these issues and pertinent facts fresh in our minds, we will revisit the issues surrounding the existence and nature of auditory objects at the end of the chapter.

6.2   Low- and High-Level Representations of the Auditory Scene: The Case of Masking

One of the classical experiments of psychoacoustics is the measurement of the detection threshold for a pure-tone "target" in the presence of a white noise "masker." In these experiments, the "target" and the "masker" are very different from each other—pure tones have pitch, while white noise obviously does not. Introspectively, that special quality of the pure tone jumps out at us. This may well be the simplest example of auditory scene analysis: There are two "objects," the tone and the noise, and as long as the tone is loud enough to exceed the detection threshold, we hear the tone as distinct from the noise (Sound Example "Masking a Tone by Noise" on the book's Web site). But is this really so?

There is an alternative explanation of masking that doesn't invoke the concept of auditory scene analysis at all. Instead, it is based on concepts guiding decisions based on noisy data, a field of research often called signal detection theory. The assumptions that are required to apply the theory are sometimes unnatural, leading to the use of the term "ideal observer" with respect to calculations based on this theory. In its simplest form, signal detection theory assumes that you know the characteristics of the signal to detect (e.g., it is a pure tone at a frequency of 1,000 Hz) and you know those of the noise (e.g., it is Gaussian white noise). You are presented with short bits of sounds that consist either of the noise by itself, or of the tone added to the noise. The problem you face consists of the fact that noise by nature fluctuates randomly, and may therefore occasionally slightly resemble, and masquerade as, the pure-tone target, especially when the target is weak. It is your role as a subject to distinguish such random fluctuations from the "real" target sound. Signal detection theory then supplies an optimal test for deciding whether an interval contains only noise or also a tone, and it even makes it possible to predict the optimal performance in situations such as a two-interval, two-alternative forced choice (2I2AFC) experiment, in which one interval consists of noise only and one interval also contains the tone.

How does this work in the case of a tone in white noise? We know (see chapter 2) that the ear filters the signal into different frequency bands, reflected in the activity of auditory nerve fibers that form synapses with hair cells at different locations along the basilar membrane. The frequency bands that are far from the tone frequency would include only noise. Bands that are close to the tone frequency would include some of the tone energy and some noise energy. It turns out that the optimal decision regarding the presence of the tone can essentially be reached by considering only a single frequency band—the one centered on the tone frequency. This band would include the highest amount of tone energy relative to the noise that goes through it. Within that band, the optimal test is essentially energetic. In a 2I2AFC trial, one simply measures the energy in the band centered on the target tone frequency during the two sound presentations, and "detects" the tone in the interval that had the higher energy in that band. Under standard conditions, no other method gives a better detection rate. In practice, we can imagine these bands evoking activity in auditory nerve fibers, and the optimal performance is achieved by simply choosing the interval that evoked the larger firing rate in the auditory nerve fibers tuned to the signal frequency.

How often would this optimal strategy correctly identify the target interval? This depends, obviously, on the level of the target tone, but performance would also depend in a more subtle way on the bandwidth of the filters. The reason is that, whereas all the energy of the tone would always be reflected in the output of the filter that is centered on the target tone frequency, the amount of noise that would also pass through this filter would be larger or smaller depending on its bandwidth. Thus, the narrower the band, the smaller the contribution of the masking noise to its output, and the more likely the interval with the higher energy would indeed be the one containing the target tone.

This argument can be reversed: Measure the threshold of a tone in broadband noise, and you can deduce the width of the peripheral filter centered at the tone frequency from the threshold. This is done by running the previous paragraph in the reverse— given the noise and tone level, the performance of the ideal observer is calculated for different filter bandwidths, until the calculated performance matches the experimental one. And indeed, it turns out that tone detection thresholds increase with frequency, as expected from the increase in bandwidth of auditory nerve fibers. This argument, originally made by Harvey Fletcher (an engineer in Bell Labs in the first half of the twentieth century), is central to much of modern psychoacoustics. The power of this argument stems from the elegant use it makes of the biology of the early auditory system (peripheral filtering) on the one hand, and of the optimality of signal detection theory on the other. It has been refined to a considerable degree by other researchers, leading to the measurement of the width of the peripheral filters (called "critical bands" in the literature) and even the shape of the peripheral filters (Unoki et al., 2006). The central finding is that, in many masking tasks, human performance is comparable to that calculated from theory, in other words, human performance approaches that of an ideal observer.

However, note that there is no mention of auditory objects, segregation, grouping, or anything else that is related to auditory scene analysis. The problem is posed as a statistical problem—signal in noise—and is solved at a very physical level, by considerations of energy measurements in the output of the peripheral filters. So, do we perform auditory scene analysis when detecting pure tones in noise, or are we merely comparing the output of the peripheral filters, or almost equivalently, firing rates of auditory nerve fibers?

As we shall see, similar questions will recur like a leitmotif throughout this chapter. Note that, for the purpose of signal detection by means of a simple comparison of spike counts, noise and tone "sensations" would seem to be a superfluous extra, nor is there any obvious need for segregation or grouping, or other fancy mechanisms. We could achieve perfect performance in the 2I2AFC test by "listening" only to the output of the correct peripheral frequency channel. However, this does not mean that we cannot also perform segregation and grouping, and form separate perceptual representations of the tone and the noise. Signal detection theory and auditory scene analysis are not mutually exclusive, but, at least in this example, it is not clear what added value scene analysis offers.

We encountered similar issues regarding high-level and low-level representations of sound before: There are physical cues, such as periodicity, formant frequencies, and interaural level differences; and then there are perceptual qualities such as pitch, speech sound identity, and spatial location. We know that we extract the physical cues (in the sense that we can record the neural activity that encodes them), but we do not perceive the physical cues directly. Rather, our auditory sensations are based on an integrated representation that takes into account multiple cues, and that, at least introspectively, is not cast in terms of the physical cues—we hear pitch rather than periodicity, vowel identity rather than formant frequencies, and spatial location rather than interaural disparities. In masking, we face a similar situation: performance is essentially determined by energy in peripheral bands, but introspectively we perceive the tone and the noise.

The presence of multiple representation levels is actually congruent with what we know about the auditory system. When discussing pitch, speech, and space, we could describe in substantial details the processing of the relevant parameters by the early auditory system: periodicity enhancement for pitch, measuring binaural disparities or estimating notch frequencies for spatial hearing, estimating formant frequencies of vowels, and so on. On the other hand, the fully integrated percept is most likely represented in cortex, often beyond the primary cortical fields.

Can we experimentally distinguish between low- and high-level representations in a more rigorous way? Merav Ahissar and Shaul Hochstein constructed a conceptual framework, called reverse hierarchy theory (RHT), to account for similar effects in vision (Hochstein & Ahissar, 2002). Recently, Nahum, Nelken, and Ahissar (2008) adapted this framework to the auditory system and demonstrated its validity to audition as well. RHT posits the presence of multiple representation levels, and also the fact (which we have emphasized repeatedly) that consciously, we tend to access the higher representation levels, with their more ecological representation of the sensory input. Furthermore, RHT also posits that the connections between different representation levels are dynamic—there are multiple low-level representations, and under the appropriate conditions we can select the most informative low-level representation for the current task. Finding the most informative low-level representation can, however, take a little while, and may require a search starting at high representation levels and proceeding backward toward the most informative low-level representations. Also, this search can find the best low-level representation only if the stimuli are presented consistently, without any variability except for the task-relevant one.

Classic psychoacoustic experiments, where the tone frequency is fixed, provide optimal conditions for a successful search for the most task-relevant representation, such as the activity of the auditory nerve fibers whose best frequency matches the frequency of the target tone. Once the task-relevant representation is accessed, behavioral performance can reach the theoretical limits set by signal detection theory. Importantly, if the high-level representation accesses the most appropriate low-level representation, the two become equivalent and we then expect a congruence of the conscious, high-level percept with the low-level, statistically limited ideal observer performance.

This theory predicts that ideal observer performance can be achieved only under limited conditions. For example, if the backward search is interrupted, performance will become suboptimal. Nahum et al. (2008) therefore performed a set of experiments whose goal was to disrupt the backward search. To do so, they needed a high-level task that pitted two low-level representations against each other. In chapter 5, we discussed the detection of tones in noise when the tones are presented to the two ears in opposite phase (binaural masking level differences, BMLDs). Similar "binaural unmasking" can also be achieved for other types of stimuli, including speech, if they are presented in opposite phase to either ear. The improvement in speech intelligibility under these circumstances is called binaural intelligibility level difference (BILD). Nahum et al. (2008) therefore used BILD to test the theory.

In the "baseline" condition of their experiment, Nahum et al. (2008) measured the discrimination thresholds separately for the case in which words were identical in the two ears (and therefore there were no binaural disparity cues), and for the case in which words were phase-inverted in one ear (and therefore had the binaural disparity cues that facilitate detection in noise). The observed thresholds matched the predictions of ideal observer theory.

The second, crucial part of the experiment introduced manipulations in aspects of the task that should be irrelevant from the point of view of ideal observer predictions, but that nevertheless significantly affected detection thresholds. For example, in one test condition, trials in which the words were identical in the two ears were presented intermixed among trials in which the words were phase-inverted in one ear. This is called "interleaved tracks" in the psychoacoustical literature. As far as statistical detection theory is concerned, whether phase-identical and phase-inverted trials are presented in separate blocks or in interleaved tracks is irrelevant—the theory predicts optimal performance either way. The results, however, showed a clear difference—the presence of binaural disparities helped subjects much less in the interleaved tracks than in the baseline condition, especially when the two words to be distinguished differed only slightly (by a single phoneme). This is exactly what RHT would predict. Presumably, the backward search failed to find the optimally informative lower-level representation because this representation changed from one trial to the next. Consequently, the optimal task-related representation of the sounds, which is presumably provided by the activity of the disparity-sensitive neurons, perhaps in the MSO or the IC, cannot be efficiently accessed, and performance becomes suboptimal.

What are the implications of this for auditory scene analysis in masking experiments? RHT suggests that optimal performance can be achieved only if the conditions in which the experiments are run allow a successful search for the optimal neural representations. In this way, it provides evidence for the multiple representation levels of sounds in the auditory system.

One way of conceptualizing what is going on is therefore to think of auditory scene analysis as operating at a high-level representation, using evidence based on neural activity at lower representation levels. Thus, the auditory scene consists of separate tone and noise objects, because it presumably reflects the evidence supplied by the peripheral auditory system: the higher energy in the peripheral band centered on the tone frequency.

Both low- and high-level representations have been studied electrophysiologically in the context of another masking paradigm, comodulation masking release (CMR). In CMR experiments, as in BILD, two masking conditions are contrasted. The first condition is a simple masking task with a noise masker and a pure tone target. As we already remarked, in this situation ideal observers, as well as well-trained humans, monitor the extra energy in the peripheral band centered on the target tone. In the second masking condition, the masker is "amplitude modulated," that is, it is multiplied by an envelope that fluctuates at a slow rate (10–20 Hz). These fluctuations in the amplitude of the masker produce a "release from masking," meaning that detecting the target tone becomes easier, so that tone detection thresholds drop. It is substantially easier for humans to hear a constant tone embedded in a fluctuating noise than one embedded in a noise of constant amplitude (Sound Example "Comodulation Masking Release" on the book's Web site).

The curious thing about CMR is that this drop in threshold is, in a sense, "too large" and depends on the bandwidth of the noise (figure 6.1). As we discussed earlier, there is an effective bandwidth, the critical band, around each tone frequency within which the noise is effective in masking the tone. In regular masking experiments, adding noise energy outside the critical band has no effect on the masking. It does not matter whether the noise energy increases if that increase is outside the critical band because the auditory nerve fibers centered on the target tone frequency "do not

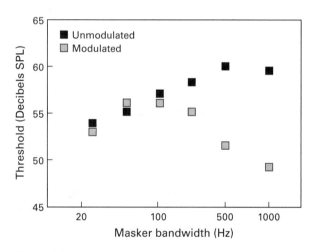

Figure 6.1
The lowest level at which a tone is detected as a function of the bandwidth of the noiseband that serves as the masker, for modulated and unmodulated noise. Whereas for unmodulated noise thresholds increase with increases in bandwidth (which causes an increase in the overall energy of the masker), broadband modulated maskers are actually less efficient in masking the tone (so that tones can be detected at lower levels). This effect is called comodulation masking release (CMR).
Adapted from Moore (1999).

hear" and are not confused by the extra noise. In contrast, when the masker is amplitude modulated, adding extra noise energy with the same amplitude modulation outside the critical band *does* affect thresholds in a paradoxical way—more noise makes the tone easier to hear. It is the effect of masker energy away from the frequency of the target tone that makes CMR interesting to both psychoacousticians and electrophysiologists, because it demonstrates that there is more to the detection of acoustic signals in noise than filtering by auditory nerve fibers.

CMR has neurophysiological correlates as early as in the cochlear nucleus. Neurons in the cochlear nucleus often follow the fluctuations of the envelope of the masker, but, interestingly, many neurons reduce their responses when masking energy is added away from the best frequency, provided the amplitude fluctuations of this extra acoustic energy follow the same rhythm. In figure 6.2, two masker conditions are contrasted: one in which the masker is an amplitude-modulated tone (left), and the other in which additional off-frequency amplitude-modulated tones are added to it, sharing the same modulation pattern as the on-frequency masker (right). The response to the masker is reduced by the addition of comodulated sidebands (compare the responses at the bottom row, left and right panels). This makes the responses to tones more salient in the comodulated condition.

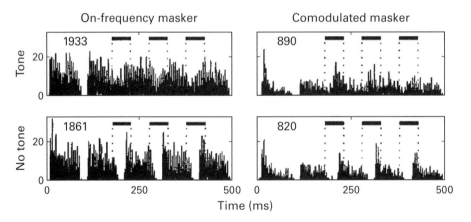

Figure 6.2
Responses of neurons in the cochlear nucleus to narrowband and wideband modulated maskers (left and right columns) with and without an added signal (top and bottom rows; in the top row, the signal consisted of three tone pips in the valleys of the masker). In the comodulated condition, when the masker had larger bandwidth, the neural responses it evoked were reduced (compare the bottom panels, left and right). As a result, adding the tone to the wideband masker results in more salient responses. (Compare the top panels, left and right; tone presentations are marked by the bars at the top of each panel.) Numbers in each panel refer to unit ID.
Adapted from figure 3 in Pressnitzer et al. (2001).

What causes this reduction in the responses to the masker when flanking bands are added? Presumably, the underlying mechanism relies on the activity of "wideband inhibitor" neurons whose activity is facilitated by increasing the bandwidth of stimuli, which in turn inhibits other neurons in the cochlear nucleus. Nelken and Young (1994) suggested the concept of wideband inhibitors to account for the complex response properties of neurons in the dorsal cochlear nucleus, and possible candidates have been identified by Winter and Palmer (1995). A model based on observing the responses of single neurons in the cochlear nucleus, using the concept of the wideband inhibitor, does indeed show CMR (Neuert, Verhey, & Winter, 2004; Pressnitzer et al., 2001).

Thus, just like a human listener, an ideal observer, observing the responses of cochlear nucleus neurons, could detect a target tone against the background of a fluctuating masker more easily if the bandwidth of the masker increases. This picture corresponds pretty much to the low-level view of tone detection in noise.

Similar experiments have been performed using intracellular recordings from auditory cortex neurons (Las et al., 2005), so that changes of the neurons' membrane potential in response to the sound stimuli could be observed. As in the cochlear nucleus, a fluctuating masker evoked responses that followed the envelope of the masker (figure 6.3, top, thick black trace). The weak tone was selected so that it did not evoke much activity by itself (figure 6.3, top, thin black trace). When the two were added together, the locking of the membrane potential to the envelope of the noise was abolished to a large extent (figure 6.3, thick gray trace). The responses to a weak tone in fluctuating noise can be compared to the responses to a strong tone presented by itself; these responses tend to be similar (compare thick gray and thin black traces in bottom panels of figure 6.3), especially after the first noise burst following tone onset.

The CMR effect seen in these data is very pronounced—whereas in the cochlear nucleus, the manipulations of masker and target caused a quantitative change in the neuronal responses (some suppression of the responses to the noise as the bandwidth of the masker is widened; some increase in the responses to the target tone), the effects in cortex are qualitative: The pattern of changes in membrane potential stopped signaling the presence of a fluctuating noise, and instead became consistent with the presence of a continuous tone alone.

Originally, the suppression of envelope locking by low-level tones in the auditory cortex was suggested as the origin of CMR (Nelken, Rotman, & Bar Yosef, 1999). However, this cannot be the case—if subcortical responses are identical with and without a tone, then the cortex cannot "see" the tone either. It is a simple matter of neuroanatomy that, for the tone to affect cortical responses, it must first affect subcortical responses. As we discussed previously, correlates of CMR at the single-neuron level are already seen in the cochlear nucleus. Las et al. (2005) suggested, instead, that neurons like those whose activity is presented in figure 6.3 encode the tone as separate

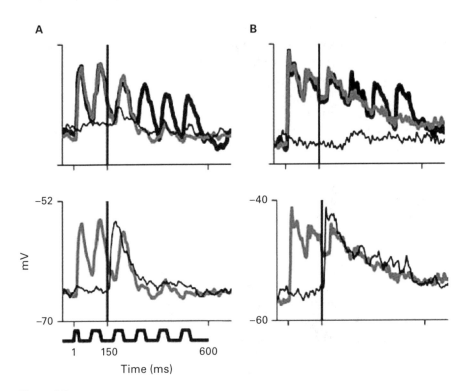

Figure 6.3
The top panels depict the responses of two cortical neurons (A and B) to noise alone (thick black line; the modulation pattern is schematically indicated at the bottom left of the figure), to a noise plus tone combination at the minimal tone level tested (gray line; tone onset is marked by the vertical line), and to a tone at the same tone level when presented alone (thin black line). The neurons responded to the noise with envelope locking—their membrane potential followed the on-off pattern of the noise. Adding a low-level tone, which by itself did not evoke much response, suppressed this locking substantially. The bottom panels depict the responses to a tone plus noise at the minimal tone level tested (gray, same as in top panel) and the response to a suprathreshold level tone presented by itself (thin black line). The responses to a low-level tone in noise and to a high-level tone in silence follow a similar temporal pattern, at least after the first noise cycle following tone onset.
From figure 6 in Las, Stern, and Nelken (2005).

from the noise—as a separate auditory object. Presumably, once it has been detected, the tone is fully represented at the level of auditory cortex in a way that is categorically different from the representation of the noise.

These experiments offer a glimpse of the way low-level and high-level representations may operate. At subcortical levels, responses reflect the physical structure of the sound waveform, and therefore small changes in the stimulus (e.g., increasing the level of a tone from below to above its masked threshold) would cause a small (but measureable) change in firing pattern. At higher levels of the auditory system (here, in primary auditory cortex), the same small change may result in a disproportionally large change in activity, because it would signal the detection of the onset of a new auditory object. Sometimes, small quantitative changes in responses can be interpreted as categorical changes in the composition of the auditory scene, and the responses of the neurons in the higher representation levels may encode the results of such an analysis, rather than merely reflect the physical structure of the sound spectrum at the eardrum.

6.3   Simultaneous Segregation and Grouping

After this detailed introduction to the different levels of representation, let us return to the basics, and specify in more detail what we mean by "elements of sounds" for the purpose of simultaneous grouping and segregation. After all, the tympanic membrane is put in motion by the pressure variations that are the sum of everything that produces sound in the environment. To understand the problem that this superposition of sounds poses, consider that the process that generates the acoustic mixture is crucially different from the process that generates a visual mixture of objects. In vision, things that are in front occlude those that are behind them. This means that occluded background objects are only partly visible and need to be "completed"; that is, their hidden bits must be inferred, but the visual images of objects rarely mix. In contrast, the additive mixing of sound waves is much more akin to the superposition of transparent layers. Analyzing such scenes brings its own special challenges.

Computationally, the problem of finding a decomposition of a sound waveform into the sum of waveforms emitted by multiple sources is ill-posed. From the perspective of the auditory brain, only the sound waveforms received at each ear are known, and these must be reconstructed as the sum of unknown waveforms emitted by an unknown number of sound sources. Mathematically, this is akin to trying to solve equations where we have only two knowns (the vibration of each eardrum) to determine an a priori unknown, and possibly quite large, number of unknowns (the vibrations of each sound source). There is no unique solution for such a problem. The problem of auditory scene analysis can be tackled only with the help of additional assumptions about the likely properties of sounds emitted by sound sources in the real world.

It is customary to start the consideration of this problem at the level of the auditory nerve representation (chapter 2). This is a representation of sounds in terms of the variation of energy in the peripheral, narrow frequency bands. We would expect that the frequency components coming from the same source would have common features—for example, the components of a periodic sound have a harmonic relationship, and all frequency components belonging to the same sound source should start at the same time and possibly end at the same time; frequency components belonging to the same sound source might grow and decline in level together; and so on and so forth. If you still recall our description of modes of vibration and impulse responses from chapter 1, you may appreciate why it is reasonable to expect that the different frequency components of a natural sound might be linked in these ways in time and frequency. We shall encounter other, possibly more subtle, grouping cues of this kind later.

The rules that specify how to select bits of sound that most likely belong together are often referred to as gestalt rules, in recognition of the importance of gestalt psychology in framing the issues governing perception of complex shapes. Thus, common onsets and common amplitude variations are akin to the common fate grouping principle in vision, according to which elements that move together in space would be perceived as parts of a single object. The so-called gestalt rules should be seen as heuristics that work reasonably well in most cases, and therefore may have been implemented as neural mechanisms.

Let us take a closer look at three of these grouping cues: common onset, harmonic structure, and common interaural time difference (ITDs), the latter being, as you may recall from chapter 5, a cue to the azimuth of a sound source. Whereas the first two turn out to be rather strong grouping cues, ITDs seem to have a somewhat different role.

6.3.1 Common Onsets

If several frequency components start at the same time, we are much more likely to perceive them as belonging to the same auditory object. This can be demonstrated in a number of ways. We will discuss one such experiment in detail here; since it used common onsets for a number of purposes, it illustrates the level of sophistication of experiments dealing with auditory scene analysis. It is also interesting because it pits a high-level and a low-level interpretation of the results against each other.

Darwin and Sutherland (1984) used the fine distinction between the vowels /I/ and /e/ in English as a tool for studying the role of common onsets in auditory perception. These vowels differ slightly in the frequency of their rather low-frequency first formant (figure 6.4A and Sound Example "Onsets and Vowels Identity" on the book's Web site;

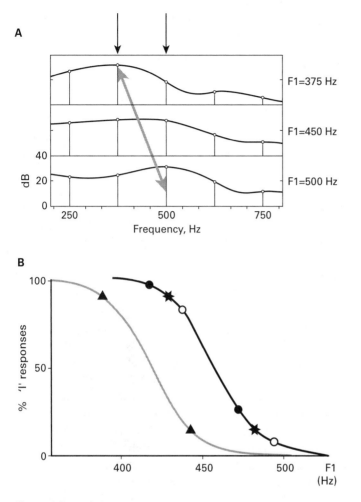

Figure 6.4

(A) Illustration of the principle of the experiment. The top and bottom spectra illustrate the first-formant region of the vowels /I/ and /e/ used in the experiment. The difference between them is in first formant frequency (375 Hz for /I/, 500 Hz for /e/). At a pitch of 125 Hz, these fall exactly on the third (top) and fourth (bottom) harmonics of the fundamental, which are therefore more intense than their neighbors. When the levels of the two harmonics are approximately equal, as in the middle spectrum, the first formant frequency is perceived between the two harmonics (here, at the category boundary between /I/ and /e/). Thus, by manipulating the relative levels of these two harmonics, it is possible to pull the perceived vowel between the extremes of /I/ and /e/. (B) Perceptual judgments for the identity of the vowel (filled circles), for the vowel with its fourth harmonic increased in level (triangles), and for the vowel with the fourth harmonic increased in level and starting before the rest of the vowel (stars and open circles). Onset asynchrony abolished the effect of the increase in level.

Based on figures 1 and 3 in Darwin and Sutherland (1984).

see also chapter 4 for background on the structure of vowels). It is possible to measure a formant boundary—a first formant frequency below which the vowel would generally be categorized as /I/ and above it as /e/. Since the boundary is somewhat below 500 Hz, Darwin and Sutherland used a sound whose fundamental frequency is 125 Hz so that the boundary lies between the third and the fourth harmonics (figure 6.4A). The perceived frequency of the first formant depends on the relative levels of the third and fourth harmonics. Figure 6.4A illustrates three cases: When the third harmonic is substantially louder than the fourth harmonic, the formant frequency is definitely 375 Hz, and an /I/ is perceived. In the opposite case, when the fourth harmonic is substantially louder than the third harmonic, the formant frequency is definitely 500 Hz and an /e/ is perceived. When both harmonics have about the same level, the perceived first formant frequency is between the two. This sound has an ambiguous quality, and listeners perceive it as an /I/ or as an /e/ with similar probabilities (Sound Example "Onsets and Vowels Identity"). In general, vowel identity judgments for such sounds were found to depend on this nominal first formant frequency, as expected, and there was a reasonably sharp transition between judgments of /I/ and /e/ as this first formant frequency increased from 375 to 500 Hz (figure 6.4B, filled circles). Darwin and Sutherland called this first formant frequency value "the nominal first formant frequency."

Darwin and Sutherland then introduced a slight modification of these stimuli. In order to shift the first formant, they increased the level of the fourth harmonic, 500 Hz, of the standard vowel by a fixed amount. By doing so, the first formant frequency that is actually perceived is pulled toward higher values, so the sound should be judged as /e/ more than as /I/. The effect is reasonably large, shifting the boundary by about 50 Hz (figure 6.4B, triangles; Sound Example "Onsets and Vowels Identity").

The heart of the experiment is a manipulation whose goal is to reverse this effect. Darwin and Sutherland's idea was to reduce the effect of the increase in the level of the fourth harmonic by supplying hints that it is not really part of the vowel. To do that, they changed its onset and offset times, starting it before or ending it after all the other harmonics composing the vowel. Thus, when the fourth harmonic started 240 ms earlier than the rest, subjects essentially disregarded its high level when they judged the identity of the vowel (figure 6.4B, open circles and stars; Sound Example "Onsets and Vowels Identity"). A similar, although smaller, perceptual effect occurred with offsets.

These results lend themselves very naturally to an interpretation in terms of scene analysis: Somewhere in the brain, the times and levels of the harmonics are registered. Note that these harmonics are resolved (chapters 2 and 3), as they are far enough from each other to excite different auditory nerve fibers. Thus, each harmonic excites a different set of auditory nerve fibers, and a process that uses common onset as a heuristic observes this neural representation of the spectrotemporal pattern. Since the fourth harmonic started earlier than the rest of the vowel, this process segregates the sounds into two components: a pure tone at the frequency of the fourth harmonic, and the vowel. As a result, the energy at 500 Hz has to be divided between the pure tone and the vowel. Only a part of it is attributed to fourth harmonic of the vowel, and the vowel is therefore perceived as more /I/-like, causing the reversal of the shift in the vowel boundary.

However, there is another possible interpretation of the same result. When the 500-Hz tone starts before the other harmonics, the neurons responding to it (the auditory nerve fibers as well as the majority of higher-order neurons throughout the auditory system) would be activated before those responding to other frequencies, and would have experienced spike rate adaptation. Consequently, their firing rates would have declined by the time the vowel started and the other harmonics came in. At the moment of vowel onset, the pattern of activity across frequency would therefore be consistent with a lower-level fourth harmonic, pulling the perception back toward /I/. We have here a situation similar to that discussed earlier in the context of masking—both high-level accounts in terms of scene analysis or low-level accounts in terms of subcortical neural firing patterns can be put forward to explain the results. Is it possible to falsify the low-level account?

Darwin and Sutherland (1984) tried to do this by adding yet another element to the game. They reasoned that, if the effect of onset asynchrony is due to perceptual grouping and segregation, they should be able to reduce the effect of an asynchronous onset by "capturing" it into yet another group, and they could then try to signal to the auditory system that this third group actually ends before the beginning of the vowel. They did this by using another grouping cue: harmonicity. Thus, they added a "captor tone" at 1,000 Hz, which started together with the 500 Hz tone before vowel onset, and ended just at vowel onset. They reasoned that the 500 Hz and the 1,000 Hz tones would be grouped by virtue of their common onset and their harmonic relationship. Ending the 1,000 Hz at vowel onset would then imply that this composite object, which includes both the 1,000- and the 500-Hz components, disappeared from the scene. Any 500-Hz sound energy remaining should then be attributed to, and grouped perceptually with, the vowel that started at the same time that the captor ended, and the 500-Hz component should exert its full influence on the vowel identity. Indeed, the captor tone reversed, at least to some degree, the effect of onset asynchrony (Sound Example "Onsets and Vowels Identity"). This indicates that more must be going on than merely spike rate adaptation at the level of the auditory nerve, since the presence or absence of the 1,000-Hz captor tone has no effect on the adaptation of 500-Hz nerve fibers.

The story doesn't end here, however, since we know today substantially more than in 1984 about the sophisticated processing that occurs in early stages of the auditory system. For example, we already encountered the wideband inhibition in the cochlear nucleus in our discussion of CMR. Wideband inhibitor neurons respond poorly to pure tones, but they are strongly facilitated by multiple tones, or sounds with a wide bandwidth. They are believed to send widespread inhibitory connections to most parts of the cochlear nucleus.

Wideband inhibition could supply an alternative low-level account of the effects of the captor tone (figure 6.5). When the captor tone is played, it could (together with the 500-Hz tone) activate wideband inhibition, which in turn would reduce the responses of cochlear nucleus neurons responding to 500 Hz, which would consequently fire less but therefore also experience less spike rate adaptation. When the 1,000-Hz captor stops, the wideband inhibition ceases, and the 500-Hz neurons would generate a "rebound" burst of activity. Because the 1,000-Hz captor ends when the vowel starts, the rebound burst in the 500-Hz neurons would be synchronized with the onset bursts of the various neurons that respond to the harmonics of the vowel, and the fact that these harmonics, including the 500-Hz tone, all fired a burst together will make it look as if they had a common onset.

Thus, once again we see that it may be possible to account for a high-level "cognitive" phenomenon in terms of relatively low-level mechanisms. Support for such low-level accounts comes from recent experiments by Holmes and Roberts (2006; Roberts & Holmes, 2006, 2007). For example, wideband inhibition is believed to be insensitive to harmonic relationships, and indeed it turns out that captor tones don't have to be harmonically related to the 500-Hz tone. They can even consist of narrow noisebands rather than pure tones. Almost any sound capable of engaging wideband inhibition will do. The captor tones can even be presented to the contralateral ear, perhaps because wideband inhibition can operate binaurally as well as monaurally. Furthermore, there are physiological results that are consistent with the role of the wideband inhibitor in this context: Bleeck et al. (2008) recorded single-neuron responses in the cochlear nucleus of guinea pigs, and demonstrated the presence of wideband inhibition, as well as the resulting rebound firing at captor offset, using harmonic complexes that were quite similar to those used in the human experiments.

But this does not mean that we can now give a complete account of these auditory grouping experiments in terms of low-level mechanisms. For example, Darwin and Sutherland (1984) already demonstrated that increasing the duration of the 500-Hz tone beyond vowel offset also changes the effect it has on the perceived vowel, and these offset effects cannot be accounted for either by adaptation or by wideband inhibition. Thus, there may be things left to do for high-level mechanisms. In this section, however, it has hopefully become clear that any such high-level mechanisms will operate on a representation that has changed from the output of the auditory nerve. For example, adaptation, wideband inhibition, and rebounds will emphasize onsets and offsets, and suppress responses to steady-state sounds. Each of the many processing stations of the auditory pathway could potentially contribute to auditory

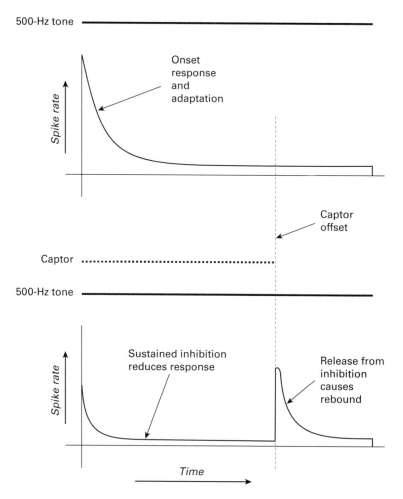

500-Hz tone

Onset
response
and
adaptation

Spike rate

Captor
offset

Captor

500-Hz tone

Sustained inhibition
reduces response

Release from
inhibition
causes
rebound

Spike rate

Time

Figure 6.5
Illustration of the effect of wideband inhibition when a captor tone is used to remove the effects of onset asynchrony. (A) Responses to the fourth harmonic (at 500 Hz) consist of an onset burst followed by adaptation to a lower level of activity. (B) In the presence of the captor, wideband inhibition would reduce the responses to the 500-Hz tone. Furthermore, at the offset of the captor tone, neurons receiving wideband inhibition tend to respond with a rebound burst (as shown in the guinea pig cochlear nucleus by Bleeck et al. 2008).
From figure 2 in Holmes and Roberts (2006).

scene analysis (and, of course, all other auditory tasks). The information that reaches the high-level mechanisms reflects the activity in all of the preceding processing stations. For a complete understanding of auditory scene analysis, we would like to understand what each of these processing stations does and how they interconnect. This is obviously an enormous research task.

6.3.2   Fundamental Frequency and Harmonicity

We will illustrate the role of pitch and harmonicity in auditory scene analysis by using a familiar task—separating the voices of two simultaneous talkers. Here we discuss a highly simplified, yet perceptually very demanding version of this, namely, the identification of two simultaneously presented vowels.

In such a double-vowel experiment, two vowels are selected at random from five or six possible vowels (e.g., /a/, /e/, /i/, /o/, /u/, or similar language-adjusted versions). The two chosen vowels are then presented simultaneously, and the subject has to identify both (Sound Example "Double Vowels" on the book's Web site). The vowels would be easily discriminated if presented one after the other, but subjects make a lot of errors when asked to identify both when they are presented together. With five possible vowels, when subjects can't make much headway by simply guessing, their performance would be only around 4% correct identification for both vowels. When both vowels have the same pitch, identification levels are in fact substantially above chance (figure 6.6): Depending on the experiment, correct identification rates may be well above 50%. Still, although well above chance, this level of performance means that, on average, at least one member of a pair is misidentified on every other stimulus presentation—identifying double vowels is a hard task.

The main manipulation we are interested in here is the introduction of a difference in the fundamental frequency (F_0) of the two vowels. When the two vowels have different F_0s, correct identification rates increase (figure 6.6), at least for F_0 differences of up to 1/2 semitone (about 3%). For larger differences in F_0, performance saturates. Thus, vowels with different F_0s are easier to discriminate than vowels with the same F_0.

What accounts for this improved performance? There are numerous ways in which pitch differences can help vowel segregation. For example, since the energy of each vowel is not distributed equally across frequency, we would expect the responses of some auditory nerve fibers to be dominated by one vowel and those of other fibers to be dominated by the other vowel. But since the activity of auditory nerve fibers in response to a periodic sound is periodic (see chapter 3), those fibers whose activity is dominated by one vowel should all fire with a common underlying rhythm, because they all phase lock to the fundamental frequency of that vowel. If the vowels differ in F_0, then each vowel will impose a different underlying rhythm on the population of nerve fibers it activates most strongly. Thus, checking the periodicity of the responses

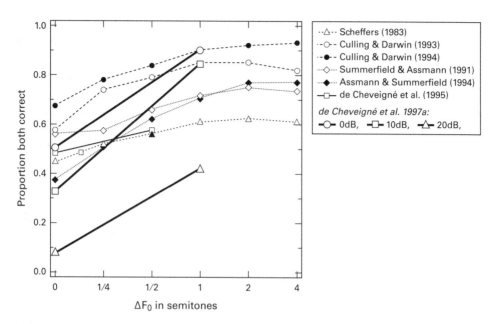

Figure 6.6
Summary of a number of studies of double vowel identification. The abscissa represents the difference between the fundamental frequencies of the two vowels. The ordinate represents the fraction of trials in which both vowels were identified correctly. The data from de Cheveigné et al. (1997a) represents experiments in which the two vowels had different sound levels (as indicated in the legend). The difference in fundamental frequency was as useful, or even more useful, for the identification of vowels with different sound levels, a result that is inconsistent with pure-channel selection and may require harmonic cancellation, as discussed in the main text.
From figure 1 of de Cheveigné et al. (1997a).

of each auditory nerve fiber should make it possible to assign different fibers to different vowels, and in this way to separate out the superimposed vowel spectra. Each vowel will dominate the activity of those fibers whose best frequency is close to the vowel's formant frequencies. Thus, the best frequencies of all the fibers that phase lock to the same underlying periodicity should correspond to the formant frequencies of the vowel with the corresponding F_0. This scheme is called "channel selection".

The plausibility of channel selection has indeed been demonstrated with neural activity in the cochlear nucleus (Keilson et al. 1997). This study looked at responses of "chopper" neurons in the cochlear nucleus to vowel sounds. Chopper neurons are known to phase lock well to the F_0 of a vowel. In this study, two different vowels were used, one /I/, and one /æ/, and these were embedded within the syllables /bIs/

or /bæs/. The /I/ had an F_0 of 88 Hz, the /æ/ a slightly higher F_0 of 112 Hz. During the experiment, the formants of the /I/ or the /æ/ sounds were tweaked to bring them close to the best frequency (BF) of the recorded chopper neuron. Figure 6.7A shows the response of the neuron to the /I/ whose second formant frequency was just above the neuron's BF. The left column shows the instantaneous firing rate of the neuron during the presentation of the syllable. The horizontal line above the firing rate histogram shows when the vowel occurred. Throughout the stimulus, the neuron appears to fire with regular bursts of action potentials, as can be seen from the peaks in the firing rate histogram. The right column shows the frequency decomposition of the firing rate during the vowel presentation. The sequence of peaks at 88 Hz and its multiples demonstrate that the neuron indeed emitted a burst of action potentials once every period of the vowel. Figure 6.7D (the bottom row), in comparison, shows the responses of the same neuron to the /ae/ sound with the slightly higher F_0. Again, we see the neuron responds with regular bursts of action potentials, which are synchronized this time to the stimulus F_0 of 112 Hz (right dot above right panel).

The two middle rows, figures 6.7B and C, show responses of the same neuron to "double vowels," that is, different mixtures of /I/ and /æ/. The firing patterns evoked by the mixed stimuli are more complex; However, the plots on the right clearly show that the neuron phase locks either to the F_0 of the /I/ of 88 Hz (figure 6.7B) or to the F_0 of the /æ/ of 112 Hz (figure 6.7C), but not to both. Which F_0 "wins" depends on which of the stimuli has more energy at the neuron's BF.

The temporal discharge patterns required to make channel selection work are clearly well developed in the cochlear nucleus. But is this the only way of using periodicity? A substantial amount of research has been done on this question, which cannot be fully reviewed here. We will discuss only a single thread of this work—the somewhat unintuitive idea that pitch is used to improve discrimination by allowing harmonic cancellation (de Cheveigné, 1997; de Cheveigné et al., 1995, 1997a, 1997b). Effectively, the idea is that the periodicity of one vowel could be used to remove it

Figure 6.7
(A and D) Responses of a chopper neuron to the syllables /bIs/ and /bæs/ with F_0 of 88 or 112 Hz, respectively. (B and C) Responses of the same neuron to mixtures of /bIs/ and /bæs/ presented at the same time. The plots on the left show poststimulus time histograms (PSTHs) of neural discharges, representing the instantaneous firing rate of the neuron during stimulus presentation. The lines above the PSTHs indicate when the vowels /I/ and /æ/ occurred during the syllables. The plots on the right are the frequency decompositions of the PSTHs during vowel presentation, measuring the locking to the fundamental frequency of the two vowels: A sequence of peaks at 88 Hz and its multiples indicates locking to the fundamental frequency of the /I/ sound, while a sequence of peaks at 112 Hz and its multiples indicates locking to the fundamental frequency of the /æ/ sound. The two fundamental frequencies are indicated by the dots above each panel. From figure 3 of Keilson et al. (1997).

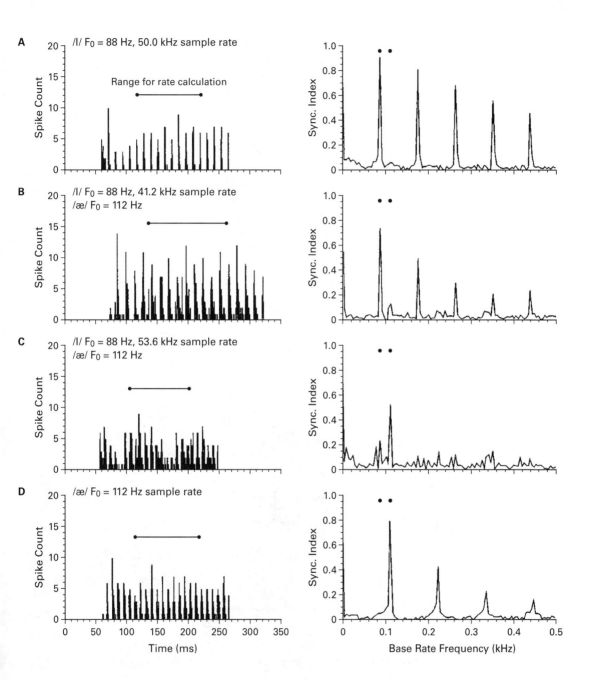

from a signal mixture, and the remainder could then be examined to identify further vowels or other background sounds. One very simple circuit that implements such a scheme is shown in figure 6.8A.

The inhibitory delay line shown in figure 6.8A acts as a filter that deletes every spike that occurs at a delay T following another spike. If the filter is excited by a periodic spike train with a period T, the output rate would be substantially reduced. If the spike train contains two superimposed trains of spikes, one with a period of T and the other with a different period, the filter would remove most of the spikes that belong to the first train, while leaving most of the spikes belonging to the other. Suppose now that two vowels are simultaneously presented to a subject. At the output of the auditory nerve, we position two cancellation filters, one at a delay corresponding to the period of one vowel, the other at the period of the other vowel. Finally,

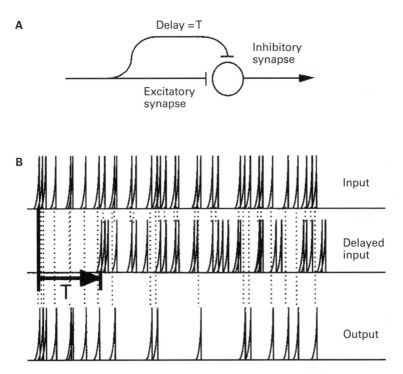

Figure 6.8
A cancellation filter. (A) Putative neural architecture. The same input is fed to the neuron through an excitatory synapse and through an inhibitory synapse, with a delay, T, between them. As a result, any spike that appears exactly T seconds following another spike is deleted from the output spike train. (B) An example of the operation of the cancellation filter. Only spikes that are not preceded by another spike T seconds earlier appear in the output.
From figure 1 of de Cheveigné (1997).

the output of each filter is simply quantified by its rate—the rate of the leftover spikes, after canceling those that presumably were evoked by the other vowel.

The results of such a process are illustrated in figure 6.9, which is derived from a simulation. The two vowels in this example are /o/ and /u/. The vowel /o/ has a rather high first formant and a rather low second formant (marked by o1 and o2 in figure 6.9), while /u/ has a lower first formant and a higher second formant (marked by u1 and u2). The thick line represents the rate of firing of the auditory nerve fiber array in response to the mixture of /o/ and /u/. Clearly, neither the formants of /o/ nor those of /u/ are apparent in this response. The dashed lines are the rates at the output of two cancellation filters, tuned to the period of each of the two vowels. The vowel /u/ had an F_0 of 125 Hz, with a period of 8 ms; /o/ had an F_0 of 132 Hz, with a period of about 7.55 ms. Thus, the cancellation filter with a period of 8 ms is expected to cancel the contribution of /u/ to the firing rate, and indeed the leftover rate shows a broad peak where the two formants of /o/ lie. Conversely, the cancellation filter with a period of 7.55 ms is expected to cancel the contribution of /o/ to the firing rate, and indeed the leftover rate has two peaks at the locations of the formant frequencies of /u/. So the cancellation scheme may actually work.

Now we have two mechanisms that may contribute to double-vowel identification: channel selection and periodicity cancellation. Do we need both? De Cheveigné and

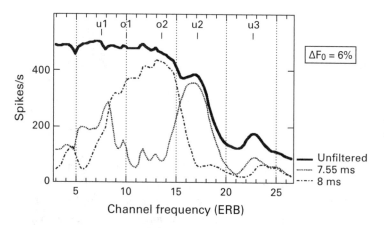

Figure 6.9
A simulation of cancellation filters. The thick black line represents the overall firing rate of auditory nerve fibers stimulated by a double vowel consisting of /o/ and /u/ played simultaneously. The thin broken lines represent the output of cancellation filters, one at the pitch of each of the two vowels, positioned at the output of each auditory nerve fiber. The representation of the formants is recovered at the output of the cancellation filters.
From figure 3a of Cheveigné et al. (1997a).

his colleagues investigated the need for periodicity cancellation in a number of experiments. One of them consisted of testing the discriminability, not just of periodic vowels, but also of nonperiodic vowels (de Cheveigné et al., 1995; De Cheveigné et al., 1997b). The latter were produced by shifting their harmonics a bit. This creates an aperiodic sound that has a poorly defined pitch, but nevertheless a clear vowel identity (Sound Example "Inharmonic Vowels" on the book's Web site). When periodic and aperiodic vowels are presented together, only the periodic vowels can be canceled with the scheme proposed in figure 6.8, but the aperiodic vowel should nevertheless be clearly represented in the "remainder." Indeed, aperiodic vowels could be more easily discriminated in double-vowel experiments with mixtures of periodic and aperiodic vowels. That result can be easily explained with the cancellation idea, but is harder to explain in terms of channel selection. The channels dominated by the aperiodic vowels would presumably lack the "tagging" by periodicity, and therefore nothing would link these channels together. Thus, channel selection alone cannot explain how inharmonic vowels can be extracted from a mixture of sounds.

Another line of evidence that supports the cancellation theory comes from experiments that introduce sound intensity differences between the vowels. A rather quiet vowel should eventually fail to dominate any channel, and the channel selection model would therefore predict that differences of F_0 would be less useful for the weaker vowel in a pair. Harmonic cancellation predicts almost the opposite: It is easier to estimate the F_0 of the higher-level vowel and hence to cancel it in the presence of F_0 differences. Consequently, the identification of the weak vowel should benefit more from the introduction of F_0 differences. Indeed, de Cheveigné and colleagues (1997a) demonstrated that the introduction of differences in F_0 produced a greater benefit for identifying the weaker than the louder vowel in a pair (see figure 6.6 for some data from that experiment). Thus, the overall pattern of double-vowel experiments seems to support the use of harmonic cancellation.

But is there any physiological evidence for harmonic cancellation operating in any station of the auditory pathway? In the cochlear nucleus, we have seen that chopper neurons tend to be dominated by the periodicity of the vowel that acoustically dominates their input. Other kinds of neurons seem to code the physical complexity of the stimulus mixture better, in that their responses carry evidence for the periodicity of both vowels. However, there is no evidence for cochlear nucleus neurons that would respond preferentially to the *weaker* vowel in a pair, as might be expected from cancellation. The same is true in the inferior colliculus (IC), as was shown by Sinex and colleagues (Sinex & Li, 2007). Neurons in the central nucleus of the IC are sensitive to the composition of the sound within a narrow frequency band around their best frequency; when this band contains harmonics of both vowels, their activity will reflect both periodicities. Although IC neurons have not been tested with the same double-vowel stimuli used by Keilson et al. (1997) in the cochlear nucleus (figure 6.7), the available data nevertheless indicate that responses of the neurons in IC follow pretty much the same rules as those followed by cochlear nucleus neurons. Thus, we would not expect IC neurons to show cancellation of one vowel or the other. Other stations of the auditory pathways have not been tested with similar stimuli. Admittedly, none of these experiments is a critical test of the cancellation filter. For example, cancellation neurons should have "notch" responses to periodicity—they should respond to sounds of all periodicities except around the period they preferentially cancel. None of the above experiments really tested this prediction.

What are we to make of all this? Clearly, two simultaneous sounds with different F_0s are easier to separate than two sounds with the same F_0. Thus, periodicity is an important participant in auditory scene analysis. Furthermore, electrophysiological data from the auditory nerve, cochlear nucleus, and the IC indicate that, at least at the level of these stations, it may be possible to improve vowel identification through channel selection by using the periodicity of neural responses as a tag for the corresponding channels. On the other hand, psychoacoustic results available to date seem to require the notion of harmonic cancellation—once you know the periodicity of one sound, you "peel" it away and study what's left. However, there is still no strong electrophysiological evidence for harmonic cancellation.

To a large degree, therefore, our electrophysiological understanding lags behind the psychophysical results. The responses we see encode the physical structure of the double-vowel stimulus, rather than the individual vowels; they do so in ways that may help disentangle the two vowels, but we don't know where and how that process ends.

Finally, none of these models offers any insight into how the spectral profiles of the two vowels are interpreted and recognized (de Cheveigné & Kawahara, 1999). That stage belongs to the phonetic processing we discussed in chapter 4, but it is worth noting here that the recovered spectra from double-vowel experiments would certainly be distorted, and could therefore pose special challenges to any speech analysis mechanisms.

6.3.3   Common Interaural Time Differences

Interaural time differences (ITDs) are a major cue for determining the azimuth of a sound source, as we have seen in chapter 5. When a sound source contains multiple frequency components, in principle all of these components share the same ITD, and therefore common ITD should be a good grouping cue. However, in contrast with common onsets and harmonicity, which are indeed strong grouping cues, common ITD appears not to be.

This is perhaps surprising, particularly since some experiments do seem to indicate a clear role for ITD in grouping sounds. For example, Darwin and Hukin (1999) simultaneously presented two sentences to their participants. The first sentence was an instruction of the type "Could you please write the word *bird* down now," and the second was a distractor like "You will also hear the sound *dog* this time." The sentences were arranged such that the words "bird" and "dog" occurred at the same time and had the same duration (Sound Example "ITD in the Perception of Speech" on the book's Web site). This created confusion as to which word (bird or dog) was the target, and which the distractor. The confusion was measured by asking listeners which word occurred in the target sentence (by pressing *b* for "bird" or *d* for "dog" on a computer keyboard), and scoring how often they got it wrong. Darwin and Hukin then used two cues, F_0 and ITD, to reduce this confusion. They found that, while rather large F_0 differences reduced the confusion by only a small (although significant) amount, even small ITDs (45 µs left ear–leading for one sentence, 45 µs right ear–leading for the other one) reduced the confusion by substantially larger amounts. Furthermore, Darwin and Hukin pitted F_0 and ITD against each other by presenting the sentences, except for the target word "dog," with different F_0s, and making the F_0 of the target word the same as that of the distractor sentence. They then played these sentences with varying ITDs, and found that ITD was actually more powerful than F_0 – in spite of the difference in F_0 between the target word and the rest of the sentence, listeners were substantially more likely to associate the word with the rest of the sentence, presumably because both had the same ITD. This experiment suggests that ITD has a powerful role in linking sequential sounds—we tend to associate together elements of sounds that occur sequentially with the same ITD. However, this is a different situation from the one we have been discussing so far, where we studied cues for grouping acoustic components that overlap in time. So what is the role of ITD in *simultaneous* grouping?

The fact that ITD is only a weak cue for simultaneous grouping was reported initially by Culling and Summerfield (1995). We will describe here a related experiment that shows the same type of effects, using a phenomenon we described earlier when discussing the role of common onsets: the shifts in the category boundary between /I/ and /e/ due to the manipulation of one harmonic. We have already discussed the role of onset asynchrony in modifying the degree of fusion of a harmonic with the rest of the tone complex. Let us now consider a similar experiment by Darwin and Hukin (1999), which shows that ITDs exercise a much smaller influence on the perceptual fusion of frequency components than common onsets.

As in the study of onset asynchrony, Darwin and Hukin (1999) generated a set of vowels spanning the range between /I/ and /e/ by modifying the first formant. The vowels had a constant pitch of 150 Hz. Then, they extracted the 600-Hz (fourth) harmonic of the vowel, and presented the vowel without its fourth harmonic at one ITD, and the missing harmonic separately with either the same or a different ITD. Perhaps surprisingly, changing the ITD of this harmonic had no effect on whether the vowel was perceived as an /I/ and /e/, even though we might have expected that changing the ITD of the fourth harmonic would separate it from the rest of the vowel, and thereby change the perceived first formant. To further demonstrate the lack of effect of ITD on simultaneous grouping, Darwin and Hukin repeated a manipulation we have already met—increasing the level of the fourth harmonic, which made more of the vowels sound like /e/, since this manipulation shifted the first formant peak to higher values. As before, they now tried to reduce the effect of the higher level of the fourth harmonic by changing its ITD (similarly to the attempt to reduce the effect of harmonic level by manipulating its onset). But the effects of increasing the level of the fourth harmonic were essentially the same, regardless of whether or not it had the same ITD as the rest of the vowel. ITD therefore seems not to operate as a simultaneous grouping cue, or at least it cannot ungroup simultaneous frequency components that have been grouped on the basis of common onset and harmonicity.

How do we understand the seemingly contradictory results of the two experiments? Darwin and Hukin suggested that the role of the sentence in the dog versus bird experiment was to direct the auditory system to process auditory objects from a specific location in space, leading to the strong effect of ITD, not so much because of its intrinsic properties, but because it suggested that the word occurred in the same spatial location. In the second experiment, there was no such cuing, and therefore other acoustic cues (e.g., harmonicity) overrode the effects of ITD.

6.3.4 Neural Correlates of Simultaneous Segregation and Grouping

Although we have presented a number of neural correlates of segregation of simultaneous sounds, as well as possible mechanisms that contribute to this goal, we did not mention many neural correlates of the actual endpoint of this process—the representation of the segregated sounds. The reason for this is simple: There are very few examples of this in the literature. One possible example is the case of CMR in auditory cortex, as described in the previous section. However, CMR is a somewhat artificial construct. We would really like to be able to show examples of mixtures of natural sounds being segregated and represented separately somewhere in the brain.

Some evidence that this may occur at the level of primary auditory cortex has been offered by Bar-Yosef and colleagues (Bar-Yosef & Nelken, 2007; Bar-Yosef, Rotman, & Nelken, 2002; Nelken & Bar-Yosef, 2008). They studied responses to birdsongs extracted from natural recordings. Because these recordings were made "in the real world," the songs were accompanied by additional acoustic components such as echoes and background noises. It is possible, however, to separate out the "foreground" birdsong from the background noise, and to present separately the cleaned "foreground only" song or the much quieter remaining background sounds to neurons (Sound Example "Birdsongs and their Backgrounds" on the book's Web site). Figure 6.10 displays the responses of four cat auditory cortex neurons to these stimuli. The top panel shows the responses of these neurons to pure tones with different

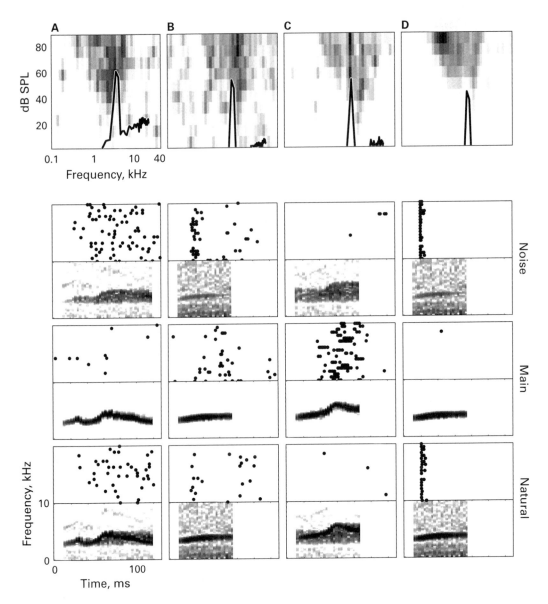

Figure 6.10

Responses of four neurons to natural bird chirps and their modifications. The top panels display in gray levels the responses of these neurons to tones of varying frequencies and levels (along the abscissa and ordinate, respectively), a representation called a frequency response area (FRA). The bottom panels represent the responses of the neurons to three stimuli: the natural bird chirp (bottom), the clean main chirp (middle), and the leftover signal (top). In each case, the spectrogram is displayed below a raster plot, using dots to indicate the time of occurrence of spikes in twenty presentations of each of the stimuli. The thick black lines on top of the FRAs represent the frequency content of the clean chirp ("Main").

From figure 13 of Bar-Yosef and Nelken (2007).

frequencies and levels. These "frequency response area" (FRA) plots reveal a typical V-shaped tuning curve with best frequencies around 4 kHz, close to the center frequency of the bird chirps that were used in these experiments. On top of the FRAs, the thick black line represents the frequency content of the clean bird chirp. Below the FRAs, the different stimuli and the resulting responses are shown. The responses are displayed as rasters—there are twenty repeats of each sound and, in each repeat, a dot represents the time of occurrence of a spike. The stimuli are shown as spectrograms (described in chapter 1).

Three stimuli are shown for each neuron. The bottom stimulus is a segment from a natural recording, including the bird chirp and all the rest of the sound, which includes echoes (the "halo" around the chirps) and rustling (apparent as a mostly uniform background at all frequencies). The middle stimulus is the "foreground only" bird chirp, and the upper stimulus is the remainder after removal of the chirp, that is, just the echoes and background. Considering that most of the sound energy of the original, natural sound is contained in the bird chirp, the responses to the original recording and the cleaned chirp (bottom and middle rows) can be surprisingly different. In fact, in the examples shown here, the responses to the background, played alone, were much more similar to the responses to the full natural stimulus than were the responses to the foreground only stimulus.

The responses of these neurons may be interpreted as correlates of the end point of a process of scene analysis—they respond to some, but not all, of the components of an auditory scene. In fact, they respond particularly well to the weaker components in the scene. Perhaps other neurons respond to the clean chirp rather than to the background, although Bar-Yosef and Nelken (2007) did not find such neurons. Alternatively, it may be that these neurons are really doing the hard part of auditory scene analysis—the foreground bird chirp is easy to hear. Hearing the background is harder, but potentially very important: The sounds of prey or predators may lie hidden in the background! Surveillance of the subtler background sounds might be a key function of auditory cortex. In fact, the same group presented data suggesting that responses in IC to these sounds are usually more closely related to the physical structure of the sounds, and therefore more strongly influenced by the high-intensity foreground. Thalamic responses, on the other hand, would appear to be more similar to the cortical responses (Chechik et al., 2006). So far, however, there are only very few such examples in the literature. Much more experimental data with additional stimuli will be required to fully assess the role of cortex in auditory scene analysis.

6.4 Nonsimultaneous Grouping and Segregation: Streaming

Simultaneous grouping and segregation is only one part of auditory scene analysis. Sound sources are often active for a long time, and the way they change (or not) as a function of time has important consequences for the way they are perceived. We already encountered an effect of this kind—the effect of ITD on grouping, which was large for sequential sounds but weak for simultaneous grouping.

A number of examples of this kind have been studied in the literature. Possibly the simplest form of streaming uses two pure tones (Sound Example "Streaming with Alternating Tones" on the book's Web site). The two tones are played alternately at a fixed rate. If the rate of presentation is slow and the interval between the two tones is small, the result is a simple melody consisting of two alternating tones. However, if the rate of presentation is fast enough and the frequency separation between the two tones is large enough, the melody breaks down into two streams, each consisting of tones of one frequency. A more interesting version of the same phenomenon, which has recently been studied intensively, is the "galloping," or "ABA" rhythm paradigm. This paradigm, first introduced by van Noorden in his PhD thesis (Van Noorden, 1975), is illustrated in figure 6.11 (Sound Example "Streaming in the Galloping Rhythm Paradigm"). The galloping rhythm is generated by playing tones of two frequencies, let's say 500 and 750 Hz, at a slow repetition rate in the pattern shown in the left side of figure 6.11. This is normally perceived as a simple "galloping" three-note melody (da di da – da di da – da di da …), as indicated in the left panel of the figure. If the melody is speeded up, however, or the frequency separation is increased, or, indeed,

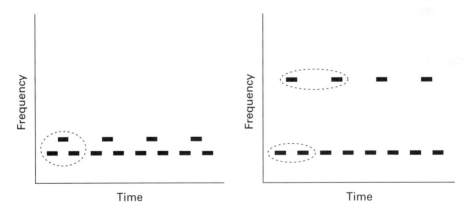

Figure 6.11
Streaming is the breakdown of a sequence of tones into two "streams." In this illustration, tones of two frequencies are presented successively, with the higher tone at half the rate of the lower one. When the frequency separation between the two is small, the result is a single stream of sounds with a basic three-tone galloping melody. When the frequency separation between the two tones is large, the sequence breaks down into two streams, one composed of the low-frequency tones, the other of the high-frequency tones.
From figure 1 of Schnupp (2008).

if you simply just keep listening to it for long enough, then the three-note melody breaks down and you perceive two streams of tones, one at the low frequency (da – da – da – da ...), and a second, with larger gaps, at the high frequency (di – – – di – – – di ...), as indicated in the right panel.

The breakdown of a sequence of sounds into two (or possibly more) things is called "streaming," and we can talk about perception of one (at slower presentation rates) or two (at faster presentation rates) streams. Later, we will discuss the relationships between these things and auditory objects, which we introduced earlier in the chapter. The study of streaming was popularized by Al Bregman in the 1970s, and is described in great detail in his highly influential book *Auditory Scene Analysis* (Bregman, 1990). Importantly, the attempts of Bregman to justify the claim that there are multiple perceptual things, which he called streams, are described in that book and will not be repeated here.

Streaming in this form has been used in classical music to create multiple musical lines with instruments that can produce only a single pitch at a time. The best known examples are probably from the Baroque period—for instance, J. S. Bach in his compositions for solo violin famously used such melodies, composed of alternating high and low tones. These melodies split apart into two separate, simultaneous melodic lines, thus enriching the musical texture. Another rather well-known example is from Liszt's *La Campanella* etude, which is a free adaptation of the main theme of the last movement of Paganini's second violin concerto (figure 6.12 and Sound Example "La Campanella" on the book's Web site).

We have already mentioned that certain conditions, such as slow rhythms with long intervals and a small pitch separation between the notes, favor the perception of a single stream, while the opposite conditions, namely, fast presentation rates and large pitch intervals (as in the *La Campanella* etude), favor the perception of two separate streams. But what happens in "intermediate" regimes? There is a tendency for the single stream to dominate perception for the first few seconds, following which the single percept may break up into two streams. Pressnitzer and Hupé (2006), who carefully measured the duration of this phase, found that for an interval of 5 semitones (the interval of a fourth, corresponding to a frequency ratio of about 4/3), and at a presentation rate of about 8 tones/s, the duration of the initial single-stream percept was on average about 20 s, corresponding to 160 tone presentations. Eventually, all subjects ended up hearing two streams. The eventual splitting of the initial single stream into two is called the "buildup of streaming."

However, the story doesn't end there. When subjects continued to listen to the sequences for even longer, the perceived organization could switch again into a single stream, and then split again, alternating between phases of one and two perceived streams. In fact, this behavior was very much the same as that found in other bistable perceptual phenomena (Pressnitzer & Hupé, 2006). Thus, the "buildup" of streaming,

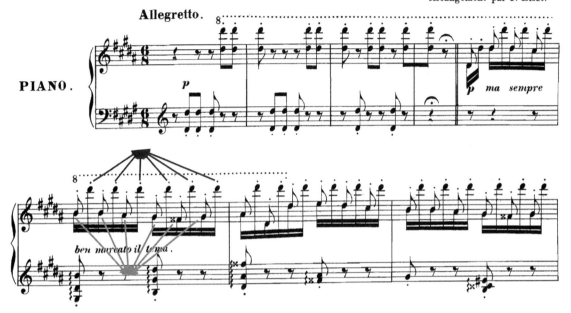

Figure 6.12

The beginning of *La Campanella* etude from Liszt's "Large Paganini Studies." The melodic line consists of the low tones in the pianist's right hand, which alternates with high tones, up to two octaves above the melodic line. The melody streams out in spite of the alternations with the high tones. The gray and black arrows indicate the notes participating in the two streams in one bar.

that is, the initial split, is only part of what neural models have to account for—it is also necessary to account for the further switching between the perception of one and two streams (Denham & Winkler, 2006).

Streaming occurs in nonhuman animals as well. Thus, MacDougall-Shackleton et al. (1998) showed streaming in a bird, the European starling, while Izumi (2002) observed an analog of streaming in Japanese macaques. In Izumi's experiment, the monkeys had to recognize short "melodies" that were played alone or with additional interleaved distracter tones. If the distracter tones were positioned in a frequency region that did not overlap that of the melodies, the monkeys were able to recognize the melodies correctly. If the distracter tones were positioned in a frequency region that did overlap with that of the melodies, the monkeys failed to recognize the melodies.

The evidence for streaming in animals is, however, patchy. Human psychophysics is often compared directly with animal electrophysiological recordings, with the hope that the operation and organization of human and animal auditory systems are similar enough to make this comparison valid and informative. While such comparisons must be handled with care, they can nevertheless be illuminating. For example, a basic model for the mechanisms behind streaming was suggested by Fishman et al. (2001), based on recordings from the auditory cortex of macaques. The macaques listened passively to a sequence of two alternating tones (as in Sound Example "Streaming with Alternating Tones"), one of which matched the BF of the neurons under study. An example of the recorded neuronal responses is illustrated in figure 6.13, which shows the responses of two multiunit clusters to such sequences. The large, transient

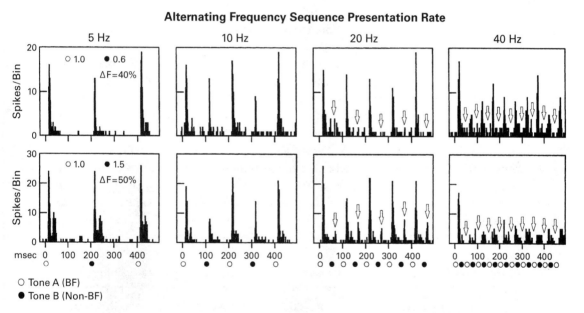

Figure 6.13

A possible neuronal correlate of streaming. The responses of two neurons to sequences of alternating tones presented at different rates. One of the two tones was always at BF, the other at an interval of 40% (top) or 50% (bottom) away. At the slower presentation rates, both tones evoked responses (e.g., the 5-Hz panels). However, at faster presentation rates, while the responses to both tones decreased, the responses to the non-BF tones (arrows) decreased to a larger degree than those of the BF tone.

From figure 8 of Fishman et al. (2001).

increases in firing rates (visible as peaks in the firing rate histograms) are the responses to the tones. The presentations of BF tones are marked by open dots and those of the non-BF tones by filled dots at the bottom of the panels (and by open arrows in the panels showing the responses to faster sequences). The crucial observation is that, as the sequence rate is increased, the responses to the non-BF tones decreased faster than the responses to the BF tones. Thus, for example, at a presentation rate of 20 Hz, the BF tones evoked large responses in both of the recording sites shown, but the non-BF tone did not evoke any responses in one of them (the upper panel) and a substantially reduced response in the other (lower panel). Fishman et al. (2001) suggested that the differential effect of presentation rate on BF and non-BF tones is the result of "forward masking"—the reduction in response to a tone due to the presentation of another tone just before.

How do these findings relate to streaming? Fishman et al. (2001) proposed the following hypothesis: As long as the majority of responsive neurons are activated by either of the two tones, a single stream is perceived. In contrast, if one tone evokes a response mostly in one neuronal population, while the other tone evokes a response mostly in a different, nonoverlapping neuronal population, two streams are perceived. Thus, when the frequency separation between the two tones is large enough, two streams are always perceived. Similarly, if the frequency separation between the two tones is very small, a single stream is always observed.

When the frequency separation between the two tones is intermediate, the rate of presentation becomes an important factor—slow presentations favor a single stream, because at low presentation rates there is less forward masking that would suppress responses to the non-BF tone. Increasing the presentation rate leads to more forward masking; in consequence, cortical neurons increasingly respond to only one tone or the other, but not to both. The neuronal populations responding to both tones tend to overlap less, which in turn favors the perception of the two tones in separate streams. The data of Fishman et al. (2001) are indeed compatible with this hypothesis.

This model is appealing, but it needs to be made quantitative. For example, one would like to know how much the two populations should overlap in order for a single stream to be perceived. Micheyl et al. (2005) used a nice twist to make this model quantitative. They decided to study the buildup of streaming—the time it takes for the initial galloping rhythm to split into two streams. First, they used ABA tone sequences at a fixed rate (8 tones/s) and measured (in humans, not macaques) which percept is present as a function of time. The results were as expected (figure 6.14B): When the interval between the two tones was 1 semitone (6%), for example, a single stream was almost always perceived, but when the interval was increased to 9 semitones, two streams were almost always heard. With 3- and 6-semitone separation, it took some time for the streams to separate, and there was some probability for hearing either one or two streams throughout the whole presentation period. Next, Micheyl et al. (2005) measured the responses of single neurons in the auditory cortex of macaque monkeys. They positioned the A tone on the BF of the neuron, so that the B tone was off-BF. Like Fishman et al. (2001), they observed a selective reduction in the response to the B tone, this time with increasing frequency separation. However, Micheyl et al. (2005) also studied how this reduction in the response to the off-BF tone (the B tone) developed with time, and found that the contrast between the responses to the A and B tones was stronger at the end than at the beginning of the sequence (figure 6.14A).

At this point, the decline in the response to the B tone mimics qualitatively the buildup of streaming, but Micheyl et al. (2005) went a step further. Remember that in this experiment, neurons always respond to the A tone, as that tone is at their BF. Micheyl and colleagues wanted to have a threshold such that if the neurons respond to the B tone above this threshold, they would also participate in the representation of the B tone and, according to the hypothesis of Fishman et al. (2001), there would be only one stream. On the other hand, when the response to the B tone is below the threshold, these neurons would not participate in the representation of the B tones, while other, similar neurons with a BF near the frequency of the B tone would presumably respond essentially only to the B tone. The A and the B tones would then be represented in the activity of nonoverlapping neural populations, which in turn should favor a two-stream percept.

How can we find such a threshold? Given a guess for the threshold, one can look back at the data and see how many times the responses to the B tone were smaller than that threshold—this would be an estimate for the probability of perceiving one stream rather than two. The question is, is it possible to find a single threshold that makes the predicted likelihoods of perceiving one stream, as derived from the neural recordings, line up with the actual likelihoods measured experimentally? The curves shown in figure 6.14B suggest that it is indeed possible to find such a threshold.

These studies show that the dynamic response properties of cortical neurons may account for streaming, but they fall someway short of a conclusive and complete account of this phenomenon. A number of critiques and open questions are still to be answered. One critique states that, while this model accounts for the buildup, it doesn't account for the bistability—the switching back and forth between one- and two-stream percepts. Unfortunately, no physiological study as yet has even attempted to account for the bistability of streaming. A second critique is that, though this model may be correct, it doesn't necessarily have to be based on cortical responses. In fact, neurons as early as the cochlear nucleus show a similar, although substantially smaller, differential adaptation effect. But while the effect is smaller, the variability in the responses in the cochlear nucleus is also much smaller, and therefore the same statistical

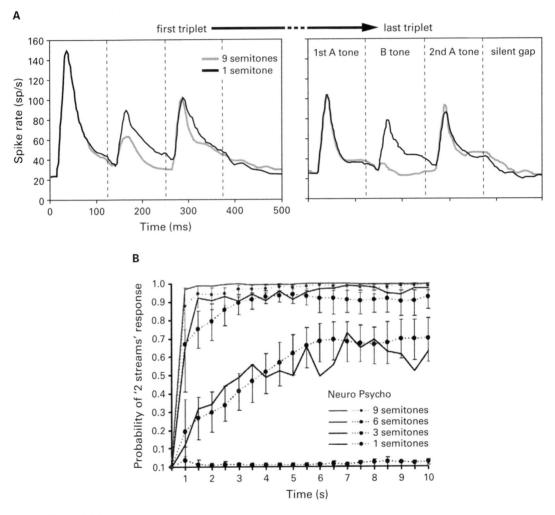

Figure 6.14
(A) Average responses of ninety-one neurons in the macaque auditory cortex to the ABA tone triplets, when the interval between the A and the B tones was 1 semitone (black) and when the interval was 9 semitones (gray). The responses to the first triplet are displayed on the left, and the responses to the last triplet on the right. Note the stronger reduction in the responses to the B tone in the 9 semitones case. (B) Buildup of streaming in humans (dashed lines) and in the neural model based on the responses in the macaque auditory cortex (continuous lines). From figures 2 and 4 of Micheyl et al. (2005).

technique used to produce the fit between monkey cortical responses and human behavior can produce a similar fit between the responses of neurons in the cochlear nucleus of the guinea pig and human behavior (Pressnitzer et al., 2008). As we have seen so often in this chapter, high-level and low-level mechanisms compete for explaining the same perceptual phenomena.

A third critique is that the Fishman model has been studied only for streaming based on frequency differences. However, streaming can be induced by many acoustic differences—for example, by amplitude modulation rate, which is only very weakly related to spectral differences (Sound Example "Streaming by Amplitude Modulation Rate" on the book's Web site). Whether the same type of increased differentiation between populations would occur for other acoustic differences is an open question. However, some initial work in this direction shows that it may be possible to generalize the Fishman model to amplitude modulation (Itatani & Klump, 2009).

With the recent intensive research into streaming, the "playground" for relating it to neural responses is now well delimited. To hazard a guess, the main weakness of all models available today is their inability to account for bistability. Thus, many puzzles remain for future work, and possibly for new conceptual models as well.

6.5 Nonsimultaneous Grouping and Segregation: Change Detection

You sit in a room preparing for an exam that is going to take place tomorrow. Music is playing in the background. Through the windows, sounds from the busy street are heard. Your roommate is walking in the next room, stepping from one end of the room to the other, but you ignore all of these sounds, concentrating on your revision. Then one of your friend's steps is different—and you are suddenly aware of it.

As we discussed in the first chapter, sounds provide information about numerous aspects of the world, and minute changes in sounds, such as the sound of a step on a different material than we expected, may be highly informative. We are very sensitive to such changes in the auditory scene. This sensitivity is often studied with a tool called Mismatch Negativity (MMN). MMN is a component of the so-called auditory event-related potentials (ERPs), the set of electrical waves that are evoked by sounds and measured by electroencephalography (EEG).

MMN is evoked by unexpected sounds embedded in a stream of expected sounds. It is preattentive: evoked even without attention. In the simplest version of an experiment for measuring MMN, the subject is distracted (e.g., by reading a book or watching a silent movie) while sounds are played by earphones and the EEG is measured. The sound sequence usually consists of two pure tones that vary in some property: They may have different frequencies, or different sound levels, or different durations. One of the two tones is played with high probability (this tone is often called the standard), while the other is rare (the deviant). The deviant tone is presented randomly in the sequence, for example, with a probability of 10%. Under these circumstances, the ERP is somewhat different in response to the standard and to the deviant: When measuring the potential between the top of the head and the bottom of the mastoids, the response to the deviant is more negative than the response to the standard in a time window around 100 to 150 ms after stimulus onset (figure 6.15).

MMN can be observed even when the changes in the sounds are quite subtle. It is sensitive to conjunction of properties or even to deviations from rather complex rules that might govern the stimulation sequence. In one of the more complex designs that have been tested, Paavilainen, Arajarvi, and Takegata (2007) used a sequence that could have tones of two frequencies, and these tones were either short or long. Each of the four possible combinations of tone frequency and tone duration (high-long, high-short, low-long, and low-short) appeared with equal probability. However, the sequence (Sound Example "A Tone Sequence Following a Complex Rule" on the book's Web site) was constructed so that short tones were almost always followed by

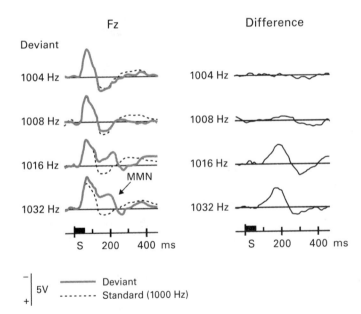

Figure 6.15
Mismatch negativity (MMN) to frequency deviants. (Left) The potential between electrode Fz (an electrode on the midline, relatively frontal) and the mastoid in response to a 1,000-Hz tone (dashed line) that serves as the standard, and deviant tones at the indicated frequencies. (Right) The difference waveforms (deviant-standard), showing a clear peak around 150 ms after stimulus onset. Note that negative potentials are plotted upward in this figure.
From figure 1 of Näätänen et al. (2007).

low-frequency tones (which could be either long or short), and long tones were always followed by high-frequency tones (which also could be either long or short). From time to time, a tone appeared that violated these rules (a high-frequency tone followed a short tone, or a low-frequency tone followed a long tone). These deviant tones evoked MMN (admittedly, a rather small one). Remarkably, in interviews following the experiment, the listeners reported that they were not aware of the rules governing the sequence, nor were they able to work out what the rules were when prompted, and when the rule was explained to them, they had great difficulty applying it to detect deviants through a conscious effort. Thus, the MMN stemmed from a presumably preattentive representation of the regularities in the sound sequence.

But what can these laboratory experiments tell us about real-world listening? Going back to the situation described at the beginning of this section, would our friend's deviant footstep evoke MMN? Apparently it does. Winkler and coworkers (2003) measured MMN in subjects who watched a movie (with sound), and were simultaneously presented with simulated street sounds. On top of this, the sounds of eleven footsteps were heard. The sounds of the steps varied a bit from one step to the next, as real steps would. One of the steps simulated walking on a different surface, and this was inserted either as the second or tenth in the sequence (Sound Example "A Naturalistic Sound Sequence with a Deviant" on the book's Web site). The subjects were engaged in a task that was related to the movie, and so they had to ignore the other two sound sources. Winkler et al. (2003) found that MMN was evoked when the deviant step was the tenth but not when it was the second in the sequence. Thus, MMN was evoked in spite of the natural variability in the sounds—presumably, when the deviant step was the tenth, a representation of the regularity of the footsteps had been generated during the preceding nine steps, so that the deviant step was detected as such. On the other hand, when the deviant step was in the second position, no representation of regularity could have been created, and no MMN occurred.

What do we know about the brain activity underlying MMN? Since MMN was defined and has been intensively studied in humans, while more fine-grained studies, such as single-neuron recordings, can usually be conducted only in nonhuman animals, it is necessary to show that MMN, or something similar, occurs in animals. And indeed, a number of studies that measured auditory evoked potentials in rats (Ruusuvirta, Penttonen, & Korhonen, 1998), cats (Csepe, Karmos, & Molnar, 1987), and monkeys (Javitt et al., 1992) reported brain responses that are similar to MMN. These results open the door to single neuron studies.

The single-neuron analogs of MMN are based on a phenomenon that has been studied in vision for some time, but was only recently imported into auditory research—stimulus-specific adaptation (SSA). We start with two stimuli, both of which evoke responses of similar strength. Next, we present one of the two stimuli repeatedly, causing a reduction in the response (adaptation). Finally, we present the other stimulus. It is possible that the neuron is really tired of responding—in that case, the response to the other stimulus would be adapted as well. However, in many cases, the response to the other stimulus is not adapted at all, or only partially adapted. In that case, we will say that the adaptation to the first stimulus is stimulus specific, or that we have SSA.

SSA is interesting, precisely because it is not really adaptation, which is usually defined as a use-dependent reduction in responses. If adaptation were really a kind of use-dependent "fatigue," then the decline in the neuron's ability to respond vigorously should affect all stimuli more or less equally. In stimulus-specific adaptation, the neuron has tired only of the repetitive, adapting stimulus, but can still fire vigorously to a different, rare stimulus. A better term would have been "habituation," which is used in the psychological literature to indicate a reduction in responses that may be stimulus specific (Dudai, 2002).

It turns out that SSA is strong in the auditory midbrain and cortex. Ulanovsky et al. (2003) used oddball sequences of pure tones, similar to those used in MMN research, and recorded single-unit responses in auditory cortex of cats. To demonstrate stimulus-specific adaptation, they used two tones that were very close in frequency—to within 10% or even 4%, which is the behavioral limit of frequency discrimination in cats. They then played one of the tones as standard with the other as deviant. As expected, the neurons adapted to the repetitive standard tone, and the deviant tone evoked relatively larger responses. However, how do we know that the neuron does not have larger responses to the deviant tone because of a preference for its frequency (it might be closer to the neuron's BF than the standard), rather than any adaptive effects? Ulanovsky et al. (2003) controlled for this issue by repeating the experiment with the roles of the standard and the deviant reversed. Since both tones served once as standard and once as deviant, any intrinsic preference for one of the tone frequencies could be discounted. Some of their results are presented in figure 6.16. The responses to a tone when it was standard (thick light gray line) were most often smaller than the responses to the same tone when it was deviant (thick dark gray line). Thus, the neuron was sensitive to the statistical structure of the sequence, producing larger responses to rare sounds.

Although the original observations of Ulanovsky et al. (2003) suggested that SSA occurs in primary auditory cortex but not in the thalamus, and would therefore be a result of cortical mechanisms, it is clear today that the situation is much more complex. SSA has since been observed as early as the inferior colliculus (Malmierca et al., 2009), although it is strong and widespread mostly outside the central nucleus, which is the core station of the inferior colliculus. Similarly, SSA has been observed in the medial geniculate body of the thalamus (Anderson, Christianson, & Linden, 2009), although there, too, it is strongest outside the core division. Within auditory cortex,

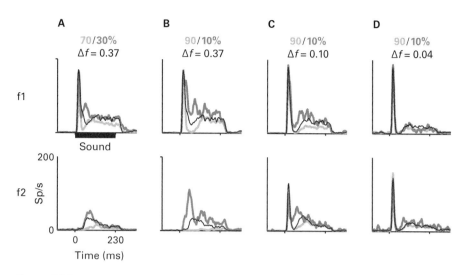

Figure 6.16

Responses of a neuron in cat auditory cortex to two frequencies (f1 and f2). The frequency difference between the tones is given at the top of each column, as well as the probabilities of the two tones. The responses are displayed as peristimulus time histograms, computed by averaging all the responses to the given frequency under three conditions: when rare (thick dark gray line), when common (thick light gray line), and when appearing randomly half the time (thin black line). From figure 1 in Ulanovsky, Las, and Nelken, (2003).

SSA appears to be more pronounced in the deeper, infragranular layers, which suggests that cortical processing may amplify it (Szymanski, Garcia-Lazaro, & Schnupp, 2009). The precise contributions of midbrain and cortical stations to the phenomenon of SSA remain to be worked out.

Is SSA the "single-neural correlate" of MMN? A number of observations suggest that the relationship between MMN and SSA is indirect. MMN occurs rather late compared to the neural responses that are usually studied in single-neuron experiments. Sometimes MMN is observed with latencies of 150 ms after stimulus onset in humans, whereas the earliest cortical responses in humans occur within 30 ms after stimulus onset (Schneider et al., 2002), and SSA is present right from the onset of the response. This temporal mismatch suggests that, in humans, too, there should be a neural signature of early deviance detection. More important, the fact that SSA in single neurons occurs so much earlier than MMN raises the possibility that it may occur, in a sense, "upstream" of MMN, and trigger a further cascade of neural processing events that ultimately produce the currents measured as MMN.

Although the relationship between SSA and MMN remains uncertain, it is clear that both share a large number of properties (Nelken & Ulanovsky, 2007) that are important for auditory scene analysis—most important, the sensitivity to sudden, unpredictable changes in the auditory scene. Thus, the auditory system comes equipped with deviance detectors, which may signal when the mental image we have created in the auditory scene needs to be updated.

6.6 Summary: Auditory Scene Analysis and Auditory Objects

Grouping and segregating multiple simultaneous and sequential sound elements to form either unified or separate "perceptual objects" is one of the most important computational tasks the auditory system performs. This task underpins, for example, our ability to understand speech under the usual adverse conditions of daily life, with competing sources and noise all around. It underpins music appreciation, particularly once we go beyond a single instrument playing a single melody. It also underlies our ability to detect subtle changes in the auditory scene, with its obvious ethological implications.

In our discussion, we referred to the formation of "auditory objects" as the result of auditory scene analysis, but also pointed out that there is as yet no consensus as to how auditory objects are to be defined. We encountered the term first in discussing masking—in that scenario, there are presumably two "things," the masker (usually some noise) and the target sound that is being masked (usually a pure tone). When we discussed simultaneous grouping and segregation, we again dealt with two things, such as two simultaneously present vowels that differ in F_0, or a vowel and a lonely harmonic that had become separated from the vowel because it started a bit early. The role of the auditory system is presumably to realize the distinction between these temporally overlapping sounds, putting bits of sounds in two baskets, one for each, well, "thing." Streaming has a similar flavor—you put the successive tones in a single stream or in two separate streams. However, when we called these things "streams," rather than baskets or objects, we were following historical convention, not applying any precise or agreed-upon definitions or distinctions. So, what are these things (objects, baskets)?

One thing they are definitely not is "sounds" in the physical sense, because there is only one sound at each moment in time—the physical pressure waveform that causes the tympanic membrane to vibrate. When we call these things sounds in the perceptual sense, as in "I heard two sounds, one of them a pure tone and the other noise," we really mean that we have somewhere in our head the idea that the physical sound we just experienced appeared to be formed by adding these individual "things" together.

It is also a bit of stretch to call these things "sound sources." They will often carry information about the sound sources, but the relationships between sound sources and the sound they emit is far from being one-to-one—when we listen to a recording of a Mahler symphony, the sound source is a loudspeaker, but the sounds we perceive are the instruments of the orchestra, alone or in combination. Classical composers perfected the art of combining different instruments together to achieve sonorities and textures that cannot be achieved by single instruments, so that multiple sound sources may appear to fuse into a single "thing." Or consider the fact that animals are sound sources that can produce very different vocalizations. Think of a cat meowing, purring, or hissing. Is the auditory object a "meow," or is it a cat?

Referring to the perceived auditory things we discussed in this chapter as "events" is also problematic. An event suggests localization in time, but the things can be rather long lasting, and they may even appear and disappear from our perception, as we have seen in the case of the bistable percept of streaming.

According to Bregman, the main importance of these things is that they serve as carriers of properties—which is precisely the purpose of objects in vision. Thus, the auditory thing may have a pitch (or not), it may have a spatial location, or it may have a phonetic quality (or not). It may have a long or short duration, be continuous or transient or rhythmic, and so on and so forth. In that respect, one might define an auditory object as a carrier of properties: a "thing" that has a specific set of values for all of these perceptual properties.

Bregman himself preferred to call these things streams, and stated that the "stream plays the same role in auditory mental experience as the object does in visual [mental experience]" (Bregman, 1990, p. 11). The term "stream" has recently been used mostly in the context of streaming—the splitting of the two-tone sequences into two streams. It has therefore acquired a more specific sense than Bregman seems to have originally intended. One could say that a stream is an auditory object, but in current usage there are auditory objects that are not streams—for example, a single burst of white noise over a background of silence wouldn't be a stream, according to current terminology.

There have been a number of attempts to define auditory objects in more precise terms. For example, an influential review by Griffiths and Warren (2004) suggested four principles for defining auditory objects. Auditory objects should pertain to things in the sensory world; object analysis is about separating information related to the object from that related to the rest of the world; it should involve abstraction of sensory information, so that different physical realizations may evoke the same auditory object; and finally it should generalize across senses (so that the voice and picture of grandma should represent the same object).

This definition is substantially more restrictive than the arguments we used (and that Bregman used before us) would require. While our rough discussion is consistent with the first two postulates of Griffiths and Warren, it certainly doesn't go as far as requiring the last two. The "things" we discuss do not necessarily have any specific relationships to material objects—they are auditory, and have to do with the sounds and not with what produced the sounds. They may represent an earlier or more primitive representation relative to the objects, as defined by Griffiths and Warren.

What does perhaps become clear in this discussion is that the vocabulary of the English language is, at present, not adequate to discuss the process of "auditory object formation," and we may have to invent, or borrow, new vocabulary to create the necessary clarity. In German, for example, the word *schall* is used exclusively for physical sound, while sound in the perceptual sense is called a *geräusch* or a *klang*. But the word "klang" would not be used to describe a stream. Rather, a stream is composed of a succession of perceptually linked "*klänge.*" The lower-level, "klang-object" is more unitary, more strongly bound perceptually. We would find it much easier to report how many klänge there were in a stream, than to guess how many harmonics there were in a klang, even if all the harmonics were resolved by the cochlear filters.

As this discussion illustrates, while auditory objects may have many meanings, these things clearly have an important place in auditory research, as they lie right at the interface between physiology and perception. In particular, we want to argue that objects (in the sense of an entity with a particular set of perceptual properties) must be formed before they are assigned properties such as pitch, spatial location, phonetic quality, and so on. This point was made more or less explicitly throughout this chapter. For example, the models we described for separating vowels in double-vowel experiments consisted of a stage in which different frequency channels that shared similar periodicity were grouped together, and only later could the phonetic quality in each group be assigned. Throughout the chapter we reviewed evidence to suggest that the "klang-objects" are already encoded in primary auditory cortex. We also reviewed evidence suggesting that the neural mechanisms that underlie streaming are expressed in primary auditory cortex, and possibly even in the cochlear nucleus, the first stage of the auditory pathway. Thus, it seems that the construction of the auditory objects begins remarkably early in the auditory system, presumably in parallel with feature extraction. These findings can be contrasted with the difficulty in finding early representations of pitch (or even just a representation of periodicity, as reviewed in chapter 3), space (as reviewed in chapter 5), and speech sound identity (as reviewed in chapter 4). Taken together, these electrophysiological findings may support the contention that objects are formed before their properties are assigned to them.

How can the brain find out about the objects in the auditory scene? The examples for auditory scene analysis that we have considered all revolved around rules that help us assign different frequency components or sound elements to different objects. The rules included grouping by common onset across frequency or grouping by common periodicity (klang formation), or segregating elements that are too far apart in frequency and too close in time (for streaming). We also saw that our auditory system is very sensitive to statistical regularities, and their violation gives rise to MMN. Thus, it is tempting to argue that objects embody such grouping and regularity rules. According to this circle of ideas, as long as the rules defining the object describe the auditory scene well, we perceive the object; once these rules are violated, we can either introduce a new object into the scene (something Bregman called the old plus new heuristic), or, if this is not a good solution, completely turn off the object— and cease to perceive it (see Winkler et al., 2009a, for a detailed presentation of these ideas).

Thus, we are left in a precarious state—we have a number of well-studied examples of auditory scene analysis, some loose terminology for describing its outcome (the formation of auditory objects), and a very rough suggestion for how this may be achieved (by finding and applying the rules that bind or separate the elements of the current auditory scene). All of this leaves a lot of room for further research, which will need to integrate electrophysiology, perception, and modeling—a perfect mix for fascinating new findings!

7 Development, Learning, and Plasticity

We have so far considered the basis by which the auditory system can detect, localize, and identify the myriad sounds that we might encounter. But how does our perception of the acoustic environment arise during development? Are we born with these abilities or do they emerge gradually during childhood? It turns out that much of the development of the auditory system takes places before birth, enabling many species, including humans, to respond to sound as soon as they are born. Nonetheless, the different parts of the ear and the central auditory pathways continue to mature for some time after that. This involves a lot of remodeling in the brain, with many neurons failing to survive until adulthood and others undergoing changes in the number and type of connections they form with other neurons. Not surprisingly, these wiring modifications can result in developmental changes in the auditory sensitivity of the neurons. As a consequence, auditory perceptual abilities mature over different timescales, in some cases not reaching the levels typically seen in adults until several years after birth.

A very important factor in the development of any sensory system is that the anatomical and functional organization of the brain regions involved is shaped by experience during so-called "sensitive" or "critical" periods of early postnatal life. These terms are often used interchangeably, but some researchers use them to describe distinct phases of development. A sensitive period would then refer to the phase during which altered experience can change behavior or neuronal response properties, whereas a critical period covers the longer phase during which these changes can be reversed if normal sensory inputs are experienced. We will therefore stick to the term sensitive period. The plasticity seen during this stage of development helps to optimize brain circuits to an individual's sensory environment. But this also means that abnormal experience—such as a loss of hearing in childhood—can have a profound effect on the manner in which neurons respond to different sounds, and therefore on how we perceive them.

Although sensitive periods of development have been described for many species and for many aspects of auditory function, including the emergence of linguistic and musical abilities, we must remember that learning is a lifelong process. Indeed, extensive plasticity is seen in the adult brain, too, which plays a vital function in enabling humans and animals to interact effectively with their acoustic environment and provides the basis on which learning can improve perceptual abilities.

7.1 When Does Hearing Start?

The development of the auditory system is a complex, multistage process that begins in early embryonic life. The embryo comprises three layers, which interact to produce the various tissues of the body. One of these layers, the ectoderm, gives rise to both neural tissue and skin. The initial stage in this process involves the formation of the otic placode, a thickening of the ectoderm in the region of the developing hindbrain. As a result of signals provided by the neural tube, from which the brain and spinal cord are derived, and by the mesoderm, the otic placode is induced to invaginate and fold up into a structure called the otocyst, from which the cochlea and otic ganglion cells—the future auditory nerve—are formed. Interestingly, the external ear and the middle ear have different embryological origins from that of the inner ear. As a consequence, congenital abnormalities can occur independently in each of these structures.

The neurons that will become part of the central auditory pathway are produced within the ventricular zone of the embryo's neural tube, from where they migrate to their final destination in the brain. Studies in animals have shown that the first auditory neurons to be generated give rise to the cochlear nucleus, superior olivary complex, and medial geniculate nucleus, with the production of neurons that form the inferior colliculus and auditory cortex beginning slightly later. In humans, all the subcortical auditory structures can be recognized by the eighth fetal week. The cortical plate, the first sign of the future cerebral cortex, also emerges at this time, although the temporal lobe becomes apparent as a distinct structure only in the twenty-seventh week of gestation (Moore & Linthicum, 2009).

To serve their purpose, the newly generated neurons must make specific synaptic connections with other neurons. Consequently, as they are migrating, the neurons start to send out axons that are guided toward their targets by a variety of chemical guidance cues those structures produce. These molecules are detected by receptors on the exploring growth cones that form the tips of the growing axons, while other molecules ensure that axons make contact with the appropriate region of the target neurons. Robust synaptic connections can be established at an early stage—by the fourteenth week of gestation in the case of the innervation of hair cells by the spiral ganglion cells. On the other hand, another seven weeks elapse before axons from the thalamus start to make connections with the cortical plate.

At this stage of development, the axons lack their insulating sheaths of myelin, which are required for the rapid and reliable conduction of action potentials that is so important in the adult auditory system. In humans, myelination of the auditory nerve and the major brainstem pathways begins at the twenty-sixth week of gestation, and it is at around this age that the first responses to sound can be measured. One way of showing this is to measure event-related potentials from the scalp of premature infants born soon after this age. But even within the womb it is possible to demonstrate that the fetus can hear by measuring the unborn baby's movements or changes in heart rate that occur in response to vibroacoustic stimulation applied to the mother's abdomen. Such measurements have confirmed that hearing onset occurs at around the end of the second trimester.

External sounds will, of course, be muffled by the mother's abdominal wall and masked by noises produced by her internal organs. A video clip showing the likely sounds the fetus will encounter is available on the book's Web site. It is therefore perhaps not immediately clear what types of sound would actually reach the fetus. Attempts to record responses from the inner ear of fetal sheep, however, suggest that low-frequency speech could be audible to human infants (Smith et al., 2003), and there is some evidence that, toward the end of pregnancy, the human fetus not only responds to but can even discriminate between different speech sounds (Shahidullah & Hepper, 1994).

7.2   Hearing Capabilities Improve after Birth

Because of the extensive prenatal development of the auditory system, human infants are born with a quite sophisticated capacity to make sense of their auditory world. They can readily distinguish between different phonemes, and are sensitive to the pitch and rhythm of their mother's voice. Within a few days of birth, babies show a preference for their mother's voice over that of another infant's mother, presumably as a result of their prenatal experience (DeCasper & Fifer, 1980). Perhaps more surprisingly, various aspects of music perception can be demonstrated early in infancy. These include an ability to distinguish different scales and chords and a preference for consonant or pleasant-sounding intervals, such as the perfect fifth, over dissonant intervals (Trehub, 2003), as well as sensitivity to the beat of a rhythmic sound pattern (Winkler et al., 2009b).

Whether these early perceptual abilities are unique to human infants or specifically related to language and music is still an open question. Mark Hauser at Harvard University and others have addressed these questions from an evolutionary perspective by investigating whether animals, and in particular nonhuman primates, can perceive speech and music in a related fashion. In one such study, Kuhl and Miller (1975) showed that adult chinchillas are able to perceive phonemes categorically in a similar fashion to human infants. But while some marked similarities certainly exist between the abilities of humans and some other species to distinguish speech sounds, pointing to the involvement of common processing mechanisms, few behavioral studies have been carried out in very young animals.

It would be wrong to conclude from this, however, that human infants can hear the world around them in the same way that adults do. Almost all auditory perceptual abilities improve gradually after birth, and the age at which adult performance is reached varies greatly with the task. For example, sounds have to be played at a greater intensity to evoke a response from an infant, and, particularly for low-frequency tones, it can take as long as a decade until children possess the same low detection thresholds seen in adults. The capacity to detect a change in the frequency of two sequentially played tones also continues to improve over several years, although frequency resolution—the detection of a tone of one frequency in the presence of masking energy at other frequencies—seems to mature earlier.

Another aspect of hearing that matures over a protracted period of postnatal development is sound localization. While parents will readily attest to the fact that newborn infants can turn toward their voices, the accuracy of these orienting responses increases with age. Figure 7.1 shows that the minimum audible angle—the smallest detectable change in sound source location—takes about 5 years to reach adult values. As we saw in chapter 5, having two ears also helps in detecting target sounds against a noisy background. The measure of this ability, the binaural masking level difference, takes

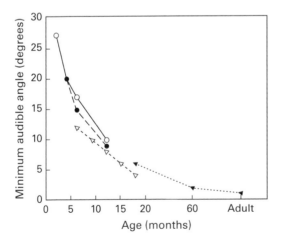

Figure 7.1
Minimum audible angles, a measure of the smallest change in the direction of a sound source that can be reliably discriminated, decrease with age in humans. Symbols represent different studies.
Based on Clifton (1992).

at least 5 years and possibly much longer to mature (Hall, Buss, & Grose, 2007). This is also the case for the precedence effect (Litovsky, 1997), indicating that the capacity to perceive sounds in the reverberant environments we encounter in our everyday lives emerges over a particularly long period.

Highly relevant to the perception of speech and music is the development of auditory temporal processing. Estimates of the minimum time period within which different acoustic events can be distinguished have been obtained using a variety of methods. These include the detection of amplitude and frequency modulation, gap detection— the smallest detectable silent interval in a sound—and nonsimultaneous masking paradigms. Although quite wide variations have been found in the age at which adult values are attained with the precise task and type of sound used, it is clear that temporal resolution also takes a long time to reach maturity. For example, "backward masking," which measures the ability of listeners to detect a tone that is followed immediately by a noise, has been reported to reach adult levels of performance as late as 15 years of age.

To make sense of all this, we need to take several factors into account. First, there is, of course, the developmental status of the auditory system. Although the ear and auditory pathways are sufficiently far advanced in their development to be able to respond to sound well before birth in humans, important and extensive changes continue to take place for several years into postnatal life. Second, "nonsensory" or cognitive factors will contribute to the performance measured in infants. These factors include attention, motivation, and memory, and they often present particular challenges when trying to assess auditory function in the very young.

We can account for the maturation of certain hearing abilities without having to worry about what might be happening in the brain at the time. This is because changes in auditory performance can be attributed to the postnatal development of the ear itself. For instance, the elevated thresholds and relatively flat audiogram seen in infancy are almost certainly due to the immature conductive properties of the external ear and the middle ear that are found at that age. As these structures grow, the resonant frequencies of the external ear decrease in value and the acoustic power transfer of the middle ear improves. In both cases, it takes several years for adult values to be reached, a timeframe consistent with age-related improvements in hearing sensitivity.

Growth of the external ears and the head also has considerable implications for sound localization. As we saw in chapter 5, the auditory system determines the direction of a sound source from a combination of monaural and binaural spatial cues. The values of those cues will change as the external ears grow and the distance between them increases (figure 7.2). As we shall see later, when we look at the maturation of the neural circuits that process spatial information, age-related differences in the cue values can account for the way in which the spatial receptive fields of auditory neurons

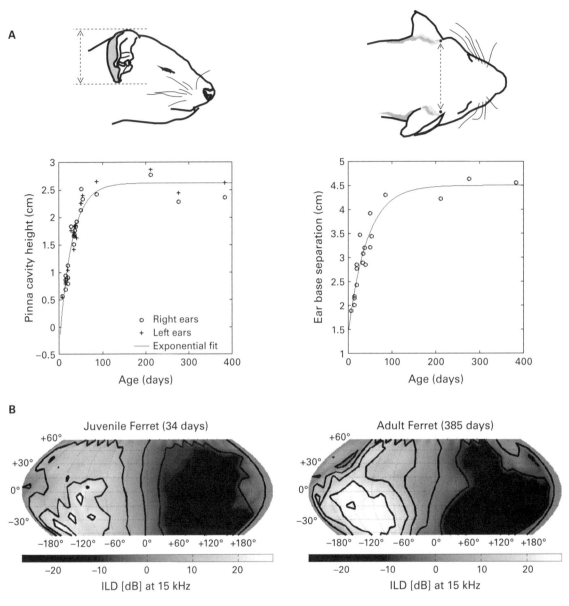

Figure 7.2

Growth of the head and external ears changes the acoustic cue values corresponding to each direction in space. (A) Age-related changes in the height of the external ear and in the distance between the ears of the ferret, a species commonly used for studying auditory development. These dimensions mature by around 4 months of age. (B) Variation in interaural level differences (ILDs) for a 15-kHz tone as a function of azimuth and elevation in a 34-day-old juvenile ferret (left) and in an adult animal at 385 days of age (right). The range of ILDs is larger and their spatial pattern is somewhat different in the older animal.

Based on Schnupp, Booth, and King (2003).

change during development. In turn, it is likely that this will contribute to the gradual emergence of a child's localization abilities.

The range of audible frequencies appears to change in early life as a result of developmental modifications in the tonotopic organization of the cochlea. You should now be very familiar with the notion that the hair cells near the base of the cochlea are most sensitive to high-frequency sounds, whereas those located nearer its apex are tuned to progressively lower frequencies. Although the basal end of the cochlea matures first, studies in mammals and chicks have shown that this region initially responds to lower sound frequencies than it does in adults. This is followed by an increase in the sound frequencies to which each region of the cochlea is most responsive, leading to an upward expansion in the range of audible sound frequencies. Such changes have not been described in humans, but it is possible that they take place before birth.

While the maturation of certain aspects of auditory perception is constrained by the development of the ear, significant changes also take place postnatally in the central auditory system. An increase in myelination of the auditory pathways results in a progressive reduction in the latency of the evoked potentials measured at the scalp in response to sound stimulation. At the level of the human brainstem, these changes are thought to be complete within the first 2 years of life. However, Nina Kraus and colleagues have recently shown that the brainstem responses evoked by speech sounds in 3- to 4-year-old children are delayed and less synchronous than those recorded in older children, whereas this difference across age is not observed with simpler sounds (Johnson et al., 2008). But it is the neural circuits at higher levels of the auditory system that mature most slowly, with sound-evoked cortical potentials taking around 12 years to resemble those seen in adults (Wunderlich & Cone-Wesson, 2006).

7.3   The Importance of Early Experience: Speech and Music

Although it remains difficult to determine how important the acoustic environment of the fetus is for the prenatal development of hearing, there is no doubt that the postnatal maturation of the central auditory pathways is heavily influenced by sensory experience. Because this process is so protracted, there is ample opportunity for the development of our perceptual faculties to be influenced by experience of the sounds we encounter during infancy. As we shall see in the following section, this also means that reduced auditory inputs, which can result, for example, from early hearing loss, and even information provided by the other senses can have a profound impact on the development of the central auditory system.

The importance of experience in shaping the maturing auditory system is illustrated very clearly by the acquisition of language during early childhood. Infants are initially able to distinguish speech sounds in any language. But as they learn from experience, this languagewide capacity quickly narrows. Indeed, during the first year of life, their ability to perceive phonetic contrasts in their mother tongue improves, while they lose their sensitivity to certain sound distinctions that occur only in foreign languages. You may remember from chapter 4 that this is nicely illustrated by the classic example of adult Japanese speakers, who struggle to distinguish the phonetic units "r" from "l," even though, at 7 months of age, Japanese infants are as adept at doing so as native English speakers (figure 7.3). In Japanese, these consonants fall within a single perceptual category, so Japanese children "unlearn" the ability to distinguish them. This process of becoming more sensitive to acoustic distinctions at phoneme boundaries of one's mother tongue, while becoming less sensitive to distinctions away from them, has been found to begin as early as 6 months of age for vowels and by 10 months for consonants (Kuhl & Rivera-Gaxiola, 2008). Perceptual narrowing based on a child's experience during infancy is not restricted to spoken language. Over the same time period, infants also become more sensitive to the correspondence between speech sounds and the talker's face in their own language, and less so for non-native language (Pons et al., 2009).

These changes in speech perception during the first year of life are driven, at least in part, by the statistical distribution of speech sounds in the language to which the infant is exposed. Thus, familiarizing infants with artificial speech sounds in which

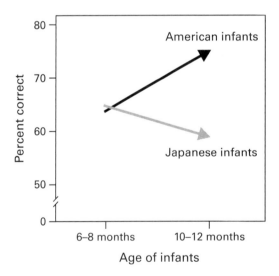

Figure 7.3
The effects of age on speech perception performance in a cross-language study of the perception of American English /r–l/ sounds by American and Japanese infants.
Based on Kuhl et al. (2006).

this distribution has been manipulated experimentally alters their subsequent ability to distinguish some of those sounds (Maye, Werker, & Gerken, 2002). But social interactions also seem to play a role. Kuhl, Tsao, and Liu (2003) showed that 9-month-old American infants readily learn phonemes and words in Mandarin Chinese, but only if they were able to interact with a live Chinese speaker. By contrast, no learning occurred if the same sounds were delivered by television or audiotape.

Not surprisingly, as a child's perceptual abilities become increasing focused on processing the language(s) experienced during early life, the capacity to learn a new language declines. In addition to the loss in the ability to distinguish phonemes in other languages during the first year of life, other aspects of speech acquisition, including the syntactic and semantic aspects of language, appear to be developmentally regulated (Ruben, 1997). The sensitive period of development during which language can be acquired with little effort lasts for about 7 years. New language learning then becomes more difficult, despite the fact that other cognitive abilities improve with age.

Sensitive periods have also been characterized for other aspects of auditory development. Perhaps the most relevant to language acquisition in humans is vocal learning in songbirds (figure 7.4). Young birds learn their songs by listening to adults during an initial sensitive period of development, the duration of which varies from one species to another and with acoustic experience and the level of hormones such as testosterone. After this purely sensory phase of learning, the birds start to make their own highly variable vocal attempts, producing what is known as "subsong," the equivalent of babbling in babies. They then use auditory feedback during a sensorimotor phase of learning to refine their vocalizations until a stable adult song is crystallized (Brainard & Doupe, 2002). Examples of the different song stages can be found on the book's Web site.

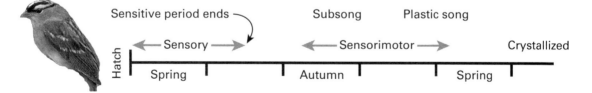

Figure 7.4
Birdsong learning stages. In seasonal species, such as the white-crowned sparrow, the sensory and sensorimotor phases of learning are separated in time. The initial vocalizations ("subsong") produced by young birds are variable and generic across individuals. Subsong gradually evolves into "plastic song," which, although still highly variable, begins to incorporate some recognizable elements of tutor songs. Plastic song is progressively refined until the bird crystallizes its stable adult song. Other songbirds show different time courses of learning.
Adapted from Brainard and Doupe (2002) with permission from Macmillan Publishers Ltd.

Thus, both human speech development and birdsong learning rely on the individual being able to hear the voices of others, as illustrated by Marler and Tamura's intriguing observation that, like humans, some songbirds possess regional dialects (Marler & Tamura, 1962). The importance of hearing the tutor song during a sensitive period of development has been demonstrated by raising songbirds with unrelated adults of the same species; as they mature, these birds start to imitate the songs produced by the tutor birds. On the other hand, birds raised in acoustic isolation—so that they are prevented from hearing the song of conspecific adults—produce abnormal vocalizations. This is also the case if songbirds are deafened before they have the opportunity to practice their vocalizations, even if they have previously been exposed to tutor songs; this highlights the importance of being able to hear their own voices as they learn to sing. In a similar vein, profound hearing loss has a detrimental effect on speech acquisition in children.

A related area where experience plays a key role is in the development of music perception. We have already pointed out that human infants are born with a remarkably advanced sensitivity to different aspects of music. As with their universal capacity to distinguish phonemes, infants initially respond in a similar way to the music of any culture. Their perceptual abilities change with experience, however, and become increasingly focused on the style of music to which they have been exposed. For example, at 6 months of age, infants are sensitive to rhythmic variations in the music of different cultures, whereas 12-month-olds show a culture-specific bias (Hannon & Trehub, 2005). The perception of rhythm in foreign music can nonetheless be improved at 12 months by brief exposure to an unfamiliar style of music, whereas this is not the case in adults.

Findings such as these again point to the existence of a sensitive period of development during which perceptual abilities can be refined by experience. As with the maturation of speech perception, passive exposure to the sounds of a particular culture probably leads to changes in neural sensitivity to the structure of music. But we also have to consider the role played by musical training. In chapter 3, we introduced the concept of absolute pitch—the ability to identify the pitch of a sound in the absence of a reference pitch. It seems likely that some form of musical training during childhood is a requirement for developing absolute pitch, and the likelihood of having this ability increases if that training starts earlier. This cannot, however, be the only explanation, as not all trained musicians possess absolute pitch. In addition, genetic factors appear to play a role in determining whether or not absolute pitch can be acquired.

There is considerable interest in being able to measure what actually goes on in the brain as auditory perceptual abilities change during development and with experience. A number of noninvasive brain imaging and electrophysiological recording methods are available to do this in humans (details of these methods are described briefly in Kuhl & Rivera-Gaxiola, 2008). Using these approaches, it has been shown that although language functions are lateralized at birth, the regions of the cerebral cortex involved are less specialized and the responses recorded from them are much slower in infants than they are in adults (Friederici, 2006; Kuhl & Rivera-Gaxiola, 2008). Event-related potentials (ERPs) are particularly suitable for studying time-locked responses to speech in young children. ERP measurements suggest that by 7.5 months of age, the brain is more sensitive to phonetic contrasts in the child's native language than in a non-native language (figure 7.5; Kuhl & Rivera-Gaxiola, 2008). This is in line with behavioral studies of phonetic learning. Intriguingly, the differences seen at this age in the ERP responses to native and non-native contrasts seem to provide an indicator of the rate at which language is subsequently acquired. Neural correlates of word learning can be observed toward the end of the first year of life, whereas violations of syntactic word order result in ERP differences at around 30 months after birth.

Some remarkable examples of brain plasticity have been described in trained musicians. Of course, speech and music both involve production (or playing, in the case of a musical instrument) as much as listening, so it is hardly surprising that motor as

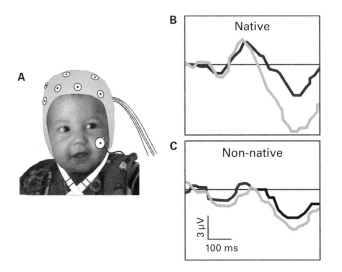

Figure 7.5
Neural correlates of speech perception in infancy. (A) Human infant wearing an ERP electrocap. (B) ERP waveforms recorded at 7.5 months of age from one sensor location in response to a native (English) and non-native (Mandarin Chinese) phonetic contrast. The black waveforms show the response to a standard stimulus, whereas the gray waveforms show the response to the deviant stimulus. The difference in amplitude between the standard and deviant waveforms is larger in the case of the native English contrast, implying better discrimination than for the non-native speech sounds.
Based on Kuhl and Rivera-Gaxiola (2008).

well as auditory regions of the brain can be influenced by musical training and experience. Neuroimaging studies have shown that musical training can produce structural and functional changes in the brain areas that are activated during auditory processing or when playing an instrument, particularly if training begins in early childhood. These changes most commonly take the form of an enlargement of the brain areas in question and enhanced musically related activity in them. One study observed structural brain plasticity in motor and auditory cortical areas of 6-year-old children who received 15 months of keyboard lessons, which was accompanied by improvements in musically relevant skills (Hyde et al., 2009). Because no anatomical differences were found before the lessons started between these children and an age-matched control group, it appears that musical training can have a profound effect on the development of these brain areas. In fact, plasticity is not restricted to the cerebral cortex, as functional differences are also found in the auditory brainstem of trained musicians (Kraus et al., 2009).

Imaging studies have also provided some intriguing insights into the basis of musical disorders. We probably all know someone who is tone deaf or unable to sing in tune. This condition may arise as a result of a reduction in the size of the arcuate fasciculus, a fiber tract that connects the temporal and frontal lobes of the cerebral cortex (Loui, Alsop, & Schlaug, 2009). Consequently, tone deafness, which is found in about 10% of the population, is likely to reflect reduced links between the brain regions involved in the processing of sound, including speech and music, and those responsible for vocal production.

7.4   Maturation of Auditory Circuits in the Brain

To track the changes that take place in the human brain during development and learning, we have to rely on noninvasive measures of brain anatomy and function. As in the mature brain, however, these methods tell us little about what is happening at the level of individual nerve cells and circuits. This requires a different approach, involving the use of more invasive experimental techniques in animals. In this section, we look at some of the cellular changes that take place during development within the central auditory pathway, and examine how they are affected by changes in sensory inputs.

The connections between the spiral ganglion cells and their targets in the cochlea and the brainstem provide the basis for the tonotopic representation of sound frequency within the central auditory system. These connections therefore have to be organized very precisely, and are thought to be guided into place at a very early stage of development by chemical signals released by the target structures (Fekete & Campero, 2007). The action potentials that are subsequently generated by the axons are not responsible just for conveying signals from the cochlea to the brain. They also influence the maturation of both the synaptic endings of the axons, including the large endbulbs of Held, which, as we saw in chapter 5, are important for transmitting temporal information with high fidelity, and the neurons in the cochlear nucleus (Rubel & Fritzsch, 2002). This is initially achieved through auditory nerve action potentials that are generated spontaneously, in the absence of sound, which are critical for the survival of the cochlear nucleus neurons until the stage at which hearing begins.

The earliest sound-evoked responses are immature in many ways. During the course of postnatal development, improvements are seen in the thresholds of auditory neurons, in their capacity to follow rapidly changing stimuli, and in phase locking, while maximum firing rates increase and response latencies decrease. Some of these response properties mature before others, and the age at which they do so varies at different levels of the auditory pathway (Hartley & King, 2010). Because it is the last structure to mature, a number of studies have focused on the development of the auditory cortex. Changes occur in the frequency selectivity of cortical neurons during infancy, a process that is greatly influenced by the acoustic environment. For example, Zhang, Bao, and Merzenich (2001) showed that exposing young rats to repeated tones of one frequency leads to a distortion of the tonotopic map, with a greater proportion of the auditory cortex now devoted to that frequency than to other values. This does not necessarily mean that the animals now hear better at these frequencies though; they actually end up being less able to discriminate sound frequencies within the enlarged representation, but better at doing so for those frequencies where the tonotopic map is compressed (Han et al., 2007). This capacity for cortical reorganization is restricted to a sensitive period of development, and different sensitive periods have been identified for neuronal sensitivity to different sound features, which coincide with the ages at which those response properties mature (Insanally et al., 2009). Linking studies such as these, in which animals are raised in highly artificial and structured environments, to the development of auditory perception in children is obviously not straightforward. It is clear, however, that the coding of different sounds by cortical neurons is very dependent on experience during infancy, and this is highly likely to influence the emergence of perceptual skills.

While the aforementioned studies emphasize the developmental plasticity of the cortex, subcortical circuits can also undergo substantial refinements under the influence of cochlear activity. These changes can have a considerable impact on the coding properties—particularly those relating to sound source localization—of auditory neurons. Neural sensitivity to ILDs and ITDs has been observed at the youngest ages examined in the lateral superior olive (LSO) (Sanes & Rubel, 1988) and medial superior olive (MSO) (Seidl & Grothe, 2005), respectively. The inhibitory projection from the medial nucleus of the trapezoid body to the LSO, which gives rise to neural sensitivity to ILDs (see chapter 5), undergoes an activity-dependent reorganization during the normal course of development (Kandler, 2004). Many of the initial connections die off and those that remain, rather bizarrely, switch from being excitatory to inhibitory before

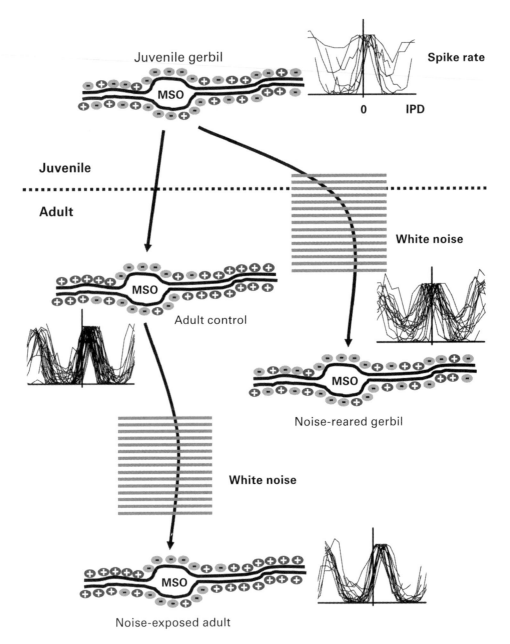

Figure 7.6

Maturation of brainstem circuits for processing interaural time differences. In juvenile gerbils, at around the time of hearing onset, excitatory (indicated by the pluses) and inhibitory inputs (the minuses) are distributed on the dendrites and somata of neurons in the medial superior olive undergoing further structural remodeling. In chapter 5, we saw that precisely timed inhibitory inputs to the gerbil MSO neurons can adjust their ITD sensitivity, so that the steepest—and therefore most informative—regions of the tuning functions lie across the range of values that can occur naturally given the size of the head. Benedikt Grothe and colleagues (Kapfer et al., 2002; Seidl and Grothe, 2005) showed that in very young gerbils these glycinergic synapses are initially distributed uniformly along each of the two dendrites of the MSO neurons. A little later in development, they disappear, leaving inhibitory inputs only on or close to the soma of the neurons, which is the pattern seen in adult gerbils (figure 7.6). This anatomical rearrangement alters the ITD sensitivity of the neurons, but occurs only if the animals receive appropriate auditory experience. If they are denied access to binaural localization cues, the infant distribution persists and the ITD functions fail to mature properly.

Changes in binaural cue sensitivity would be expected to shape the development of the spatial receptive fields of auditory neurons and the localization behaviors to which they contribute. Recordings from the superior colliculus (Campbell et al., 2008) and auditory cortex (Mrsic-Flogel, Schnupp, & King, 2003) have shown that the spatial tuning of the neurons is indeed much broader in young ferrets than it is in adult animals. But it turns out that this is due primarily to the changes in the localization cue values that take place as the head and ears grow. Thus, presenting infant animals with stimuli through "virtual adult ears" led to an immediate sharpening in the spatial receptive fields. This demonstrates that both peripheral and central auditory factors have to be taken into account when assessing how adult processing abilities are reached.

Nevertheless, it is essential that the neural circuits involved in sound localization are shaped by experience. As we have seen, the values of the auditory localization cues depend on the size and shape of the head and external ears, and consequently will vary from one individual to another. Each of us therefore has to learn to localize with our own ears. That this is indeed the case has been illustrated by getting listeners to localize sounds through someone else's ears. Once again, this can be achieved using virtual acoustic space stimuli. They fare much better when the stimuli are generated from acoustical measurements made from their own ears—the ones they have grown up with (Wenzel et al., 1993).

(MSO). At this age, neurons prefer interaural phase differences (IPD) around 0. By contrast, in adult gerbils, glycinergic inhibition is restricted to the cell soma and is absent from the dendrites and IPD response curves are shifted away from 0, so that the maximal slope lies within the physiological range. This developmental refinement depends on acoustic experience, as demonstrated by the effects of raising gerbils in omnidirectional white noise to eliminate spatial cues, which preserves the juvenile state. Exposing adults to noise has no effect on either the distribution of glycinergic synapses on the MSO neurons or their IPD functions.

From Seidl and Grothe (2005) with permission from the American Physiological Society.

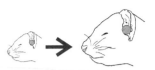

A Behavior

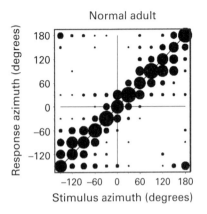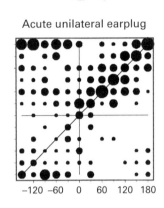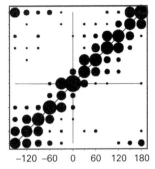

B Physiology

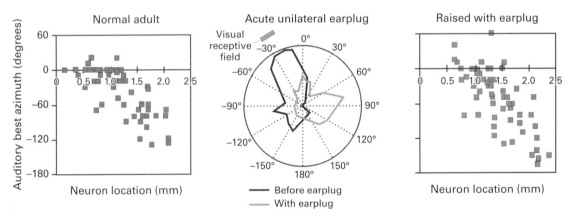

Figure 7.7
Auditory experience shapes the maturation of sound localization behavior and the map of auditory space in the superior colliculus. (A) Stimulus-response plots showing the combined data of three normally reared ferrets (normal adults), another three animals just after inserting an earplug into the left ear (adult unilateral earplug), and three ferrets that had been raised and tested with the left ear occluded with a plug that produced 30- to 40-dB attenuation (raised with earplug). These plots illustrate the distribution of approach-to-target responses (ordinate) as a function of stimulus location (abscissa). The stimuli were bursts of broadband noise. The size of the dots indicates, for a given speaker angle, the proportion of responses made to different response

Plasticity of auditory spatial processing has been demonstrated by manipulating the sensory cues available. For example, inducing a reversible conductive hearing loss by plugging one ear will alter the auditory cue values corresponding to different directions in space. Consequently, both sound localization accuracy and the spatial tuning of auditory neurons will be disrupted. However, if barn owls (Knudsen, Esterly, & Knudsen, 1984) or ferrets (King, Parsons, & Moore, 2000) are raised with a plug inserted in one ear, they learn to localize sounds accurately (figure 7.7A). Corresponding changes are seen in the optic tectum (Knudsen, 1985) and superior colliculus (King et al., 2000), where, despite the abnormal cues, a map of auditory space emerges in register with the visual map (figure 7.7B).

At the end of chapter 5, we discussed the influence that vision can have over judgments of sound source location in humans. A similar effect is also seen during development if visual and auditory cues provide spatially conflicting information. This has been demonstrated most clearly by providing barn owls with spectacles containing prisms that shift the visual world representation relative to the head. A compensatory shift in the accuracy of sound-evoked orienting responses and in the auditory spatial receptive fields of neurons in the optic tectum occurs in response to the altered visual inputs, which is brought about by a rewiring of connections in the midbrain (figure 7.8; Knudsen, 1999). A video clip of barn owl localization behavior during prism learning is available on the book's Web site. This experiment was possible because barn owls have a very limited capacity to move their eyes. In mammals, compensatory eye movements would likely confound the results of using prisms. Nevertheless, other approaches suggest that vision also plays a guiding role in aligning the different sensory representations in the mammalian superior colliculus (King et al., 1988). Studies in barn owls have shown that experience-driven plasticity is most pronounced during development, although the sensitive period for visual refinement of both the auditory space map and auditory localization behavior can be extended under certain conditions (Brainard & Knudsen, 1998).

Finally, we need to consider how complex vocalizations are learned. This has so far been quite difficult to investigate in nonhuman species, but studies of birdsong learning have provided some intriguing insights into the neural processing of complex

locations. Occluding one ear disrupts sound localization accuracy, but adaptive changes take place during development that enable the juvenile plugged ferrets to localize sound almost as accurately as the controls. (B) The map of auditory space in the ferret SC, illustrated by plotting the best azimuth of neurons versus their location within the nucleus. Occluding one ear disrupts this spatial tuning (in the example shown, by shifting the azimuth response profile to a different region of space), but, as with the behavioral data, near-normal spatial tuning is present in ferrets that were raised with one ear occluded. This indicates that adaptive plasticity is also seen in the neural responses.
Based on King, Parsons, and Moore (2000).

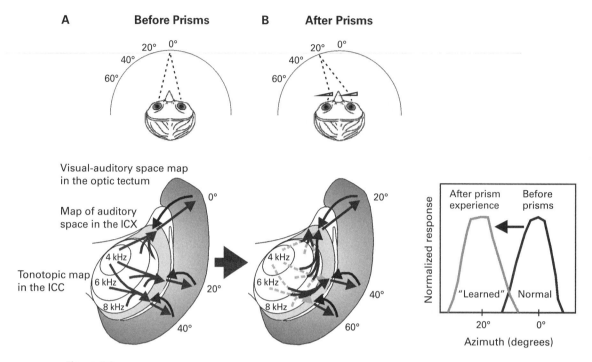

Figure 7.8

Visual experience shapes the map of auditory space in the midbrain of the barn owl. (A) The owl's inferior colliculus (ICX) contains a map of auditory space, which is derived from topographic projections that combine spatial information across different frequency channels in the central nucleus of the inferior colliculus (ICC). The ICX map of auditory space is then conveyed to the optic tectum, where it is superimposed on a map of visual space. (B) The auditory space maps in both the optic tectum and the ICX can be refined by visual experience during development. This has been demonstrated by chronically shifting the visual field in young owls by mounting prisms in front of their eyes. The same visual stimulus now activates a different set of neurons in the optic tectum. The auditory space maps in the ICX and tectum gradually shift by an equivalent amount in prism-reared owls, thereby reestablishing the alignment with the optically displaced visual map in the tectum. This involves growth of novel projections from the ICC to the ICX (black arrows); the original connections remain in place but are suppressed (dashed gray arrows). (C) Illustration for one neuron of the shift in auditory spatial tuning produced by prism rearing.

signals that evolve over time, and there is every reason to suppose that similar principles will apply to the development of sensitivity to species-specific vocalizations in mammals. In section 7.3, we described how vocal learning in songbirds is guided by performance feedback during a sensitive period of development. Several forebrain areas are thought to be involved in the recognition of conspecific song. In juvenile zebra finches, neurons in field L, the avian equivalent of the primary auditory cortex, are less acoustically responsive and less selective for natural calls over statistically equivalent synthetic sounds than they are in adult birds (Amin, Doupe, & Theunissen, 2007). Neuronal selectivity for conspecific songs emerges at the same age at which the birds express a behavioral preference for individual songs (Clayton, 1988), implicating the development of these response properties in the maturation of song recognition. The auditory forebrain areas project to a cluster of structures, collectively known as the "song system," which have been shown to be involved in vocal learning. Recording studies have shown that certain neurons of the song system prefer the bird's own song or the tutor's song over other complex sounds, including songs from other species (Margoliash, 1983), and that these preferences emerge following exposure to the animal's own vocal attempts (Solis & Doupe, 1999).

7.5   Plasticity in the Adult Brain

We have seen that many different aspects of auditory processing and perception are shaped by experience during sensitive periods of development. While the length of those periods can vary with sound property, brain level, and species, and may be extended by hormonal or other factors, it is generally accepted that the potential for plasticity declines with age. That would seem to make sense, since more stability may be desirable and even necessary in the adult brain to achieve the efficiency and reliability of a mature nervous system. But it turns out that the fully mature auditory system shows considerable adaptive plasticity that can be demonstrated over multiple timescales.

Numerous examples have been described where the history of stimulation can determine the responsiveness or even the tuning properties of auditory neurons. For example, if the same stimulus, say a tone of a particular frequency, is presented repeatedly, neurons normally show a decrease in response strength. However, the response can be restored if a different frequency is presented occasionally (Ulanovsky, Las, & Nelken, 2003). As we discussed in chapter 6, this phenomenon is known as stimulus-specific adaptation, and facilitates the detection of rare events and sudden changes in the acoustic environment. On the other hand, the sensitivity of auditory neurons can be adjusted so that the most frequently occurring stimuli come to be represented more precisely. A nice example of this "adaptive coding" was described by Dean and colleagues (2005), who showed that the relationship between the firing rate of inferior colliculus neurons and sound level can change to improve the coding of those levels that occur with the highest probability (figure 7.9). One important consequence of this is that a greater range of sound levels can be encoded, even though individual neurons have a relatively limited dynamic range.

These changes occur in passive hearing conditions and are therefore caused solely by adjustments in the statistics of the stimulus input. If a particular tone frequency is given behavioral significance by following it with an aversive stimulus, such as a mild electric shock, the responses of cortical neurons to that frequency can be enhanced (Weinberger, 2004). Responses to identical stimuli can even change over the course of a few minutes in different ways in a task-dependent fashion (Fritz, Elhilali, &

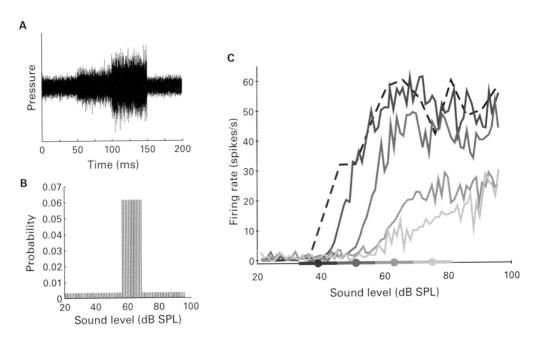

Figure 7.9

Adaptive coding of sound level by neurons in the guinea pig inferior colliculus. (A) Changes in the sensitivity of these neurons can be induced by presenting broadband stimuli for several seconds in which the sound level varies every 50 ms, but with a high-probability region centered on different values. (B) Distribution of sound levels in a stimulus with a high-probability region centered on 63 dB SPL. (C) Rate-level functions for one neuron for four different sound level distributions (indicated by the filled circles and thick lines on the x axis) plus the baseline function (dashed line). The functions shift as the high-probability region changes, so that maximum sensitivity is maintained over the range of sound levels that are most commonly encountered. Adapted from Dean, Harper, and McAlpine (2005) with permission from Macmillan Publishers Ltd.

Shamma, 2005), implying that this plasticity may reflect differences in the meaning of the sound according to the context in which it is presented.

Over a longer time course, the tonotopic organization of the primary auditory cortex of adult animals can change following peripheral injury. If the hair cells in a particular region of the cochlea are damaged as a result of exposure to a high-intensity sound or some other form of acoustic trauma, the area of the auditory cortex in which the damaged part of the cochlea would normally be represented becomes occupied by an expanded representation of neighboring sound frequencies (Robertson & Irvine, 1989). A similar reorganization of the cortex has been found to accompany improvements in behavioral performance that occur as a result of "perceptual learning." Recanzone, Schreiner, and Merzenich (1993) trained monkeys on a frequency discrimination task and reported that the area of cortex representing the tones used for training increased in parallel with improvements in discrimination performance. Since then, a number of other changes in cortical response properties have been reported as animals learn to respond to particular sounds. This does not necessarily involve a change in the firing rates or tuning properties of the neurons, as temporal firing patterns can be altered as well (Bao et al., 2004; Schnupp et al., 2006).

There is a key difference between the cortical changes observed following training in adulthood and those resulting from passive exposure to particular sounds during sensitive periods of development, in that the sounds used for training need to be behaviorally relevant to the animals. This was nicely demonstrated by Polley, Steinberg, and Merzenich (2006), who trained rats with the same set of sounds on either a frequency or a level recognition task. An enlarged representation of the target frequencies was found in the cortex of animals that learned the frequency recognition task, whereas the representation of sound level in these animals was unaltered. By contrast, training to respond to a particular sound level increased the proportion of neurons tuned to that level without affecting their tonotopic organization. These findings suggest that attention or other cognitive factors may dictate how auditory cortical coding changes according to the behavioral significance of the stimuli, which is thought to be signaled by the release in the auditory cortex of "neuromodulators" such as acetylcholine. Indeed, simply coupling the release of acetylcholine with the repeated presentation of a sound stimulus in untrained animals is sufficient to induce a massive reorganization of the adult auditory cortex (Kilgard, 2003).

Training can also dramatically improve the auditory perceptual skills of humans, and the extent to which learning generalizes to other stimuli or tasks can provide useful insights into the underlying neural substrates (Wright & Zhang, 2009). As in the animal studies, perceptual learning in humans can be accompanied by enhanced responses in the auditory cortex (Alain et al., 2007; van Wassenhove & Nagarajan, 2007). It is not, however, necessarily the case that perceptual learning directly reflects changes in brain areas that deal with the representation of the sound attribute in

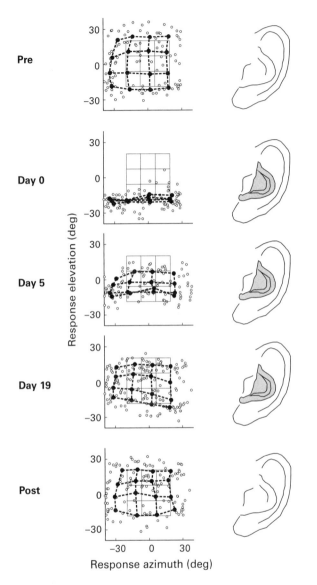

Figure 7.10

Learning to localize sounds with new ears in adult humans. In this study, the accuracy of sound localization was assessed by measuring eye movements made by human listeners toward the location of broadband sound sources. The stimuli were presented at random locations encompassed by the black grid in each of the middle panels. The end points of all the saccadic eye movements made by one subject are indicated by the small circles. The black dots and connecting lines represent the average eye movement vectors for targets located within neighboring sectors of the question. Thus, a substantial part of the improvement seen in pitch discrimination during perceptual learning tasks is nonspecific—for example, subjects playing a computer game while hearing pure tones (but not explicitly attending to these sounds) improve in pitch discrimination. The same was shown to be true even for subjects who played a computer game without hearing any pure tones (Amitay, Irwin, & Moore, 2006)! Such improvement must be due to general factors governing task performance rather than to specific changes in the properties of neurons in the auditory system.

In addition to improving the performance of subjects with normal hearing, training can promote the capacity of the adapt brain to adjust to altered inputs. This has been most clearly demonstrated in the context of sound localization. In the previous section, we saw that the neural circuits responsible for spatial hearing are shaped by experience during the phase of development when the localization cues are changing in value as a result of head growth. Perhaps surprisingly, the mature brain can also relearn to localize sound in the presence of substantially altered auditory spatial cues. Hofman, Van Riswick, and Van Opstal (1998) showed that adult humans can learn to use altered spectral localization cues. To do this, they inserted a mold into each external ear, effectively changing its shape and therefore the spectral cues corresponding to different sound directions. This led to an immediate disruption in vertical localization, with performance gradually recovering over the next few weeks (figure 7.10).

Because it relies much more on binaural cues, localization in the horizontal plane becomes inaccurate if an earplug is inserted in one ear. Once again, however, the mature auditory system can learn to accommodate the altered cues. This has been shown in both humans (Kumpik, Kacelnik, & King, 2010) and ferrets (Kacelnik et al., 2006), and seems to involve a reweighting away from the abnormal binaural cues so that greater use is made of spectral-shape information. This rapid recovery of sound localization accuracy occurs only if appropriate behavioral training is provided (figure 7.11). It is also critically dependent on the descending pathways from the auditory cortex to the midbrain (Bajo et al., 2010), which can modulate the responses of

stimulus grid. The overlap between the response and target matrices under normal listening conditions (pre) shows that saccadic eye movements are quite accurate in azimuth and elevation. Molds were then fitted to each external ear, which altered the spatial pattern of spectral cues. Measurements made immediately following application of the molds (day 0) showed that elevation judgments were severely disrupted, whereas azimuth localization within this limited region of space were unaffected. The molds were left in place for several weeks, and, during this period, localization performance gradually improved before stabilizing at a level close to that observed before the molds were applied. Interestingly, no aftereffect was observed after the molds were removed (post), as the subjects were able to localize sounds as accurately as they did in the precontrol condition. Adapted from Hofman, Van Riswick, and Van Opstal (1998) with permission from Macmillan Publishers Ltd.

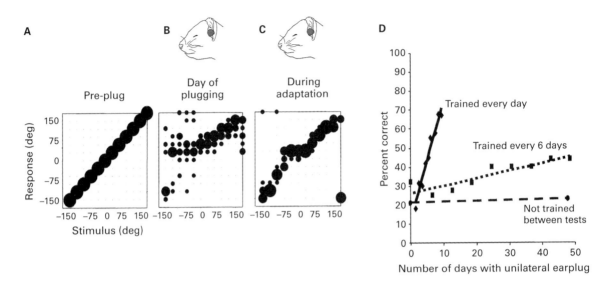

Figure 7.11

Plasticity of spatial hearing in adult ferrets. (A–C) Stimulus-response plots showing the distribution of responses (ordinate) made by a ferret as a function of stimulus location in the horizontal plane (abscissa). The size of the dots indicates, for a given speaker angle, the proportion of responses made to different locations. Correct responses are those that fall on the diagonal, whereas all other responses represent errors of different magnitude. Prior to occlusion of the left ear, the animal achieved 100% correct scores at all stimulus directions (A), but performed poorly, particularly on the side of the earplug, when the left ear was occluded (B). Further testing with the earplug still in place, however, led to a recovery in localization accuracy (C). (D) Mean change in performance (averaged across all speaker locations) over time in three groups of ferrets with unilateral earplugs. No change was found in trained ferrets ($n = 3$) that received an earplug for 7 weeks, but were tested only at the start and end of this period (circles and dashed regression line). These animals therefore received no training between these tests. Two other groups of animals received an equivalent amount of training *while* the left ear was occluded. Although the earplug was in place for less time, a much faster rate of improvement was observed in the animals that received daily training ($n = 3$; diamonds and solid regression line) compared to those that were tested every 6 days ($n = 6$; squares and dotted regression line).
From Kacelnik et al. (2006).

the neurons found there in a variety of ways (Suga & Ma, 2003). This highlights a very important, and often ignored, aspect of auditory processing, namely, that information passes down as well as up the pathway. As a consequence of this, plasticity in subcortical as well as cortical circuits is likely to be involved in the way humans and other species interact with their acoustic environments.

7.6   Summary: The Pros and Cons of Plasticity

We have seen in this chapter that the auditory system possesses a truly remarkable and often underestimated capacity to adapt to the sensory world. This is particularly the case in the developing brain, when newly formed neural circuits are refined by experience during specific and often quite narrow time windows. But the capacity to learn and adapt to the constantly changing demands of the environment is a lifelong process, which requires that processing in certain neural circuits can be modified in response to both short-term and long-term changes in peripheral inputs. The value of this plasticity is clear: Without it, it would not be possible to customize the brain to the acoustical cues that underlie our ability to localize sound or for the processing of native language. But the plasticity of the central auditory system comes at a potential cost, as this means that a loss of hearing, particularly during development, can induce a rewiring of connections and alterations in the activity of neurons, which might give rise to conditions such as tinnitus, in which phantom sounds are experienced in the absence of acoustic stimulation (Eggermont, 2008). At the same time, however, experience-dependent learning provides the auditory system with the capacity to accommodate the changes in input associated with hearing loss and its restoration, a topic that we shall return to in the final chapter.

8 Auditory Prostheses: From the Lab to the Clinic and Back Again

Hearing research is one of the great scientific success stories of the last 100 years. Not only have so many interesting discoveries been made about the nature of sound and the workings of the ear and the auditory brain, but these discoveries have also informed many immensely useful technological developments in entertainment and telecommunications as well as for clinical applications designed to help patients with hearing impairment.

Having valiantly worked your way through the previous chapters of the book, you will have come to appreciate that hearing is a rather intricate and subtle phenomenon. And one sad fact about hearing is that, sooner or later, it will start to go wrong in each and every one of us. The workings of the middle and inner ears are so delicate and fragile that they are easily damaged by disease or noise trauma or other injuries, and even those who look after their ears carefully cannot reasonably expect them to stay in perfect working order for over 80 years or longer. The consequences of hearing impairment can be tragic. No longer able to follow conversations with ease, hearing impaired individuals can all too easily become deprived of precious social interaction, stimulating conversation, and the joy of listening to music. Also, repairing the auditory system when it goes wrong is not a trivial undertaking, and many early attempts at restoring lost auditory function yielded disappointing results. But recent advances have led to technologies capable of transforming the lives of hundreds of thousands of deaf and hearing impaired individuals. Improved hearing aid and cochlear implant designs now enable many previously profoundly deaf people to pick up the phone and call a friend.

And just as basic science has been immensely helpful in informing design choices for such devices, the successes, limitations, or failures of various designs are, in turn, scientifically interesting, as they help to confirm or disprove our notions of how the auditory system operates. We end this book with a brief chapter on hearing aids and cochlear implants in particular. This chapter is not intended to provide a systematic or comprehensive guide to available devices, or to the procedures for selecting or fitting them. Specialized audiology texts are available for that purpose. The aim of this chapter is rather to present a selection of materials chosen to illustrate how the fundamental science that we introduced in the previous chapters relates to practical and clinical applications.

8.1   Hearing Aid Devices Past and Present

As we mentioned in chapter 2, by far the most common cause of hearing loss is damage to cochlear hair cells, and in particular to outer hair cells whose purpose seems to be to provide a mechanical amplification of incoming sounds. Now, if problems stem from damage to the ear's mechanical amplifier, it would make sense to try to remedy the situation by providing alternative means of amplification. Hearing loss can also result from pathologies of the middle ear, such as otosclerosis, a disease in which slow, progressive bone growth on the middle ear ossicles reduces the efficiency with which airborne sounds are transmitted to the inner ear. In such cases of conductive hearing loss, amplification of the incoming sound can also be beneficial.

The simplest and oldest hearing aid devices sought to amplify the sound that enters the ear canal by purely mechanical means. So-called ear trumpets were relatively widely used in the 1800s. They funneled collected sound waves down a narrowing tube to the ear canal. In addition to providing amplification by collecting sound over a large area, they had the advantage of fairly directional acoustic properties, making it possible to collect sound mostly from the direction of the sound source of interest.

Ear trumpets do, of course, have many drawbacks. Not only are they fairly bulky, awkward, and technologically rather limited, many users would also be concerned about the "cosmetic side effects." Already in the 1800s, many users of hearing aids were concerned that these highly conspicuous devices might not exactly project a very youthful and dynamic image. Developing hearing aids that could be hidden from view therefore has a long history. King John VI of Portugal, who reigned from 1816 to 1826 and was very hard of hearing, had a particularly curious solution to this problem. He had a throne constructed in which an ear trumpet was worked into one of the arm rests, disguised as an elaborately carved lion head. This ear trumpet was then connected to the enthroned King's ear via a tube (see figure 8.1). Subjects wishing to address the King were required to kneel and speak directly into the lion's mouth.

The design of King John VI's chair is certainly ingenious, but not very practical. Requiring anyone who wishes to speak with you to kneel and address you through the jaws of your carved lion might be fun for an hour or so, but few psychologically well-balanced individuals would choose to hold the majority of their conversations in that manner. It is also uncertain whether the hearing aid chair worked all that well for King John VI. His reign was beset by intrigue, both his sons rebelled against him,

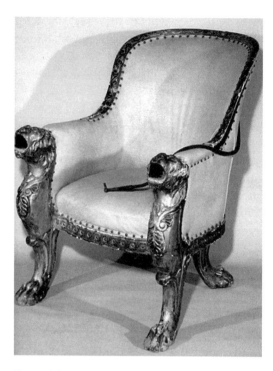

Figure 8.1
A chair with in-built ear trumpet, which belonged to King John VI of Portugal.

and he ultimately died from arsenic poisoning. Thus, it would seem that the lion's jaws failed to pick up on many important pieces of court gossip.

Modern hearing aids are thankfully altogether more portable, and they now seek to overcome their cosmetic shortcomings not by intricate carving, but through miniaturization, so that they can be largely or entirely concealed behind the pinna or in the ear canal. And those are not the only technical advances that have made modern devices much more useful. A key issue in hearing aid design is the need to match and adapt the artificial amplification provided by the device to the specific needs and deficits of the user. This is difficult to do with simple, passive devices such as ear trumpets. In cases of conductive hearing loss, all frequencies tend to be affected more or less equally, and simply boosting all incoming sounds can be helpful. But in the countless patients with sensorineural hearing loss due to outer hair cell damage, different frequency ranges tend to be affected to varying extents. It is often the case that sensorineural hearing loss affects mostly high frequencies. If the patient is supplied with a device that amplifies all frequencies indiscriminately, then such a device would most likely overstimulate the patient's still sensitive low-frequency hearing before it amplifies the higher frequencies enough to bring any benefit. The effect of such a device would be to turn barely comprehensible speech into unpleasantly loud booming noises. It would not make speech clearer.

You may also remember from section 2.3 that the amplification provided by the outer hair cells is highly nonlinear and "compressive," that is, the healthy cochlea amplifies very quiet sounds much more than moderately loud ones, which gives the healthy ear a very wide "dynamic range," allowing it to process sounds over an enormous amplitude range. If this nonlinear biological amplification is replaced by an artificial device that provides simple linear amplification, users often find environmental sounds transition rather rapidly from barely audible to uncomfortably loud. Adjusting such devices to provide a comfortable level of loudness can be a constant struggle. To address this, modern electronic hearing aids designed for patients with sensorineural hearing loss offer nonlinear compressive amplification and "dynamic gain control."

Thus, in recent years, hearing aid technology has become impressively sophisticated, and may incorporate highly directional microphones, as well as digital signal processing algorithms that transpose frequency bands, allowing information in the high-frequency channels in which the patient has a deficit to be presented to the still intact low-frequency part of the cochlea. And for patients who cannot receive the suitably amplified, filtered, and transposed sound through the ear canal, perhaps because of chronic or recurrent infections, there are even bone-anchored devices that deliver the sound as mechanical vibration of a titanium plate embedded in the skull, or directly vibrate the middle ear ossicles by means of a small transducer system implanted directly in the middle ear.

With such a wide variety of technologies available, modern hearing aid devices can often bring great benefit to patients, but only if they are carefully chosen and adjusted to fit each patient's particular needs. Otherwise they tend to end up in a drawer, gathering dust. In fact, this still seems to be the depressingly common fate of many badly fitted hearing aids. It has been estimated (Kulkarni & Hartley, 2008) that, of the 2 million hearing aids owned by hearing impaired individuals in the UK in 2008, as many as 750,000, more than one third, are not being used on a regular basis, presumably because they fail to meet the patient's needs. Also, a further 4 million hearing impaired individuals in the UK who could benefit from hearing aids do not own one, most likely because they lack faith in the devices or are unaware of the benefits they could bring. This is unfortunate, given that a suitably chosen and well-fitted modern device can often bring great benefits even to very severely hearing impaired patients (Wood & Lutman, 2004).

To work at their best, hearing aids should squeeze as much useful acoustic information as possible into the reduced frequency and dynamic range that remains available to the patient. As we shall see in the following sections, the challenges for cochlear implant technology are similar, but tougher, as cochlear implants have so far been used predominantly in patients with severe or profound hearing loss (thresholds above 75 dB SPL) over almost the entire frequency range, so very little normal functional hearing is left to work with.

8.2 The Basic Layout of Cochlear Implants

Cochlear implants are provided to the many patients who are severely deaf due to extensive damage to their hair cells. Severe hearing loss caused by middle ear disease can often be remedied surgically. Damaged tympanic membranes can be repaired with skin grafts, and calcified ossicles can be trimmed or replaced. But at present there is no method for regenerating or repairing damaged or lost sensory hair cells in the mammalian ear. And when hair cells are lost, the auditory nerve fibers that normally connect to them are themselves at risk and may start to degenerate. It seems that auditory nerve fibers need to be in contact with hair cells to stay in the best of health. But while this anterograde degeneration of denervated auditory nerve fibers is well documented, and can even lead to cell death and shrinkage in the cochlear nuclei, it is a very slow process and rarely leads to a complete degeneration of the auditory afferents. Also, a patient's hearing loss is often attributable to outer hair cell damage. Without the amplification provided by these cells, the remaining inner hair cells are incapable of providing sensitive hearing, but they nevertheless survive and can exercise their beneficial trophic influences on the many type I auditory nerve fibers that contact them. Consequently, even after many years of profound deafness, most hearing impaired patients still retain many thousand auditory nerve fibers, waiting for auditory input. Cochlear implants are, in essence, simple arrays of wires that stimulate these nerve fibers directly with pulses of electrical current.

Of course, the electrical stimulation of the auditory nerve needs to be as targeted and specific as one can make it. Other cranial nerves, such as the facial nerve, run close to the auditory branch of the vestibulocochlear nerve, and it would be unfortunate if electrical stimulus pulses delivered down the electrodes, rather than evoking auditory sensations, merely caused the patient's face to twitch. To achieve highly targeted stimulation with an extracellular electrode, it is necessary to bring the electrode contacts into close proximity to the targeted auditory nerves. And to deliver lasting benefits to the patient, they need to stay there, for many years. At present, practically all cochlear implant devices in clinical use achieve this by inserting the electrode contacts into the canals of the cochlea.

Figure 8.2 shows the layout of a typical modern cochlear implant. The intracochlear electrode is made of a plastic sheath fitted with electrode contacts. It is threaded into the cochlea, either through the round window or through a small hole drilled into the bony shell of the cochlea just next to the round window. The electrode receives

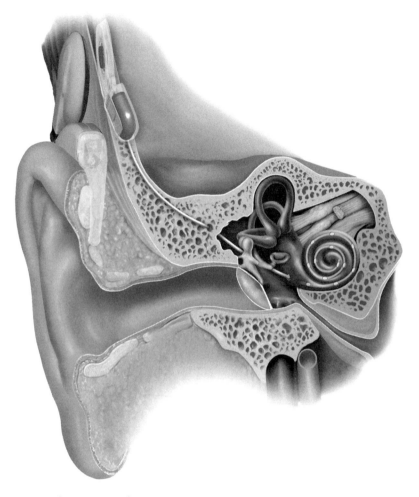

Figure 8.2
A modern cochlear implant.
Image kindly provided by MedEl, Austria.

its electrical signals from a receiver device, which is implanted under the scalp, on the surface of the skull, somewhat above and behind the outer ear. This subcutaneous device in turn receives its signals and its electrical energy via an induction coil from a headpiece radio transmitter. Small, strong magnets fitted into the subcutaneous receiver and the transmitter coil hold the latter in place on the patient's scalp. The transmitter coil in turn is connected via a short cable to a "speech processor," which is usually fitted behind the external ear. This speech processor collects sounds from the environment through a microphone and encodes them into appropriate electrical signals to send to the subcutaneous receiver. It also supplies the whole circuitry with electrical power from a battery. We will have a lot more to say about the signal processing that occurs in the speech processor in just a moment, but first let's look in a bit more detail at how the intracochlear electrode is meant to interface with the structures of the inner ear.

When implanting the device, the surgeon threads the electrode through a small opening at or near the round window, up along the scala tympani, so as to place the electrode contacts as close as possible to the modiolus (the center of the cochlear helix). Getting the electrode to "hug the modiolus" is thought to have two advantages: First, it reduces the risk that the electrode might accidentally scratch the stria vascularis, which runs along the opposite external wall of the cochlear coil, and could bleed easily and cause unnecessary trauma. Second, it is advantageous to position the electrode contacts very close to the auditory nerve fibers, whose cell bodies, the spiral ganglion cells, live in a cavity inside the modiolus known as Rosenthal's canal.

Inserting an electrode into the cochlea is a delicate business. For example, it is thought to be important to avoid pushing the electrode tip through the basilar membrane and into the scala media or scala vestibuli, as that could damage auditory nerve fiber axons running into the organ of Corti. And, it is also thought that electrode contacts that are pushed through into the scala media or scala vestibuli are much less efficient at stimulating auditory nerve fibers than those that sit on the modiolar wall of the scala tympani. You may recall that the normal human cochlea helix winds through two and a half turns. Threading an electrode array from the round window through two and a half turns all the way up to the cochlear apex is not possible at present. Electrode insertions that cover the first, basal-most one to one and a quarter turns are usually as much as can reasonably be achieved. Thus, after even a highly successful CI operation, the electrode array will not cover the whole of the cochlea's tonotopic range, as there will be no contacts placed along much of the apical, low-frequency end.

Through its electrode contacts, the cochlear implant then aims to trigger patterns of activity in the auditory nerve fibers, which resemble, as much as possible, the activity that would be set up by the synaptic inputs from the hair cells if the organ of Corti on the basilar membrane were functional. What such normal patterns of activity should look like we have discussed in some detail in chapter 2. You may recall that, in addition to the tonotopic place code for sound frequency and the spike rate coding for sound intensity, a great deal of information about a sound's temporal structure is conveyed through the phase locked discharge patterns of auditory nerve fibers. This spike pattern information encodes the sound's amplitude envelope, its periodicity, and even the submillisecond timing of features that we rely on to extract interaural time differences for spatial hearing. Sadly, the intracochlear electrode array cannot hope to reproduce the full richness of information that is encoded by a healthy organ of Corti. There are quite serious limitations of what is achievable with current technology, and many compromises must be made. Let us first consider the place coding issue.

8.3   Place Coding with Cochlear Implants

If the electrodes can only cover the first of the two and a half turns of the cochlea, then you might expect that less than half of the normal tonotopic range is covered by the electrode array. Indeed, if you look back at figure 2.3, which illustrated the tonotopy of the normal human basilar membrane, you will see that the first, basal-most turn of the human cochlea covers the high-frequency end, from about 20 to 1.2 kHz or so. The parts of the basilar membrane that are most sensitive to frequencies lower than that are beyond the reach of current cochlear implant designs. This high-frequency bias could be problematic. You may recall that the formants of human speech, which carry much of the phonetic information, all evolve at relatively low frequencies, often as low as just a few hundred hertz.

Poor coverage of the low-frequency end is an important limitation for cochlear implants, but it is not as big a problem as it may seem at first glance, for two reasons. First, Rosenthal's canal, the home of the cell bodies of the auditory nerve fibers, runs alongside the basilar membrane for only about three quarters of its length, and does not extend far into the basilar membrane's most apical turn. The spiral ganglion cells that connect to the low-frequency apical end of the basilar membrane cover the last little stretch with axons that fan out over the last turn, rather than positioning themselves next to the apical points on the basilar membrane they innervate (Kawano, Seldon, & Clark, 1996). Consequently, there is a kind of anatomical compression of the tonotopy of the spiral ganglion relative to that of the organ of Corti, and an electrode array that runs along the basilar membrane for 40% of its length from the basal end may nevertheless come into close contact with over 60% of spiral ganglion cells. Second, it seems that our auditory system can learn to understand speech fairly well even if formant contours are shifted up in frequency. In fact, implantees who had previous experience of normal hearing often describe the voices they hear through the implants as "squeaky" or "Mickey Mouse-like" compared to the voices they used to experience, but they can nevertheless understand the speech well enough to hold a telephone conversation.

Trying to get cochlear implants to cover a wide range of the inner ear's tonotopy is one issue. Another technical challenge is getting individual electrode contacts to target auditory nerve fibers so that small parts of the tonotopic array can be activated selectively. It turns out that electrical stimuli delivered at one point along the electrode array tend to spread sideways and may activate not just one or a few, but many neighboring frequency channels. This limits the frequency resolution that can be achieved with cochlear implants, and constitutes another major bottleneck of this technology.

Obviously, the number of separate frequency channels that a cochlear implant delivers can never be greater than the number of independent electrode contacts that can be fitted on the implant. The first ever cochlear implants fitted to human patients in the 1950s had just a single channel (Djourno & Eyries, 1957), and were intended to provide a lip-reading aid and generate a basic sound awareness. They were certainly not good enough to allow the implantees to understand speech. At the time of writing, the number of channels in implants varies with the manufacturer, but is usually less than twenty five. This is a very small number given that the device is aimed to replace tonotopically organized input from over 3,000 separate inner hair cells in the healthy human cochlea. You might therefore think that it would be desirable to increase this number further.

However, simply packing greater and greater numbers of independent contacts onto the device is not enough. Bear in mind that the electrode contacts effectively float in the perilymphatic fluid that fills the scala tympani, and any voltage applied to the contacts will provoke current flows that may spread out in all directions, and affect auditory nerve fibers further afield almost as much as those in the immediate vicinity. There is little point in developing electrodes with countless separate contacts if the "cross talk" between these contacts is very high and the electrodes cannot deliver independent information because each electrode stimulates very large, and largely overlapping, populations of auditory nerve fibers. Somehow the stimulating effect of each electrode contact must be kept local.

One strategy that aims to achieve this is the use of so-called bipolar, or sometimes even tripolar, rather than simple monopolar electrode configurations. A bipolar configuration, rather than delivering voltage pulses to each electrode contact independently, delivers voltage pulses of opposite polarity in pairs of neighboring electrode sites. Why would that be advantageous? An electrode influences neurons in its vicinity by virtue of the electric field it generates when a charge is applied to it (compare figure 8.3). The field will cause any charged particles in the vicinity, such as sodium ions in the surrounding tissue, to feel forces of electrostatic attraction toward or repulsion away from the electrode. These forces will cause the charges to move, thus setting up electric currents, which in turn may depolarize the membranes of neurons in the vicinity to the point where these neurons fire action potentials. The density of the induced currents will be proportional to the voltage applied, but will fall off with distance from the electrode according to an inverse square law. Consequently, monopolar electrodes will excite nearby neurons more easily than neurons that are further away, and while this decrease with distance is initially dramatic, it does "level off" to an extent at greater distances. This is illustrated in figure 8.3A. The little arrows point in the direction of the electric force field, and their length

A   B

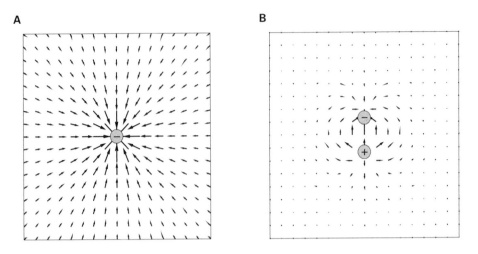

Figure 8.3
Electric fields created by monopolar (A) and bipolar (B) electrodes.

is proportional to the logarithm of the size of the electric forces available to drive currents at each point.

In a bipolar electrode arrangement, as illustrated in figure 8.3B, equal and opposite charges are present at a pair of electrode contacts in close vicinity. Each of these electrodes produces its own electrostatic field, which conforms to the inverse square law, and a nearby charged particle will be attracted to one and repelled by the other electrode in the pair. However, seen from points a little further afield, the two electrodes with their opposite charges may seem to lie "more or less equally far away," and in "more or less the same direction," and the attractive and repulsive forces exercised by the two electrodes will therefore cancel each other at these more distant points. Over distances that are large compared to the separation of the electrodes, the field generated by a bipolar electrode therefore declines much faster than one generated by a monopolar electrode. (Note that the electric field arrows around the edges of figure 8.3B are shorter than those in panel A.) In theory, it should therefore be possible to keep the action of cochlear implant electrodes more localized when the electrode contacts are used in pairs to produce bipolar stimulation, rather than driving each electrode individually.

We say "in theory," because experimental evidence suggests that, in practice, the advantage bipolar electrode arrangements offer tends to be modest. For example, Bierer and Middlebrooks (2002) examined the activation of cortical neurons achieved in a guinea pig that had received a scaled-down version of a human cochlear implant. The implant had six distinct stimulating electrode sites, and brief current pulses were delivered, either in a monopolar configuration, each site being activated in isolation, or in a bipolar mode, with pairs of adjacent electrodes being driven in opposite polarities. Cortical responses to the electrical stimuli were recorded through an array of sixteen recording electrodes placed along a 1.5-mm-long stretch of the guinea pig cortex, a stretch that covers the representation of about two to three octaves of the tonotopic axis in this cortical field. Figure 8.4 shows a representative example of the data they obtained.

The gray scale shows the normalized spike rate observed at the cortical location, shown on the y-axis at the time following stimulus onset on the x-axis. Cortical neurons responded to the electrical stimulation of the cochlea with a brief burst of nerve impulses. And while any one stimulating electrode caused a response over a relatively wide stretch of cortical tissue, the "center of gravity" of the neural activity pattern (shown by the black arrow heads) nevertheless shifts systematically as a function of the site of cortical stimulation. The activation achieved in bipolar mode is somewhat more focal than that seen with monopolar stimulation, but the differences are not dramatic.

Experiments testing the level of speech comprehension that can be achieved by implanted patients also fail to show substantial and consistent advantages of bipolar stimulation (Wilson, 2004). While patients tend to understand speech with monopolar or bipolar stimulation more or less equally well, there are very large differences in how well individual patients can understand speech at all, regardless of the stimulation mode. Much more important than the electrode configuration appears to be how

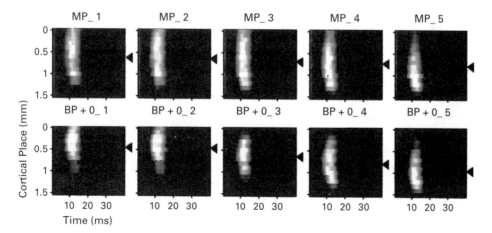

Figure 8.4
Activation of guinea pig auditory cortex in response to stimulation at five different sites on a cochlear implant with either monopolar (MP) or bipolar (BP) electrode configuration.
Adapted from figure 4 of Bierer and Middlebrooks (2002) with permission from the American Physiological Society.

many spiral ganglion cells survive, and how successfully the electrode can be implanted to bring the contacts into close proximity with these remaining nerve fibers. Even in monopolar configurations, the field strength initially drops off very rapidly due to the inverse square law, and if the electrodes are well positioned, the voltage delivered to the electrode can be adjusted so that only a limited set of neurons in the closer vicinity receive suprathreshold currents. If the electrode sites are quite distant from the spiral ganglion cells, however, selective stimulation cannot be achieved with either monopolar or bipolar stimulation.

Of course, for electrodes inserted into the scala tympani, the partition wall between the scala tympani and Rosenthal's canal sets absolute limits on how close the contacts can get to the neurons they are meant to stimulate, and this in turn limits the number of distinct channels of acoustic information that can be delivered through a cochlear implant. If electrodes could be implanted in the modiolus or the auditory nerve trunk to contact the auditory nerve fibers directly, this might increase the number of well-separated channels that could be achieved, and possible designs are being tested in animal experiments (Middlebrooks & Snyder, 2007). But the surgery involved in implanting these devices is somewhat riskier, and whether such devices would work well continuously for decades is at present uncertain. Also, in electrode arrays that target the auditory nerve directly, working out the tonotopic order of the implanted electrodes is less straightforward.

With any stimulating electrode, larger voltages will cause stronger currents, and the radius over which neurons are excited by the electrode will grow accordingly. The duration of a current pulse also plays a role, as small currents may be sufficient to depolarize a neuron's cell membrane to threshold provided that they are applied for long enough. To keep the effect of a cochlear implant electrode localized to a small set of spiral ganglion cells, one would therefore want to keep the stimulating currents weak and brief, but that is not always possible because cochlear implants signal changes in sound level by increasing or decreasing stimulus current, and implantees perceive larger currents (or longer current pulses) as "louder" (McKay, 2004; Wilson, 2004). In fact, quite modest increases in stimulus current typically evoke substantially louder sensations.

In normal hearing, barely audible sounds would typically be approximately 90 dB weaker than sounds that might be considered uncomfortably loud. In cochlear implants, in contrast, electrical stimuli grow from barely audible to uncomfortably loud if the current amplitude increases by only about 10 dB or so (McKay, 2004; Niparko, 2004). One of the main factors contributing to these differences between natural and electrical hearing is, of course, that the dynamic range compression achieved by the nonlinear amplification of sounds through the outer hair cells in normal hearing, which we discussed in section 2.3, is absent in direct electrical stimulation. Cochlear implants, just like many digital hearing aids, must therefore map sound amplitude onto stimulus amplitude in a highly nonlinear fashion.

Stronger stimulating currents, which signal louder sounds, will, of course, not just drive nearby nerve fibers more strongly, but also start to recruit nerve fibers increasingly further afield. In other words, louder sounds may mean poorer channel separation. To an extent this is a natural state of affairs, since, as we have seen in section 2.4, louder sounds also produce suprathreshold activation over larger stretches of the tonotopic array in natural hearing. However, we have also seen that, in natural hearing, temporal information provided through phase locking may help disambiguate place-coded frequency information at high sound levels (compare, for example, sections 2.4 and 4.3). In this manner, phase-locked activity with an underlying 500-Hz rhythm in a nerve fiber with a characteristic frequency of 800 Hz would be indicative of a loud 500-Hz tone. As we discuss further below, contemporary cochlear implants are sadly not capable of setting up similar temporal fine structure codes.

A lateral spread of activation with higher stimulus intensities could become particularly problematic if several electrode channels are active simultaneously. As we have just seen in discussing bipolar electrodes, cancellation of fields from nearby electrode channels can be advantageous (even if the benefits are in practice apparently not very large). Conversely, it has been argued that "vector addition" of fields generated by neighboring electrodes with the same polarity could be deleterious (McKay, 2004; Wilson & Dorman, 2009). Consequently, a number of currently available speech processors for cochlear implants are set up to avoid such potentially problematic channel interactions by never stimulating more than one electrode at a time. You may wonder how that can be done; after all, many sounds we hear are characterized by their distribution of acoustic energy across several frequency bands. So how is it possible to convey fairly complex acoustic spectra, such as the multiple formant peaks of a vowel, without ever activating more than one channel at a time? Clearly, this involves some trickery and some compromises, as we shall see in the next sections, where we consider the encoding of speech, pitch, and sound source location through cochlear implants.

8.4 Speech Processing Strategies Used in Cochlear Implants

You will recall from chapter 4 that, at least for English and most other Indo-European languages, semantic meaning in speech is carried mostly by the time-varying pattern of formant transitions, which are manifest as temporal modulations of between 1 and 7 Hz and spectral modulations of less than 4 cycles/kHz. Consequently, to make speech comprehensible, neither the spectral nor the temporal resolutions need to be very high. Given the technical difficulties involved in delivering a large number of well-separated spectral channels through a cochlear implant, this is a distinct advantage.

In fact, a paper by Bob Shannon and colleagues (1995) described a nice demonstration that as few as four suitably chosen frequency channels can be sufficient to achieve good speech comprehension. This was done by using a signal-processing technique known as "noise vocoding," which bears some similarity to the manner in which speech signals are processed for cochlear implants. Thus, when clinicians or scientists wish to give normally hearing individuals an idea of what the world would sound like through a cochlear implant, they usually use noise vocoded speech for these demonstrations. (You can find examples of noise vocoded sounds on the Web site that accompanies this book.) Further work by Dorman, Loizou, and Rainey (1997) has extended Shannon's vocoder results, and demonstrated that increasing the number of vocoded channels beyond six brings little additional benefit for the comprehension of speech in quiet situations. Consequently, if a cochlear implant device can deliver at least half a dozen or so reasonably well-separated frequency channels, there is a good chance that the implantee will be able to learn to use the device to understand speech well enough to use a telephone unaided.

The first step in noise vocoding, as well as in speech processing for cochlear implants, is to pass the recorded sound through a series of bandpass filters. This process is fundamentally similar to the gamma-tone filtering we described in sections 1.5 and 2.4 as a method for modeling the function of the basilar membrane, only speech processors and noise vocoders tend to use fewer, more broadly tuned, nonoverlapping filters. Figure 8.5C illustrates the output of such a filter bank, comprising six bandpass filters, in response to the acoustic waveform shown in figure 8.5A and B.

Bandpass filtering similar to that shown in figure 8.5 is the first step in the signal processing for all cochlear implant speech processors, but processors differ in what they then do with the output of the filters. One of the simplest processing strategies, referred to as the *simultaneous analog signal* (SAS) strategy, uses the filter outputs more or less directly as the signal that is fed to the stimulating electrodes. The filter outputs (shown by the gray lines in figure 8.5C) are merely scaled to convert them into alternating currents of an amplitude range that is appropriate for the particular electrode site they are sent to. The appropriate amplitude range is usually determined when the devices are fitted, simply by delivering a range of amplitudes to each site and asking the patient to indicate when the signal becomes uncomfortably loud. A close cousin of the SAS strategy, known as *compressive analog* (CA), differs from SAS only in the details of the amplitude scaling step.

Given that speech comprehension usually requires only modest levels of spectral resolution, SAS and CA speech processing can support good speech comprehension even though these strategies make no attempt to counteract potentially problematic channel interactions. But speech comprehension with SAS declines dramatically if there is much background noise, particularly if the noise is generated by other people speaking in the background, and it was thought that more refined strategies that

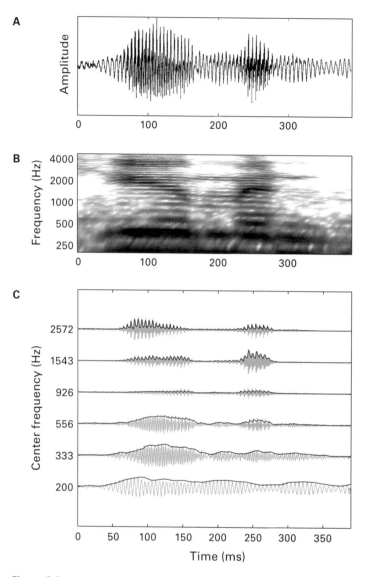

Figure 8.5

(A) Waveform of the word "human" spoken by a native American speaker. (B) Spectrogram of the same word. (C) Gray lines: Output of a set of six bandpass filters in response to the same word. The filter spacing and bandwidth in this example are two-thirds of an octave. The center frequencies are shown in the y-axis. Black lines: amplitude envelopes of the filter outputs, as estimated with half-wave rectification and bandpass filtering.

aim to achieve a better separation of a larger number of channels might be beneficial. The first strategy to work toward this goal is known as *continuous interleaved sampling* (CIS). A CIS device sends a train of continuous pulses to each of the electrode channels (Wilson, 2004). These pulses occur at a fixed rate of typically close to 1 kHz (but sometimes considerably higher, as in some modern "HiRes" devices), and the rate is the same on each channel; the pulses are offset in time ("interleaved"), however, so that adjacent electrode channels never receive exactly synchronized pulses. These interleaved pulse trains then serve as a carrier signal, and their amplitudes are modulated to follow the (again suitably scaled and compressed) amplitude envelope of the output of the corresponding bandpass filter (shown by the black lines in figure 8.5C). The resulting CIS signals are illustrated by the gray lines shown in figure 8.6.

Note, by the way, that the pulses used in CIS, and indeed in all pulsatile stimulation for cochlear implants, are "biphasic," meaning that each current pulse is always followed by a pulse of opposite polarity, so that, averaged over time, the net charge outflow out of the electrodes is zero. This is done because, over the long term, net currents flowing from or into the electrodes can have undesirable electrochemical consequences, and provoke corrosion of the electrode channels or toxic reactions in the tissue.

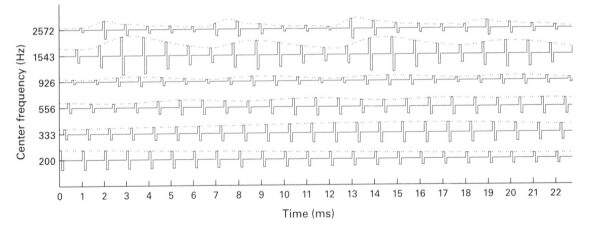

Figure 8.6
The continuous interleaved sampling (CIS) speech coding strategy. Amplitude envelopes from the output of a bank of bandpass filters (black dotted lines; compare figure 8.5C) are used to modulate the amplitude of regular biphasic pulse trains. The pulses for different frequency bands are offset in time so that no two pulses are on at the same time. The modulated pulses are then delivered to the cochlear implant electrodes.

Because in CIS, no two electrode channels are ever on simultaneously, there is no possibility of unwanted interactions of fields from neighboring channels. The basic CIS strategy delivers pulse trains, like those shown in figure 8.6, to each of the electrode contacts in the implant. A number of implants now have more than twenty channels, and the number of available channels is bound to increase as technology develops. One reaction to the availability of an increasing number of channels has been the emergence of numerous variants of the CIS strategy which, curiously, deliberately choose not to use all the available electrode channels. These strategies, with names like n-of-m, ACE ("advanced combinatorial encoder"), and SPEAK ("spectral peak"), use various forms of "dynamic peak picking" algorithms. Effectively, after amplitude extraction, the device uses only the amplitude envelopes of a modest number of frequency bands that happened to be associated with the largest amplitudes, and switches the low-amplitude channels off. The rationale is to increase the contrast between the peaks and troughs of the spectral envelopes of the sound, which could help create, for example, a particularly salient representation of the formants of a speech signal.

While all of these variants of CIS still use asynchronous, temporally interleaved pulses to reduce channel interactions, there are also algorithms being developed that deliberately synchronize current pulses out of adjacent electrodes in an attempt to create "virtual channels" by "current steering" (Wilson & Dorman, 2009). At its simplest, by simultaneously activating two adjacent channels, the developers are hoping to produce a peak of activity at the point between the two electrodes. However, the potential to effectively "focus" electrical fields onto points between the relatively modest number of contacts on a typical electrode is, of course, limited, and such approaches have so far failed to produce substantial improvements in speech recognition scores compared to older techniques. For a more detailed description of the various speech-processing algorithms in use today, the interested reader may turn to reviews by Wilson and colleagues (2004; 2009), which also discuss the available data regarding the relative effectiveness of these various algorithms.

One thing we can conclude from the apparent proliferation of speech-processing algorithms in widespread clinical use is that, at present, none of the available algorithms is clearly superior to any of the others. As Wilson (2004) pointed out, implantees who score highly on speech comprehension tasks with SAS also tend to do well with CIS, and vice versa. The key predictors for how well patients will hear with their implants remain the health of their auditory nerves, the age at implantation, whether the surgery went smoothly, and whether the patients are willing and able to adapt to the very different acoustic experience provided by an electrical device compared to natural hearing. Which of the many speech algorithms is used seems much less important, and is more a matter of personal preference. Some modern devices can be reprogrammed to offer the user a choice of algorithms. Even the number of electrode channels seems less critical than one might think, as long as the number is seven or more (Fishman, Shannon, & Slattery, 1997).

8.5 Pitch and Music Perception Through Cochlear Implants

As we have just seen, the majority of cochlear implant speech-processing strategies in use today rely on pulsatile stimulation, where pulses are delivered at a relatively high rate (1 kHz or more) to each stimulating electrode. The pulse rate is the same on each electrode, and is constant, independent of the input sound. The rationale behind this choice of pulse train carriers is to deliver sufficiently well-resolved spectral detail to allow speech recognition through a modest array of electrode contacts, which suffer from high levels of electrical cross-talk. But when you cast your mind back to our discussions of phase locking in chapter 2, and recall from chapter 3 that phase locking provides valuable temporal cues to the periodicity, and hence the pitch, of a complex sound, you may appreciate that the constant-rate current pulse carriers used in many cochlear implant coding strategies are in some important respects very unnatural. CIS or similar stimulation strategies provide the auditory nerve fibers with very little information about the temporal fine structure of the sound. Phase locking to the fixed-rate pulsatile carrier itself would transmit no information about the stimulus at all. Some fibers might conceivably be able to phase lock to some extent to the ampli- tude envelopes in the various channels (rounded to the nearest multiple of the carrier pulse rate), but the amplitude envelopes used in CIS to modulate the pulse trains are low-pass filtered at a few hundred hertz to avoid a phenomenon called "aliasing." Consequently, no temporal cues to the fundamental frequency of a complex sound above about 300 Hz survive after the sound has been processed with CIS or a similar strategy. And to infer the fundamental frequency from the harmonic structure of the sound would, as you may recall, require a very fine spectral resolution, which even a healthy cochlea may struggle to achieve, and which is certainly beyond what cochlear implants can deliver at present or in the foreseeable future. With these facts in mind, you will not be surprised to learn that the ability of implantees to distinguish the pitches of different sounds tends to be very poor indeed, with many implantees strug- gling to discriminate even pitch intervals as large as half an octave or greater (Sucher & McDermott, 2007).

   Against this background, you may wonder to what extent it even makes sense to speak about pitch perception at all in the context of electrical hearing with cochlear implants. This is a question worth considering further, and in its historical context (McKay, 2004). As you may recall from chapter 3, the American National Standards Institute (1994) defines pitch as "that auditory attribute of sound according to which sounds can be ordered on a scale from low to high." As soon as cochlear implants with multiple electrode sites became available, researchers started delivering stimulus pulses to either an apical or a basal site, asking the implantees which electrical stimulus "sounded higher." In such experiments, many implantees would reliably rank more basal stimulation sites as "higher sounding" than apical sites. These reported percepts were therefore in line with the normal cochlear tonotopic order. However, if, instead of delivering isolated pulses to various points along the cochlea, one stimulates just a single point on the cochlea with regular pulse trains and varies the pulse rates over a range from 50 to 300 Hz, implantees will also report higher pulse rates as "higher sounding," even if the place of stimulation has not changed (McKay, 2004; Moore and Carlyon, 2005; Shannon, 1983).

If you find these observations hard to reconcile, then you are in good company. Moving the site of stimulation toward a more basal location is a very different manipulation from increasing the stimulus pulse rate. How can they both have the same effect, and lead to a higher sounding percept? One very interesting experiment by Tong and colleagues (1983) suggests how this conundrum might be solved: Fast pulse rates and basal stimulation sites may both sound "high," but the "direction" labeled as "up" is not the same in both cases. Tong et al. (1983) presented nine different electrical pulse train stimuli to their implantee subjects. The stimuli encompassed all combinations of three different pulse rates and three different cochlear places, as shown in the left of figure 8.7. But instead of presenting the electrical stimuli in pairs and asking "which one sounds higher," the stimuli were presented in triplets, and the

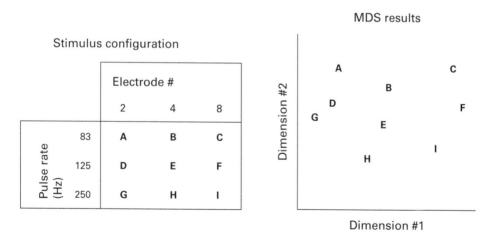

Figure 8.7
Perceptual multidimensional scaling (MDS) experiment by Tong and colleagues (1983). Cochlear implant users were asked to rank the dissimilarity of nine different stimuli (A–I), which differed in pulse rates and cochlear locations, as shown in the table on the left. MSD analysis results of the perceptual dissimilarity (distance) ratings, shown on the right, indicate that pulse rate and cochlear place change the implantee's sound percept along two independent dimensions.

subjects were asked "which two of the three stimuli sound most alike." By repeating this process many times with many different triplets of sounds, it is possible to measure the "perceptual distance" or perceived dissimilarity between any two of the sounds in the stimulus set. Tong and colleagues then subjected these perceptual distance estimates to a multidimensional scaling (MDS) analysis.

The details of MDS are somewhat beyond the scope of this book, but let us try to give you a quick intuition of the ideas behind it. Imagine you were asked to draw a map showing the locations of three towns—A, B, and C—and you were told that the distance from A to C is 200 miles, while the distances from A to B and from B to C are 100 miles each. In that case, you could conclude that towns A, B, and C must lie on a single straight line, with B between A and C. The map would therefore be "one-dimensional." But if the A–B and B–C distances turned out to be 150 miles each (in general, if the sum of the A–B and B–C distances is larger than the A–C distance), then you can conclude that A, B, and C cannot lie on a single (one-dimensional) straight line, but rather must be arranged in a triangle in a (two-dimensional) plane. Using considerations of this sort, MDS measures whether it is possible to "embed" a given number of points into a space of a low number of dimensions without seriously distorting ("straining") their pairwise distances.

If cochlear place and pulse rate both affected the same single perceptual variable, that is, "pitch," then it ought to be possible to arrange all the perceptual distances between the stimuli used in the experiment by Tong et al. (1983) along a single, one-dimensional "perceptual pitch axis." However, the results of the MDS analysis showed this not to be possible. Only a two-dimensional perceptual space (shown on the right in figure 8.7) can accommodate the observed pairwise perceptual distances between the stimuli used by Tong and colleagues. The conclusion from this experiment is clear: When asked to rank stimuli from "high" to "low," implantees might report both changes in the place of stimulation to more basal locations and increases in the pulse rate as producing a "higher" sound, but there seem to be two different directions in perceptual space along which a stimulus can "become higher."

A number of authors writing on cochlear implant research have taken to calling the perceptual dimension associated with the locus of stimulation "place pitch," and that which is associated with the rate of stimulation "periodicity pitch." Describing two demonstrably independent (orthogonal) perceptual dimensions as two different "varieties" of pitch seems to us an unfortunate choice. If we present normal listeners with a range of artificial vowels, keep the fundamental frequency constant but shift some of the formant frequencies upward to generate something resembling a /u/ to /i/ transition, and then pressed our listeners to tell us which of the two vowels sounded "higher," most would reply that the /i/, with its larger acoustic energy content at higher formant frequencies, sounds "higher" than the /u/. If we then asked the same listeners to compare a /u/ with a fundamental frequency of 440 Hz with another /u/ with a fundamental frequency of 263 Hz, the same listeners would call the first one higher. But only in the second case, the "periodicity pitch" case where the fundamental frequency changes from the note C_4 to A_4 while the formant spectrum remains constant, are we dealing with "pitch" in the sense of the perceptual quality that we use to appreciate musical melody. The "place pitch" phenomenon, which accompanies spectral envelope changes rather than changes in fundamental frequency, is probably better thought of as an aspect of timbre, rather than a type of pitch.

The use of the term "place pitch" has nevertheless become quite widespread, and as long as this term is used consistently and its meaning is clear, such usage, although in our opinion not ideal, is nevertheless defensible. Perhaps more worrying is the fact that one can still find articles in the cochlear implant literature that simply equate the term "pitch" with place of cochlear stimulation, without any reference to temporal coding or further qualification. Given the crucial role temporal discharge patterns play in generating musical pitch, that is simply wrong.

With the concepts of "place pitch" and "periodicity pitch" now clear and fresh in our minds, let us return to the question of why pitch perception is generally poor in cochlear implant recipients, and what might be done to improve it. An inability to appreciate musical melody is one of the most common complaints of implantees, although their ability to appreciate musical rhythms is very good. (On the book's Web site you can find examples of noise vocoded pieces of music, which may give you an impression of what music might sound like through a cochlear implant.) Furthermore, speakers of tonal languages, such as Mandarin, find it harder to obtain good speech recognition results with cochlear implants (Ciocca et al., 2002). However, melody appreciation through electrical hearing is bound to stay poor unless the technology evolves to deliver more detailed temporal fine structure information about a sound's periodicity. Indeed, a number of experimental speech processor strategies are being developed and tested, which aim to boost temporal information by increasing the signals' depth of modulation, as well as synchronizing stimulus pulses relative to the sound's fundamental frequency across all electrode channels (Vandali et al., 2005). These do seem to produce a statistically significant but nevertheless modest improvement over conventional speech processing algorithms.

What exactly needs to be done to achieve good periodicity pitch coding in cochlear implants remains somewhat uncertain. As we mentioned earlier, electrical stimulation of the cochlea with regular pulse trains of increasing frequency from 50 to 300 Hz produces a sensation of increasing pitch (McKay, 2004; Shannon, 1983), but unfortunately, increasing the pulse rates beyond 500 Hz usually does not increase the perceived pitch further (Moore & Carlyon, 2005). In contrast, as we saw in chapter 3, the normal ("periodicity") pitch range of healthy adults extends up to about 4 kHz. Why is the limit of periodicity pitch that can be easily achieved with direct electrical stimulation through cochlear implants so much lower than that obtained with acoustic click-trains in the normal ear?

One possibility that was considered, but discounted on the basis of psychoacoustical evidence, is that the basal, and hence normally high-frequency, sites stimulated by cochlear implants may simply not be as sensitive to temporal patterning in the pitch range as their low-frequency, apical neighbors (Carlyon & Deeks, 2002). One likely alternative explanation is that electrical stimulation may produce an excessive level of synchronization of activity in the auditory nerve, which prevents the transmission of temporal fine structure at high rates. Recall that, in the normal ear, each inner hair cell connects to about ten or so auditory nerve fibers, and hair cells sit so closely packed that several hundred auditory nerve fibers would all effectively serve more or less the same "frequency channel." This group of several hundred fibers operates according to the "volley principle," that is, while they phase lock to the acoustic signal, an individual auditory nerve fiber need not respond to every period of the sound. If it skips the odd period, the periods it misses will very likely be marked by the firing of some other nerve fiber that forms part of the assembly. Being able to skip periods is important, because physiological limitations such as refractoriness mean that no nerve fiber can ever fire faster than a theoretical maximum of 1,000 Hz, and few are able to maintain firing rates greater than a few hundred hertz for prolonged periods. Consequently, the temporal encoding of the periodicity of sounds with fundamental frequencies greater than a few hundred hertz relies on effective operation of the volley principle, so that nerve fibers can "take it in turns" to mark the individual periods. In other words, while we want the nerve fibers to lock to the periodicity of the sound, we do not want them to be synchronized to each other.

It is possible that the physiology of the synapses that connect the nerve fibers to the inner hair cells may favor such an asynchronous activation. In contrast, electrical current pulses from extracellular electrodes that, relative to the spatial scale of individual nerve fibers, are both very large and far away, can only lead to a highly synchronized activation of the nerve fibers, and would make it impossible for the auditory nerve to rely on the volley principle for the encoding of high pulse rates. Recordings from the auditory nerve of implanted animals certainly indicate highly precise time locking to every pulse in a pulse-train, as well as an inability to lock to rates higher than a few hundred hertz (Javel et al., 1987), and recordings in the central nervous system in response to electrical stimulation of the cochlea also provide indirect evidence for a hypersynchronization of auditory nerve fibers (Hartmann & Kral, 2004).

If this hypersynchronization is indeed the key factor limiting pitch perception through cochlear implants, then technical solutions to this problem may be a long way off. There have been attempts to induce a degree of "stochastic resonance" to desynchronize the activity of the auditory nerve fibers by introducing small amounts of noise or jitter into the electrode signals, but these have not yet produced significant improvements in pitch perception through cochlear implants (Chen, Ishihara, & Zeng, 2005). Perhaps the contacts of electrodes designed for insertion into the scala tympani are simply too few, too large, and too far away from the spiral ganglion to allow the activation of auditory nerve fibers in a manner that favors the stimulus-locked yet desynchronized activity necessary to transmit temporal fine structure information at high rates. In that case, "proper" pitch perception through cochlear implants may require a radical redesign of the implanted electrodes, so that many hundreds, rather than just a few dozen, distinct electrical channels can be delivered in a manner that allows very small groups of auditory nerve fibers to be targeted individually and activated independently of their neighbors.

You may have got the impression that using cochlear implants to restore hearing, or, in the case of the congenitally deaf, to introduce it for the first time, involves starting with a blank canvas in which the patient has no auditory sensation. This is not always the case, however, as some residual hearing, particularly at low frequencies (1 kHz or less), is often still present. Given the importance of those low frequencies in pitch perception, modified cochlear electrode arrays are now being used that focus on stimulating the basal, dead high-frequency region of the cochlea while leaving hearing in the intact low-frequency region to be boosted by conventional hearing aids.

8.6 Spatial Hearing with Cochlear Implants

Until recently, cochlear implantation was reserved solely for patients with severe hearing loss in both ears, and these patients would typically receive an implant in one ear only. The decision to implant only one ear was motivated partly from considerations of added cost and surgical risk, but also from doubts about the added benefit a second device might bring, and the consideration that, at a time when implant technology was developing rapidly, it might be worth "reserving" the second ear for later implantation with a more advanced device. While unilateral implantation remains the norm at the time of writing this book, attitudes are changing rapidly in favor of bilateral implantation. Indeed, in 2009, the British National Institute for Health and Clinical Excellence (NICE) changed its guidelines, and now recommends that profoundly deaf children and certain groups of adult patients should routinely be considered for bilateral implantation.

You may recall from chapter 5 that binaural cues play a key role in our ability to localize sounds in space and to pick out sounds of interest among other competing sounds. Any spatial hearing that humans are capable of with just one ear stems from a combination of head-shadow effects and their ability to exploit rather subtle changes at the high end of the spectrum, where direction-dependent filtering by the external ear may create spectral-shape localization cues. Contrast this with the situation for most cochlear implant patients who will receive monaural stimulation via a microphone located above and behind the ear, which conveys very limited spectral detail because, for the reasons discussed earlier, typically not much more than half a dozen or so effectively separated frequency channels are available at any time. Moreover, the position of the microphone means that no benefit can be obtained from spectral localization cues. It is therefore unsurprising that, with just a single implant, patients are effectively unable to localize sound sources or to understand speech in noisy environments. Communicating in a busy restaurant or bar is therefore particularly difficult for individuals with unilateral cochlear implants.

Their quality of life can, however, sometimes be improved considerably by providing cochlear implants in both ears, and patients with bilateral cochlear implants show substantially improved sound localization compared to their performance with either implant alone (Litovsky et al., 2006; van Hoesel & Tyler, 2003). Sensitivity to ILDs can be as good as that seen in listeners with normal hearing, although ITD thresholds tend to be much worse, most likely because of the lack of temporal fine structure information provided by the implants (van Hoesel & Tyler, 2003). Speech-in-noise perception can also improve following bilateral cochlear implantation. In principle, such benefits may accrue solely from "better ear" effects: The ear on the far side of a noise source will be in a sound shadow produced by the head, which can improve the signal-to-noise ratio if the sounds of interest originate from a different direction than the distracting noise. A listener with two ears may be able to benefit from the better ear effect simply by attending to the more favorably positioned ear (hence the name), but a listener with only one functional ear may have to turn his or her head in awkward and uncomfortable ways depending on the directions of the target and noise sources. However, Long and colleagues (2006) showed that patients with bilateral cochlear implants can experience binaural unmasking on the basis of envelope-based ITDs, suggesting that they should be able to use their binaural hearing to improve speech perception in noisy environments beyond what is achievable by the better ear effect alone.

8.7   Brain Plasticity and Cochlear Implantation

You may recall from chapter 7 that the auditory system is highly susceptible to long-term changes in input. A very important issue for the successful outcome of cochlear implantation is therefore the age at which hearing is lost and the duration of deafness prior to implantation. We know, for example, that early sensorineural hearing loss can cause neurons in the central auditory system to degenerate and die (Shepherd & Hardie, 2000), and can alter the synaptic and membrane properties of those neurons that survive (Kotak, Breithaupt, & Sanes, 2007). Neural pathways can also be rewired, especially if hearing is lost on one side only (Hartley & King, 2010). Since bilateral cochlear implantees often receive their implants at different times, their auditory systems will potentially have to endure a period of complete deafness followed by deafness in one ear. This can have profound consequences for the organization of the central auditory pathway.

A number of studies highlight the importance of early implantation for maximizing the benefits of electrical hearing. The latencies of cortical auditory evoked potentials fall to normal values only if children are implanted before a certain age (Sharma & Dorman, 2006), while studies in deaf cats fitted with a cochlear implant have also shown that cortical response plasticity declines with age (Kral & Tillein, 2006). Another complication is that the absence of sound-evoked inputs, particularly during early development, results in the auditory cortex being taken over by other sensory modalities (Doucet et al., 2006; Lee et al., 2007). Now cross-modal reorganization can be very useful, making it possible, for example, for blind patients to localize sounds more accurately (Röder et al., 1999), or for deaf people to make better use of visual speech. On the other hand, if auditory areas of the brain in the deaf are taken over by other sensory inputs, the capacity of those areas to process restored auditory inputs provided by cochlear implants may be limited.

We have discussed several examples in this book where auditory and visual information is fused in ways that can have profound effects on perception. A good example of this is the McGurk effect, in which viewing someone articulating one speech sound while listening to another sound can change what we hear (see chapter 4 and accompanying video clip on the book's Web site). If congenitally deaf children are fitted with cochlear implants within the first two and a half years of life, they go on to experience the McGurk effect. However, after this age, auditory and visual speech cues can no longer be fused (Schorr et al., 2005), further emphasizing the importance of implantation within a sensitive period of development. Interestingly, patients who received cochlear implants following postlingual deafness—who presumably benefitted from multisensory experience early in life—are better than listeners with normal hearing at fusing visual and auditory signals, which improves their understanding of speech in situations where both sets of cues are present (Rouger et al., 2007).

On the basis of the highly dynamic way in which the brain processes auditory information, it seems very likely that the capacity of patients to interpret the distorted signals provided by cochlear implants will be enhanced by experience and training strategies that encourage their use in specific auditory tasks. Indeed, it is almost certainly only because the brain possesses such remarkable adaptive capabilities that cochlear implants work at all.

Notes

Chapter 1

1. Fourier was not 100% correct, as it is possible to conceive some "not square integrable functions" for which his rule does not apply, but these are quite extreme examples that could never occur in everyday physical signals like sound waves.

2. Digital music recordings typically use 44,100 samples per second.

3. Systems engineers may choose to model such a system either as an FIR or as in infinite impulse response (IIR) filter. These are equivalent descriptions. IIRs are sometimes more efficient, but conceptually much less intuitive, and we shall not discuss them here.

4. For certain types of sound, under certain conditions, there are small but significant deviations from Weber's law, known as the "near miss," about which we will say a little more later.

Chapter 2

1. The word "cochlea" appears to be misspelled more often than that of almost any other anatomical structure. What seems to confuse a lot of people is that the noun "cochlea" is spelled without an "r" at the end, in contrast to the adjective "cochlear," meaning "belonging to the cochlea."

2. But don't count on that being sufficient. If you have to shoot guns or trigger other loud, explosive noises, you should also get a pair of ear plugs or mufflers.

3. Note, however, that the cochleagram contains much "temporal structure," visible as a fine vertical banding in the right panel of figure 2.6. We shall see in chapter 3 that this allows the brain to make deductions about the sound's harmonic structure even if individual harmonics are not resolved in the cochlear place code.

Chapter 4

1. Pinyin is a system for writing Chinese speech with the Latin alphabet, which is widely used and endorsed by the government of the People's Republic of China.

2. While VOT is the main feature that distinguishes stop consonants, it is not the only one. Another is "aspiration noise." Thus, before the onset of a stop consonant, air pressure builds up in the mouth. This escapes in a brief burst of turbulent airflow when the consonant is released. The air pressure build-up is higher in /t/ or /p/ than in /d/ or /b/, so that the former have more aspiration noise.

References

Ahissar, M., Lubin, Y., Putter-Katz, H., & Banai, K. (2006). Dyslexia and the failure to form a perceptual anchor. *Nature Neuroscience, 9*, 1558–1564.

Alain, C., Arnott, S. R., Henevor , S., Graham, S., & Grady, C. L. (2001). "What" and "where" in the human auditory system. *Proceedings of the National Academy of Sciences of the United States of America, 98*, 12301–12306.

Alain, C., Snyder, J., He, Y., & Reinke, K. (2007). Changes in auditory cortex parallel rapid perceptual learning. *Cerebral Cortex, 17*, 1074–1084.

Amin, N., Doupe, A., & Theunissen, F. E. (2007). Development of selectivity for natural sounds in the songbird auditory forebrain. *Journal of Neurophysiology, 97*, 3517–3531.

Amitay, S., Irwin, A., & Moore, D. (2006). Discrimination learning induced by training with identical stimuli. *Nature Neuroscience, 9*, 1446–1448.

Anderson, L. A., Christianson, G. B., & Linden, J. F. (2009). Stimulus-specific adaptation occurs in the auditory thalamus. *Journal of Neuroscience, 29*, 7359–7363.

ANSI (1994). *American National Standard Acoustical Terminology*. ANSI S1.1-1994. New York: American National Standards Institute.

Ashida, G., Abe, K., Funabiki, K., & Konishi, M. (2007). Passive soma facilitates submillisecond coincidence detection in the owl's auditory system. *Journal of Neurophysiology, 97*, 2267–2282.

Ashmore, J. (2008). Cochlear outer hair cell motility. *Physiological Reviews, 88*, 173–210.

Bajo, V. M., Nodal, F. R., Moore, D. R., & King, A. J., (2010). The descending corticocollicular pathway mediates learning-induced auditory plasticity. *Nature Neuroscience, 13*, 253–260.

Bao, S., Chang, E. F., Woods, J., & Merzenich, M. M. (2004). Temporal plasticity in the primary auditory cortex induced by operant perceptual learning. *Nature Neuroscience, 7*, 974–981.

Bar-Yosef, O., Nelken, I. (2007). The effects of background noise on the neural responses to natural sounds in cat primary auditory cortex. *Frontiers in Computational Neuroscience 1*, 3.

Bar-Yosef, O., Rotman, Y., & Nelken, I. (2002). Responses of neurons in cat primary auditory cortex to bird chirps: Effects of temporal and spectral context. *Journal of Neuroscience, 22,* 8619–8632.

Barrett, D. J. K., & Hall, D. A. (2006). Response preferences for "what" and "where" in human non-primary auditory cortex. *Neuroimage, 32,* 968–977.

Bendor, D., & Wang, X. (2005). The neuronal representation of pitch in primate auditory cortex. *Nature, 436,* 1161–1165.

Bertelson, P., & Radeau, M. (1981). Cross-modal bias and perceptual fusion with auditory-visual spatial discordance. *Perception & Psychophysics, 29,* 578–584.

Bierer, J. A., & Middlebrooks, J. C. (2002). Auditory cortical images of cochlear-implant stimuli: Dependence on electrode configuration. *Journal of Neurophysiology, 87,* 478–492.

Bizley, J. K., & King, A. J. (2009). Visual influences on ferret auditory cortex. *Hearing Research, 258,* 55–63.

Bizley, J. K., Nodal, F. R., Bajo, V. M., Nelken, I., & King, A. J. (2007). Physiological and anatomical evidence for multisensory interactions in auditory cortex. *Cerebral Cortex, 17,* 2172–2189.

Bizley, J. K., Walker, K. M., Silverman, B. W., King, A. J., & Schnupp, J. W. (2009). Interdependent encoding of pitch, timbre, and spatial location in auditory cortex. *Journal of Neuroscience, 29,* 2064–2075.

Blackburn, C. C., & Sachs, M. B. (1990). The representations of the steady-state vowel sound /e/ in the discharge patterns of cat anteroventral cochlear nucleus neurons. *Journal of Neurophysiology, 63,* 1191–1212.

Blauert, J. (1997). *Spatial hearing: The psychophysics of human sound localization.* Rev. ed. Cambridge, MA: MIT Press.

Bleeck, S., Ingham, N. J., Verhey, J. L., & Winter, I. M. (2008). Rebound depolarization in single units of the ventral cochlear nucleus: A contribution to grouping by common onset? *Neuroscience, 154,* 139–146.

Boatman, D. (2004). Cortical bases of speech perception: Evidence from functional lesion studies. *Cognition, 92,* 47–65.

Brainard, M. S., & Doupe, A. J. (2002). What songbirds teach us about learning. *Nature, 417,* 351–358.

Brainard, M. S., & Knudsen, E. I. (1998). Sensitive periods for visual calibration of the auditory space map in the barn owl optic tectum. *Journal of Neuroscience, 18,* 3929–3942.

Brand, A., Behrend, O., Marquardt, T., McAlpine, D., & Grothe, B. (2002). Precise inhibition is essential for microsecond interaural time difference coding. *Nature, 417,* 543–547.

Bregman, A. S. (1990). *Auditory scene analysis: The perceptual organization of sound.* Cambridge, MA: MIT Press.

Bronkhorst, A. W., & Houtgast, T. (1999). Auditory distance perception in rooms. *Nature, 397,* 517–520.

Brosch, M., Selezneva, E., & Scheich, H. (2005). Nonauditory events of a behavioral procedure activate auditory cortex of highly trained monkeys. *Journal of Neuroscience, 25,* 6797–6806.

Brugge, J. F., Reale, R. A., & Hind, J. E. (1996). The structure of spatial receptive fields of neurons in primary auditory cortex of the cat. *Journal of Neuroscience, 16,* 4420–4437.

Brugge, J. F., Reale, R. A., Jenison, R. L., & Schnupp, J. (2001). Auditory cortical spatial receptive fields. *Audiology & Neuro-Otology, 6,* 173–177.

Butler, R. A. (1986). The bandwidth effect on monaural and binaural localization. *Hearing Research, 21,* 67–73.

Callan, D. E. C. A., Jones, J. A., Munhall, K., Callan, A. M., Kroos, C., & Vatikiotis-Bateson, E. (2003). Neural processes underlying perceptual enhancement by visual speech gestures. *Neuroreport, 14,* 2213–2218.

Calvert, G. A., Bullmore, E. T., Brammer, M. J., Campbell, R., Williams, S. C. R., McGuire, P. K., et al. (1997). Activation of auditory cortex during silent lipreading. *Science, 276,* 593–596.

Campbell, R. A., King, A. J., Nodal, F. R., Schnupp, J. W., Carlile, S., & Doubell, T. P. (2008). Virtual adult ears reveal the roles of acoustical factors and experience in auditory space map development. *Journal of Neuroscience, 28,* 11557–11570.

Cariani, P. A., & Delgutte, B. (1996a). Neural correlates of the pitch of complex tones. I. Pitch and pitch salience. *Journal of Neurophysiology, 76,* 1698–1716.

Cariani, P. A., & Delgutte, B. (1996b). Neural correlates of the pitch of complex tones. II. Pitch shift, pitch ambiguity, phase invariance, pitch circularity, rate pitch, and the dominance region for pitch. *Journal of Neurophysiology, 76,* 1717–1734.

Carlyon, R. P., & Deeks, J. M. (2002). Limitations on rate discrimination. *Journal of the Acoustical Society of America, 112,* 1009–1025.

Carr, C. E., & Konishi, M. (1988). Axonal delay lines for time measurement in the owl's brainstem. *Proceedings of the National Academy of Sciences of the United States of America, 85,* 8311–8315.

Chase, S. M., & Young, E. D. (2008). Cues for sound localization are encoded in multiple aspects of spike trains in the inferior colliculus. *Journal of Neurophysiology, 99,* 1672–1682.

Chechik, G., Anderson, M. J., Bar-Yosef, O., Young, E. D., Tishby, N., & Nelken, I. (2006). Reduction of information redundancy in the ascending auditory pathway. *Neuron, 51,* 359–368.

Chen, H., Ishihara, Y. C., & Zeng, F. G. (2005). Pitch discrimination of patterned electric stimulation. *Journal of the Acoustical Society of America, 118,* 338–345.

Christensen-Dalsgaard, J. (2005). Directional hearing in non-mammalian tetrapods. In A. N. Popper & R. R. Fay (Eds.), *Sound source localization* (pp. 67–123). New York: Springer.

Ciocca, V., Francis, A. L., Aisha, R., & Wong, L. (2002). The perception of Cantonese lexical tones by early-deafened cochlear implantees. *Journal of the Acoustical Society of America, 111,* 2250–2256.

Clayton, N. (1988). Song discrimination learning in zebra finches. *Animal Behaviour, 36,* 1016–1024.

Clifton, R. (1992). The development of spatial hearing in human infants. *Developmental Psychoacoustics,* 135–157.

Cody, A. R., & Russell, I. J. (1987). The response of hair cells in the basal turn of the guinea-pig cochlea to tones. *Journal of Physiology, 383,* 551–569.

Coleman, P. D. (1963). An analysis of cues to auditory depth perception in free space. *Psychological Bulletin, 60,* 302–315.

Cooper, N. P. (1996). Two-tone suppression in cochlear mechanics. *Journal of the Acoustical Society of America, 99,* 3087–3098.

Csepe, V., Karmos, G., & Molnar, M. (1987). Evoked potential correlates of stimulus deviance during wakefulness and sleep in cat—animal model of mismatch negativity. *Electroencephalography and Clinical Neurophysiology, 66,* 571–578.

Culling, J. F., & Summerfield, Q. (1995). Perceptual separation of concurrent speech sounds: Absence of across-frequency grouping by common interaural delay. *Journal of the Acoustical Society of America, 98,* 785–797.

Cynx, J., & Shapiro, M. (1986). Perception of missing fundamental by a species of songbird (*Sturnus vulgaris*). *Journal of Comparative Psychology (Washington, D.C.), 100,* 356–360.

Dallos, P. (1996). Overview: Cochlear neurobiology. In P. Dallos, A. N. Popper, & R. R. Fay (Eds.), *The cochlea* (pp. 1–43). New York: Springer.

Darwin, C. J., & Hukin, R. W. (1999). Auditory objects of attention: The role of interaural time differences. *Journal of Experimental Psychology, 25,* 617–629.

Darwin, C. J., & Sutherland, N. S. (1984). Grouping frequency components of vowels: When is a harmonic not a harmonic? *Quarterly Journal of Experimental Psychology Section A, 36,* 193–208.

Dean, I., Harper, N., & McAlpine, D. (2005). Neural population coding of sound level adapts to stimulus statistics. *Nature Neuroscience, 8,* 1684–1689.

DeCasper, A., & Fifer, W. (1980). Of human bonding: Newborns prefer their mothers' voices. *Science, 208,* 1174–1176.

de Cheveigné, A. (1997). Concurrent vowel identification. III. A neural model of harmonic interference cancellation. *Journal of the Acoustical Society of America, 101,* 2857–2865.

de Cheveigné, A., & Kawahara, H. (1999). Missing-data model of vowel identification. *Journal of the Acoustical Society of America, 105,* 3497–3508.

de Cheveigné, A., Kawahara, H., Tsuzaki, M., & Aikawa, K. (1997a). Concurrent vowel identification. I. Effects of relative amplitude and F_0 difference. *Journal of the Acoustical Society of America, 101,* 2839–2847.

de Cheveigné, A., McAdams, S., Laroche, J., & Rosenberg, M. (1995). Identification of concurrent harmonic and inharmonic vowels: A test of the theory of harmonic cancellation and enhancement. *Journal of the Acoustical Society of America, 97,* 3736–3748.

de Cheveigné, A., McAdams, S., & Marin, C. M. H. (1997b). Concurrent vowel identification. II. Effects of phase, harmonicity, and task. *Journal of the Acoustical Society of America, 101,* 2848–2856.

de Cheveigné, A., & Pressnitzer, D. (2006). The case of the missing delay lines: Synthetic delays obtained by cross-channel phase interaction. *Journal of the Acoustical Society of America, 119,* 3908–3918.

Delgutte, B. (1997). Auditory neural processing of speech. In W. J. Hardcastle & J. Laver, Eds., *The handbook of phonetic sciences* (pp. 507–538). Oxford: Blackwell.

Denham, S. L., & Winkler, I. (2006). The role of predictive models in the formation of auditory streams. *Journal of Physiology, Paris, 100,* 154–170.

Devore, S., Ihlefeld, A., Hancock, K., Shinn-Cunningham, B., & Delgutte, B. (2009). Accurate sound localization in reverberant environments is mediated by robust encoding of spatial cues in the auditory midbrain. *Neuron, 62,* 123–134.

Diehl, R. L. (2008). Acoustic and auditory phonetics: The adaptive design of speech sound systems. *Philosophical Transactions of the Royal Society B. Biological Sciences, 363,* 965–978.

Djourno, A., & Eyries, C. (1957). Prothèse auditive par excitation électrique à distance du nerf sensoriel à l'aide d'un bobinage inclus à demeure. *La Presse Medicale, 35,* 14–17.

Dorman, M. F., Loizou, P. C., & Rainey, D. (1997). Speech intelligibility as a function of the number of channels of stimulation for signal processors using sine-wave and noise-band outputs. *Journal of the Acoustical Society of America, 102,* 2403–2411.

Doucet, M., Bergeron, F., Lassonde, M., Ferron, P., & Lepore, F. (2006). Cross-modal reorganization and speech perception in cochlear implant users. *Brain, 129,* 3376–3383.

Doupe, A. J., & Konishi, M. (1991). Song-selective auditory circuits in the vocal control system of the zebra finch. *Proceedings of the National Academy of Sciences of the United States of America, 88,* 11339–11343.

Dudai, Y. (2002). *Memory from A to Z.* Oxford: Oxford University Press.

Eggermont, J. J. (2008). The role of sound in adult and developmental auditory cortical plasticity. *Ear and Hearing, 29,* 819-829.

Eggermont, J. J. (1995). Representation of a voice onset time continuum in primary auditory cortex of the cat. *Journal of the Acoustical Society of America, 98,* 911–920.

Elliott, T. M., & Theunissen, F. E. (2009). The modulation transfer function for speech intelligibility. *PLoS Computational Biology, 5,* e1000302.

Engineer, C. T., Perez, C. A., Chen, Y. H., Carraway, R. S., Reed, A. C., Shetake, J. A., et al. (2008). Cortical activity patterns predict speech discrimination ability. *Nature Neuroscience, 11,* 603–608.

Fay, R. R. (2005). Perception of pitch by goldfish. *Hearing Research, 205,* 7–20.

Fekete, D., & Campero, A. (2007). Axon guidance in the inner ear. *International Journal of Developmental Biology, 51,* 549–556.

Fettiplace, R., & Fuchs, P. A. (1999). Mechanisms of hair cell tuning. *Annual Review of Physiology, 61,* 809–834.

Fishman, K. E., Shannon, R. V., & Slattery, W. H. (1997). Speech recognition as a function of the number of electrodes used in the SPEAK cochlear implant speech processor. *Journal of Speech, Language, and Hearing Research: JSLHR, 40,* 1201–1215.

Fishman, Y. I., Reser, D. H., Arezzo, J. C., & Steinschneider, M. (2001). Neural correlates of auditory stream segregation in primary auditory cortex of the awake monkey. *Hearing Research, 151,* 167–187.

Fitch, W. T. (2006). Production of vocalizations in mammals. In K. Brown (Ed.), *Encyclopedia of language and linguistics* (pp. 115–121). Oxford: Elsevier.

Fitzpatrick, D. C., Kuwada, S., Kim, D. O., Parham, K., & Batra, R. (1999). Responses of neurons to click-pairs as simulated echoes: Auditory nerve to auditory cortex. *Journal of the Acoustical Society of America, 106,* 3460–3472.

Friederici, A. (2006). The neural basis of language development and its impairment. *Neuron, 52,* 941–952.

Fritz, J., Elhilali, M., & Shamma, S. (2005). Differential dynamic plasticity of A1 receptive fields during multiple spectral tasks. *Journal of Neuroscience, 25,* 7623–7635.

Ghazanfar, A. A., Maier, J. X., Hoffman, K. L., & Logothetis, N. K. (2005). Multisensory integration of dynamic faces and voices in rhesus monkey auditory cortex. *Journal of Neuroscience, 25,* 5004–5012.

Ghazanfar, A. A., & Rendall, D. (2008). Evolution of human vocal production. *Current Biology, 18,* R457–R460.

Glendenning, K. K., Baker, B. N., Hutson, K. A., & Masterton, R. B. (1992). Acoustic chiasm V: Inhibition and excitation in the ipsilateral and contralateral projections of LSO. *Journal of Comparative Neurology, 319,* 100–122.

Goblick, T. J., Jr., & Pfeiffer, R. R. (1969). Time-domain measurements of cochlear nonlinearities using combination click stimuli. *Journal of the Acoustical Society of America, 46,* 924–938.

Greenberg, S. (2006). A multi-tier framework for understanding spoken language. In S. Greenberg & W. A. Ainsworth, Eds., *Listening to speech: An auditory perspective* (p. 411). Mahwah, NJ: Lawrence Erlbaum Associates.

Griffiths, T. D., & Warren, J. D. (2004). What is an auditory object? *Nature Reviews Neuroscience*, 5, 887–892.

Groh, J., Trause, A., Underhill, A., Clark, K., & Inati, S. (2001). Eye position influences auditory responses in primate inferior colliculus. *Neuron, 29*, 509–518.

Hall, D. A., & Plack, C. J. (2009). Pitch processing sites in the human auditory brain. *Cerebral Cortex, 19*, 576–585.

Hall, J., III, Buss, E., & Grose, J. (2007). The binaural temporal window in adults and children. *Journal of the Acoustical Society of America, 121*, 401–410.

Han, Y., Kover, H., Insanally, M., Semerdjian, J., & Bao, S. (2007). Early experience impairs perceptual discrimination. *Nature Neuroscience, 10*, 1191–1197.

Hannon, E., & Trehub, S. (2005). Tuning in to musical rhythms: Infants learn more readily than adults. *Proceedings of the National Academy of Sciences of the United States of America, 102*, 12639–12643.

Harper, N. S., & McAlpine, D. (2004). Optimal neural population coding of an auditory spatial cue. *Nature, 430*, 682–686.

Hartley, D. E., & King, A. J., (2010). Development of the auditory pathway. In A. Palmer & A. Rees (Eds.), *The auditory brain* (pp. 361–386). Oxford: Oxford University Press.

Hartline, P. H., Vimal, R. L., King, A. J., Kurylo, D. D., & Northmore, D. P. (1995). Effects of eye position on auditory localization and neural representation of space in superior colliculus of cats. *Experimental Brain Research, 104*, 402–408.

Hartmann, R., & Kral, A. (2004). Central responses to electrical hearing. In F.-G. Zeng, A. N. Popper, & R. R. Fay (Eds.), *Cochlear implants: Auditory prostheses and electric hearing* (pp. 213–285). New York: Springer.

Hartmann, W. M., & Wittenberg, A. (1996). On the externalization of sound images. *Journal of the Acoustical Society of America, 99*, 3678–3688.

Hartung, K., & Trahiotis, C. (2001). Peripheral auditory processing and investigations of the "precedence effect" which utilize successive transient stimuli. *Journal of the Acoustical Society of America, 110*, 1505–1513.

Heffner, H. E., & Heffner, R. S. (1990). Effect of bilateral auditory cortex lesions on sound localization in Japanese macaques. *Journal of Neurophysiology, 64*, 915–931.

Heffner, H., & Whitfield, I. C. (1976). Perception of the missing fundamental by cats. *Journal of the Acoustical Society of America, 59*, 915–919.

Heffner, R. S., & Heffner, H. E. (1992). Visual factors in sound localization in mammals. *Journal of Comparative Neurology, 317*, 219–232.

Henning, G. B. (1974). Detectability of interaural delay in high-frequency complex waveforms. *Journal of the Acoustical Society of America, 55*, 84–90.

Hickok, G., & Poeppel, D. (2004). Dorsal and ventral streams: A framework for understanding aspects of the functional anatomy of language. *Cognition, 92,* 67–99.

Hine, J. E., Martin, R. L., & Moore, D. R. (1994). Free-field binaural unmasking in ferrets. *Behavioral Neuroscience, 108,* 196–205.

Hochstein, S., & Ahissar, M. (2002). View from the top: Hierarchies and reverse hierarchies in the visual system. *Neuron, 36,* 791–804.

Hofman, M., & Van Opstal, J. (2003). Binaural weighting of pinna cues in human sound localization. *Experimental Brain Research, 148,* 458–470.

Hofman, P. M., & Van Opstal, A. J. (2002). Bayesian reconstruction of sound localization cues from responses to random spectra. *Biological Cybernetics, 86,* 305–316.

Hofman, P., Van Riswick, J., & Van Opstal, A. (1998). Relearning sound localization with new ears. *Nature Neuroscience, 1,* 417–421.

Holmes, S. D., & Roberts, B. (2006). Inhibitory influences on asynchrony as a cue for auditory segregation. *Journal of Experimental Psychology, 32,* 1231–1242.

Huang, A. Y., & May, B. J. (1996). Spectral cues for sound localization in cats: Effects of frequency domain on minimum audible angles in the median and horizontal planes. *Journal of the Acoustical Society of America, 100,* 2341–2348.

Hyde, K. L., Lerch, J., Norton, A., Forgeard, M., Winner, E., Evans, A. C., et al. (2009). Musical training shapes structural brain development. *Journal of Neuroscience, 29,* 3019–3025.

Insanally, M. N., Köver, H., Kim, H., & Bao, S. (2009). Feature-dependent sensitive periods in the development of complex sound representation. *Journal of Neuroscience, 29,* 5456–5462.

Irvine, D. R., Park, V. N., & McCormick, L. (2001). Mechanisms underlying the sensitivity of neurons in the lateral superior olive to interaural intensity differences. *Journal of Neurophysiology, 86,* 2647–2666.

Itatani, N., & Klump, G. M. (2009). Auditory streaming of amplitude-modulated sounds in the songbird forebrain. *Journal of Neurophysiology, 101,* 3212–3225.

Izumi, A. (2002). Auditory stream segregation in Japanese monkeys. *Cognition, 82,* B113–B122.

Javel, E., Tong, Y. C., Shepherd, R. K., & Clark, G. M. (1987). Responses of cat auditory nerve fibers to biphasic electrical current pulses. *Annals of Otology, Rhinology, and Laryngology, 96,* 26–30.

Javitt, D. C., Schroeder, C. E., Steinschneider, M., Arezzo, J. C., & Vaughan, H. G., Jr. (1992). Demonstration of mismatch negativity in the monkey. *Electroencephalography and Clinical Neurophysiology, 83,* 87–90.

Jay, M. F., & Sparks, D. L. (1984). Auditory receptive fields in primate superior colliculus shift with changes in eye position. *Nature, 309,* 345–347.

Jeffress, L. (1948). A place theory of sound localization. *Journal of Comparative and Physiological Psychology, 41*, 35–39.

Jenison, R. L. (1998). Models of direction estimation with spherical-function approximated cortical receptive fields. In P. Poon & J. Brugge (Eds.), *Central auditory processing and neural modeling* (pp. 161–174). New York: Plenum Press.

Jenison, R. L., Schnupp, J. W., Reale, R. A., & Brugge, J. F. (2001). Auditory space-time receptive field dynamics revealed by spherical white-noise analysis. *Journal of Neuroscience, 21*, 4408–4415.

Jenkins, W. M., & Masterton, R. B. (1982). Sound localization: Effects of unilateral lesions in central auditory system. *Journal of Neurophysiology, 47*, 987–1016.

Jenkins, W. M., & Merzenich, M. M. (1984). Role of cat primary auditory cortex for sound-localization behavior. *Journal of Neurophysiology, 52*, 819–847.

Jia, S., & He, D. Z. (2005). Motility-associated hair-bundle motion in mammalian outer hair cells. *Nature Neuroscience, 8*, 1028–1034.

Jiang, D., McAlpine, D., & Palmer, A. R. (1997). Responses of neurons in the inferior colliculus to binaural masking level difference stimuli measured by rate-versus-level functions. *Journal of Neurophysiology, 77*, 3085–3106.

Johnson, K., Nicol, T., Zecker, S., & Kraus, N. (2008). Developmental plasticity in the human auditory brainstem. *Journal of Neuroscience, 28*, 4000–4007.

Joris, P. X., Smith, P. H., & Yin, T. C. T. (1998). Coincidence detection in the auditory system: 50 years after Jeffress. *Neuron, 21*, 1235–1238.

Kacelnik, O., Nodal, F. R., Parsons, C. H., & King, A. J. (2006). Training-induced plasticity of auditory localization in adult mammals. *PLoS Biology, 4*, e71.

Kandler, K. (2004). Activity-dependent organization of inhibitory circuits: Lessons from the auditory system. *Current Opinion in Neurobiology, 14*, 96–104.

Kanold, P. O., & Young, E. D. (2001). Proprioceptive information from the pinna provides somatosensory input to cat dorsal cochlear nucleus. *Journal of Neuroscience, 21*, 7848–7858.

Kapfer, C., Seidl, A. H., Schweizer, H., & Grothe, B. (2002). Experience-dependent refinement of inhibitory inputs to auditory coincidence-detector neurons. *Nature Neuroscience, 5*, 247–253.

Kawano, A., Seldon, H. L., & Clark, G. M. (1996). Computer-aided three-dimensional reconstruction in human cochlear maps: Measurement of the lengths of organ of Corti, outer wall, inner wall, and Rosenthal's canal. *Annals of Otology, Rhinology, and Laryngology, 105*, 701–709.

Keilson, S. E., Richards, V. M., Wyman, B. T., & Young, E. D. (1997). The representation of concurrent vowels in the cat anesthetized ventral cochlear nucleus: Evidence for a periodicity-tagged spectral representation. *Journal of the Acoustical Society of America, 102*, 1056–1071.

Kemp, D. T. (2002). Otoacoustic emissions, their origin in cochlear function, and use. *British Medical Bulletin, 63,* 223–241.

Kennedy, H. J., Crawford, A. C., & Fettiplace, R. (2005). Force generation by mammalian hair bundles supports a role in cochlear amplification. *Nature, 433,* 880–883.

Kilgard, M. (2003). Cholinergic modulation of skill learning and plasticity. *Neuron, 38,* 678–680.

King, A. J. (1999). Sensory experience and the formation of a computational map of auditory space in the brain. *Bioessays, 21,* 900–911.

King, A. J., Hutchings, M. E., Moore, D. R., & Blakemore, C. (1988). Developmental plasticity in the visual and auditory representations in the mammalian superior colliculus. *Nature, 332,* 73–76.

King, A. J., Parsons, C. H., & Moore, D. R. (2000). Plasticity in the neural coding of auditory space in the mammalian brain. *Proceedings of the National Academy of Sciences of the United States of America, 97,* 11821–11828.

King, A. J., Schnupp, J. W., & Doubell, T. P. (2001). The shape of ears to come: Dynamic coding of auditory space. *Trends in Cognitive Sciences, 5,* 261–270.

Kluender, K. R., Diehl, R. L., & Killeen, P. R. (1987). Japanese quail can learn phonetic categories. *Science, 237,* 1195–1197.

Knudsen, E. I. (1985). Experience alters the spatial tuning of auditory units in the optic tectum during a sensitive period in the barn owl. *Journal of Neuroscience, 5,* 3094–3109.

Knudsen, E. I. (1999). Mechanisms of experience-dependent plasticity in the auditory localization pathway of the barn owl. *Journal of Comparative Physiology A. Neuroethology, Sensory, Neural, and Behavioral Physiology, 185,* 305–321.

Knudsen, E., Esterly, S., & Knudsen, P. (1984). Monaural occlusion alters sound localization during a sensitive period in the barn owl. *Journal of Neuroscience, 4,* 1001–1011.

Knudsen, E. I. (1982). Auditory and visual maps of space in the optic tectum of the owl. *Journal of Neuroscience, 2,* 1177–1194.

Knudsen, E. I., & Konishi, M. (1978). A neural map of auditory space in the owl. *Science, 200,* 795–797.

Köppl, C., & Carr, C. E. (2008). Maps of interaural time difference in the chicken's brainstem nucleus laminaris. *Biological Cybernetics, 98,* 541–559.

Kotak, V., Breithaupt, A., & Sanes, D. (2007). Developmental hearing loss eliminates long-term potentiation in the auditory cortex. *Proceedings of the National Academy of Sciences of the United States of America, 104,* 3550–3555.

Kral, A., & Tillein, J. (2006). Brain plasticity under cochlear implant stimulation. *Advances in Oto-Rhino-Laryngology, 64,* 89–108.

Kraus, N., Skoe, E., Parbery-Clark, A., & Ashley, R. (2009). Experience-induced malleability in neural encoding of pitch, timbre, and timing. *Annals of the New York Academy of Sciences, 1169,* 543–557.

Krishna, B. S., & Semple, M. N. (2000). Auditory temporal processing: responses to sinusoidally amplitude-modulated tones in the inferior colliculus. *Journal of Neurophysiology, 84,* 255–273.

Krumbholz, K., Patterson, R. D., Seither-Preisler, A., Lammertmann, C., & Lutkenhoner, B. (2003). Neuromagnetic evidence for a pitch processing center in Heschl's gyrus. *Cerebral Cortex, 13,* 765–772.

Kuhl, P. K., Conboy, B. T., Coffey-Corina, S., Padden, D., Rivera-Gaxiola, M., & Nelson, T. (2008). Phonetic learning as a pathway to language: New data and native language magnet theory expanded (NLM-e). *Philosophical Transactions of the Royal Society of London. Series B, Biological Sciences, 363,* 979–1000.

Kuhl, P. K., & Miller, J. D. (1975). Speech perception by the chinchilla: Voiced-voiceless distinction in alveolar plosive consonants. *Science, 190,* 69–72.

Kuhl, P. K., & Miller, J. D. (1978). Speech perception by the chinchilla: Identification function for synthetic VOT stimuli. *Journal of the Acoustical Society of America, 63,* 905–917.

Kuhl, P., & Rivera-Gaxiola, M. (2008). Neural substrates of language acquisition. *Annual Review of Neuroscience, 31,* 511–534.

Kuhl, P. K., Stevens, E., Hayashi, A., Deguchi, T., Kiritani, S., & Iverson, P. (2006). Infants show a facilitation effect for native language phonetic perception between 6 and 12 months. *Developmental Science, 9,* F13–F21.

Kuhl, P., Tsao, F., & Liu, H. (2003). Foreign-language experience in infancy: Effects of short-term exposure and social interaction on phonetic learning. *Proceedings of the National Academy of Sciences of the United States of America, 100,* 9096–9101.

Kulkarni, K., & Hartley, D. E. (2008). Recent advances in hearing restoration. *Journal of the Royal Society of Medicine, 101,* 116–124.

Kumpik, D. P., Kacelnik, O., & King, A. J. (2010). Adaptive plasticity of human auditory localization in response to altered binaural cues. *Journal of Neuroscience, 30,* 4883–4894.

Langendijk, E. H., & Bronkhorst, A. W. (2002). Contribution of spectral cues to human sound localization. *Journal of the Acoustical Society of America, 112,* 1583–1596.

Las, L., Stern, E. A., & Nelken, I. (2005). Representation of tone in fluctuating maskers in the ascending auditory system. *Journal of Neuroscience, 25,* 1503–1513.

Lee, H., Truy, E., Mamou, G., Sappey-Marinier, D., & Giraud, A. (2007). Visual speech circuits in profound acquired deafness: A possible role for latent multimodal connectivity. *Brain, 130,* 2929–2941.

Lewicki, M. S. (2002). Efficient coding of natural sounds. *Nature Neuroscience, 5,* 356–363.

Liberman, M. C. (1982). Single-neuron labeling in the cat auditory nerve. *Science, 216,* 1239–1241.

Licklider, J. C. R. (1948). The influence of interaural phase relations upon the masking of speech by white noise. *Journal of the Acoustical Society of America, 20,* 150–159.

Liljencrants, J. & Lindblom, B. (1972). Numerical simulation of vowel quality systems: The role of perceptual contrast. *Language, 48,* 839–862.

Lisker, L., & Abramson, A. S. (1964). Across-language study of voicing in initial stops: Acoustical measurements. *Word, 20,* 384–422.

Litovsky, R. (1997). Developmental changes in the precedence effect: Estimates of minimum audible angle. *Journal of the Acoustical Society of America, 102,* 1739–1745.

Litovsky, R. Y. (1998). Physiological studies of the precedence effect in the inferior colliculus of the kitten. *Journal of the Acoustical Society of America, 103,* 3139–3152.

Litovsky, R., Parkinson, A., Arcaroli, J., & Sammeth, C. (2006). Simultaneous bilateral cochlear implantation in adults: A multicenter clinical study. *Ear and Hearing, 27,* 714–731.

Loftus, W. C., Bishop, D. C., Saint Marie, R. L., & Oliver, D. L. (2004). Organization of binaural excitatory and inhibitory inputs to the inferior colliculus from the superior olive. *Journal of Comparative Neurology, 472,* 330–344.

Lomber, S. G., & Malhotra, S. (2008). Double dissociation of "what" and "where" processing in auditory cortex. *Nature Neuroscience, 11,* 609–616.

Long, C., Carlyon, R., Litovsky, R., & Downs, D. (2006). Binaural unmasking with bilateral cochlear implants. *Journal of the Association for Research in Otolaryngology, 7,* 352–360.

Loui, P., Alsop, D., & Schlaug, G. (2009). Tone deafness: A new disconnection syndrome? *Journal of Neuroscience, 29,* 10215–10220.

Lutfi, R. A., & Liu, C. J. (2007). Individual differences in source identification from synthesized impact sounds. *Journal of the Acoustical Society of America, 122,* 1017–1028.

MacDougall-Shackleton, S. A., Hulse, S. H., Gentner, T. Q., & White, W. (1998). Auditory scene analysis by European starlings (*Sturnus vulgaris*): Perceptual segregation of tone sequences. *Journal of the Acoustical Society of America, 103,* 3581–3587.

Maeder, P. P., Meuli, R. A., Adriani, M., Bellmann, A., Fornari, E., Thiran, J. P., Pillet, A. & Clark, S. (2001). Distinct pathways involved in sound recognition and localization: a human fMRI study. *Neuroimage, 14,* 802–816.

Malhotra, S., Hall, A. J., & Lomber, S. G. (2004). Cortical control of sound localization in the cat: unilateral cooling deactivation of 19 cerebral areas. *Journal of Neurophysiology, 92,* 1625–1643.

Malmierca, M. S., Cristaudo, S., Perez-Gonzalez, D., & Covey, E. (2009). Stimulus-specific adaptation in the inferior colliculus of the anesthetized rat. *Journal of Neuroscience, 29*, 5483–5493.

Manley, G. A., Koppl, C., & Konishi, M. (1988). A neural map of interaural intensity differences in the brain stem of the barn owl. *Journal of Neuroscience, 8*, 2665–2676.

Margoliash, D. (1983). Acoustic parameters underlying the responses of song-specific neurons in the white-crowned sparrow. *Journal of Neuroscience, 3*, 1039–1057.

Marler, P., & Tamura, M. (1962). Song "dialects" in three populations of white-crowned sparrows. *Condor, 64*, 368–377.

May, B. J. (2000). Role of the dorsal cochlear nucleus in the sound localization behavior of cats. *Hearing Research, 148*, 74–87.

Maye, J., Werker, J., & Gerken, L. (2002). Infant sensitivity to distributional information can affect phonetic discrimination. *Cognition, 82*, 101–111.

McAlpine, D. (2004). Neural sensitivity to periodicity in the inferior colliculus: Evidence for the role of cochlear distortions. *Journal of Neurophysiology, 92*, 1295–1311.

McAlpine, D. (2005). Creating a sense of auditory space. *Journal of Physiology, 566*, 21–28.

McAlpine, D., Jiang, D., & Palmer, A. R. (2001). A neural code for low-frequency sound localization in mammals. *Nature Neuroscience, 4*, 396–401.

McGurk, H., & MacDonald, J. (1976). Hearing lips and seeing voices. *Nature, 264*, 746–748.

McKay, C. (2004). Psychophysics and electrical stimulation. In F.-G. Zeng, A. N. Popper, & R. R. Fay (Eds.), *Cochlear implants: Auditory prostheses and electric hearing* (pp. 287–333). New York: Springer.

Micheyl, C., Tian, B., Carlyon, R. P., & Rauschecker, J. P. (2005). Perceptual organization of tone sequences in the auditory cortex of awake macaques. *Neuron, 48*, 139–148.

Mickey, B. J., & Middlebrooks, J. C. (2005). Sensitivity of auditory cortical neurons to the locations of leading and lagging sounds. *Journal of Neurophysiology, 94*, 979–989.

Middlebrooks, J. C., & Pettigrew, J. D. (1981). Functional classes of neurons in primary auditory cortex of the cat distinguished by sensitivity to sound location. *Journal of Neuroscience, 1*, 107–120.

Middlebrooks, J. C., & Snyder, R. L. (2007). Auditory prosthesis with a penetrating nerve array. *Journal of the Association for Research in Otolaryngology, 8*, 258–279.

Middlebrooks, J. C., Xu, L., Eddins, A. C., & Green, D. M. (1998). Codes for sound-source location in nontonotopic auditory cortex. *Journal of Neurophysiology, 80*, 863–881.

Miller, G. A. (1947). Sensitivity to changes in the intensity of white noise and its relation to masking and loudness. *Journal of the Acoustical Society of America, 19*, 609.

Miller, L. M., Escabi, M. A., Read, H. L., & Schreiner, C. E. (2002). Spectrotemporal receptive fields in the lemniscal auditory thalamus and cortex. *Journal of Neurophysiology, 87*, 516–527.

Miller, L. M., & Recanzone, G. H. (2009). Populations of auditory cortical neurons can accurately encode acoustic space across stimulus intensity. *Proceedings of the National Academy of Sciences of the United States of America, 106*, 5931–5935.

Mills, A. W. (1958). On the minimum audible angle. *Journal of the Acoustical Society of America, 30*, 237–246.

Mills, A. W. (1960). Lateralization of high-frequency tones. *Journal of the Acoustical Society of America, 32*, 132–134.

Moore, B. C. J. (1999). Neurobiology: Modulation minimizes masking. *Nature, 397*, 108–109.

Moore, B. C. J., & Carlyon, R. P. (2005). Perception of pitch by people with cochlear hearing loss and by cochlear implant users. In C. J. Plack, A. J. Oxenham, & R. R. Fay (Eds.), *Pitch: Neural coding and perception* (pp. 234–277). New York, London: Springer.

Moore, J. K., & Linthicum, F. H. (2009). The human auditory system: A timeline of development. *International Journal of Audiology, 46*, 460–478.

Morimoto, M. (2001). The contribution of two ears to the perception of vertical angle in sagittal planes. *Journal of the Acoustical Society of America, 109*, 1596–1603.

Mrsic-Flogel, T. D., King, A. J., Jenison, R. L., & Schnupp, J. W. (2001). Listening through different ears alters spatial response fields in ferret primary auditory cortex. *Journal of Neurophysiology, 86*, 1043–1046.

Mrsic-Flogel, T. D., King, A. J., & Schnupp, J. W. (2005). Encoding of virtual acoustic space stimuli by neurons in ferret primary auditory cortex. *Journal of Neurophysiology, 93*, 3489–3503.

Mrsic-Flogel, T. D., Schnupp, J. W., & King, A. J. (2003). Acoustic factors govern developmental sharpening of spatial tuning in the auditory cortex. *Nature Neuroscience, 6*, 981–988.

Musicant, A. D., & Butler, R. A. (1984). The psychophysical basis of monaural localization. *Hearing Research, 14*, 185–190.

Näätänen, R., Paavilainen, P., Rinne, T., & Alho, K. (2007). The mismatch negativity (MMN) in basic research of central auditory processing: A review. *Clinical Neurophysiology, 118*, 2544–2590.

Nahum, M., Nelken, I., & Ahissar, M. (2008). Low-level information and high-level perception: the case of speech in noise. *PLoS Biology, 6*, e126.

Nakamoto, K. T., Zhang, J., & Kitzes, L. M. (2004). Response patterns along an isofrequency contour in cat primary auditory cortex (AI) to stimuli varying in average and interaural levels. *Journal of Neurophysiology, 91*, 118–135.

Nelken, I., & Bar-Yosef, O. (2008). Neurons and objects: The case of auditory cortex. *Front Neuroscience, 2*, 107–113.

Nelken, I., Bizley, J. K., Nodal, F. R., Ahmed, B., King, A. J., & Schnupp, J. W. (2008). Responses of auditory cortex to complex stimuli: Functional organization revealed using intrinsic optical signals. *Journal of Neurophysiology, 99,* 1928–1941.

Nelken, I., Chechik, G., Mrsic-Flogel, T. D., King, A. J., & Schnupp, J. W. (2005). Encoding stimulus information by spike numbers and mean response time in primary auditory cortex. *Journal of Computational Neuroscience, 19,* 199–221.

Nelken, I., Rotman, Y., & Bar Yosef, O. (1999). Responses of auditory-cortex neurons to structural features of natural sounds. *Nature, 397,* 154–157.

Nelken, I., & Ulanovsky, N. (2007). Change detection, mismatch negativity and stimulus-specific adaptation in animal models. *Journal of Psychophysiology, 21,* 214–223.

Nelken, I., & Young, E. D. (1994). Two separate inhibitory mechanisms shape the responses of dorsal cochlear nucleus type IV units to narrowband and wideband stimuli. *Journal of Neurophysiology, 71,* 2446–2462.

Neuert, V., Verhey, J. L., & Winter, I. M. (2004). Responses of dorsal cochlear nucleus neurons to signals in the presence of modulated maskers. *Journal of Neuroscience, 24,* 5789–5797.

Niparko, J. K. (2004). Cochlear implants: Clinical applications. In F.-G. Zeng, A. N. Popper, & R. R. Fay (Eds.), *Cochlear implants: Auditory prostheses and electric hearing* (pp. 53–100). New York: Springer.

Oldfield, S. R., & Parker, S. P. (1984). Acuity of sound localisation: A topography of auditory space. II. Pinna cues absent. *Perception, 13,* 601–617.

Oliver, D. L., Beckius, G. E., Bishop, D. C., & Kuwada, S. (1997). Simultaneous anterograde labeling of axonal layers from lateral superior olive and dorsal cochlear nucleus in the inferior colliculus of cat. *Journal of Comparative Neurology, 382,* 215–229.

Paavilainen, P., Arajärvi, P., & Takegata, R. (2007). Preattentive detection of nonsalient contingencies between auditory features. *Neuroreport, 18,* 159–163.

Palmer, A. R., & King, A. J. (1982). The representation of auditory space in the mammalian superior colliculus. *Nature, 299,* 248–249.

Palmer, A. R., & King, A. J. (1985). A monaural space map in the guinea-pig superior colliculus. *Hearing Research, 17,* 267–280.

Palmer, A. R., & Russell, I. J. (1986). Phase-locking in the cochlear nerve of the guinea-pig and its relation to the receptor potential of inner hair-cells. *Hearing Research, 24,* 1–15.

Patterson, R. D., Uppenkamp, S., Johnsrude, I. S., & Griffiths, T. D. (2002). The processing of temporal pitch and melody information in auditory cortex. *Neuron, 36,* 767–776.

Pecka, M., Brand, A., Behrend, O., & Grothe, B. (2008). Interaural time difference processing in the mammalian medial superior olive: The role of glycinergic inhibition. *Journal of Neuroscience, 28,* 6914–6925.

Peña, J. L., & Konishi, M. (2002). From postsynaptic potentials to spikes in the genesis of auditory spatial receptive fields. *Journal of Neuroscience, 22,* 5652–5658.

Pinker, S. (1994). *The language instinct: The new science of language and mind.* London: Allen Lane.

Plack, C. J., & Oxenham, A. J. (2005). The psychophysics of pitch. In C. J. Plack, A. J. Oxenham, R. R. Fay, & A. N. Popper (Eds.), *Pitch: Neural coding and perception* (pp. 7–55). New York: Springer.

Poeppel, D., & Hickok, G. (2004). Towards a new functional anatomy of language. *Cognition, 92,* 1–12.

Polley, D., Steinberg, E., & Merzenich, M. (2006). Perceptual learning directs auditory cortical map reorganization through top-down influences. *Journal of Neuroscience, 26,* 4970–4982.

Pons, F., Lewkowicz, D., Soto-Faraco, S., & Sebastián-Gallés, N. (2009). Narrowing of intersensory speech perception in infancy. *Proceedings of the National Academy of Sciences of the United States of America, 106,* 10598–10602.

Pressnitzer, D., & Hupé, J. M. (2006). Temporal dynamics of auditory and visual bistability reveal common principles of perceptual organization. *Current Biology, 16,* 1351–1357.

Pressnitzer, D., Meddis, R., Delahaye, R., & Winter, I. M. (2001). Physiological correlates of comodulation masking release in the mammalian ventral cochlear nucleus. *Journal of Neuroscience, 21,* 6377–6386.

Pressnitzer, D., Sayles, M., Micheyl, C., & Winter, I. M. (2008). Perceptual organization of sound begins in the auditory periphery. *Current Biology, 18,* 1124–1128.

Qin, L., Sakai, M., Chimoto, S., & Sato, Y. (2005). Interaction of excitatory and inhibitory frequency-receptive fields in determining fundamental frequency sensitivity of primary auditory cortex neurons in awake cats. *Cerebral Cortex, 15,* 1371–1383.

Quian Quiroga, R., Kraskov, A., Koch, C., & Fried, I. (2009). Explicit encoding of multimodal percepts by single neurons in the human brain. *Current Biology, 19,* 1308–1313.

Rajan, R., Aitkin, L. M., Irvine, D. R., & McKay, J. (1990). Azimuthal sensitivity of neurons in primary auditory cortex of cats. I. Types of sensitivity and the effects of variations in stimulus parameters. *Journal of Neurophysiology, 64,* 872–887.

Reale, R. A., Jenison, R. L., & Brugge, J. F. (2003). Directional sensitivity of neurons in the primary auditory (AI) cortex: Effects of sound-source intensity level. *Journal of Neurophysiology, 89,* 1024–1038.

Recanzone, G., Schreiner, C., & Merzenich, M. (1993). Plasticity in the frequency representation of primary auditory cortex following discrimination training in adult owl monkeys. *Journal of Neuroscience, 13,* 87–103.

Rice, J. J., May, B. J., Spirou, G. A., & Young, E. D. (1992). Pinna-based spectral cues for sound localization in cat. *Hearing Research, 58,* 132–152.

Robert, D. (2005). Directional hearing in insects. In A. N. Popper & R. R. Fay (Eds.), *Sound source localization* (pp. 6–66). New York: Springer.

Roberts, B., & Holmes, S. D. (2006). Asynchrony and the grouping of vowel components: Captor tones revisited. *Journal of the Acoustical Society of America, 119*, 2905–2918.

Roberts, B., & Holmes, S. D. (2007). Contralateral influences of wideband inhibition on the effect of onset asynchrony as a cue for auditory grouping. *Journal of the Acoustical Society of America, 121*, 3655–3665.

Robertson, D., & Irvine, D. R. (1989). Plasticity of frequency organization in auditory cortex of guinea pigs with partial unilateral deafness. *Journal of Comparative Neurology, 282*, 456–471.

Röder, B., Teder-Sälejärvi, W., Sterr, A., Rösler, F., Hillyard, S., & Neville, H. (1999). Improved auditory spatial tuning in blind humans. *Nature, 400*, 162–166.

Romanski, L. M., Tian, B., Fritz, J., Mishkin, M., Goldman Rakic, P. S., & Rauschecker, J. P. (1999). Dual streams of auditory afferents target multiple domains in the primate prefrontal cortex. *Nature Neuroscience, 2*, 1131–1136.

Rose, J. E., Brugge, J. F., Anderson, D. J., & Hind, J. E. (1967). Phase-locked response to low-frequency tones in single auditory nerve fibers of the squirrel monkey. *Journal of Neurophysiology, 30*, 769–793.

Rouger, J., Lagleyre, S., Fraysse, B., Deneve, S., Deguine, O., & Barone, P. (2007). Evidence that cochlear-implanted deaf patients are better multisensory integrators. *Proceedings of the National Academy of Sciences of the United States of America, 104*, 7295–7300.

Rubel, E., & Fritzsch, B. (2002). Auditory system development: Primary auditory neurons and their targets. *Annual Review of Neuroscience, 25*, 51–101.

Ruben, R. (1997). A time frame of critical/sensitive periods of language development. *Acta Oto-Laryngologica, 117*, 202–205.

Ruggero, M. A., Narayan, S. S., Temchin, A. N., & Recio, A. (2000). Mechanical bases of frequency tuning and neural excitation at the base of the cochlea: Comparison of basilar-membrane vibrations and auditory-nerve-fiber responses in chinchilla. *Proceedings of the National Academy of Sciences of the United States of America, 97*, 11744–11750.

Ruggero, M. A., Rich, N. C., Recio, A., Narayan, S. S., & Robles, L. (1997). Basilar-membrane responses to tones at the base of the chinchilla cochlea. *Journal of the Acoustical Society of America, 101*, 2151–2163.

Russ, B. E., Ackelson, A. L., Baker, A. E., & Cohen, Y. E. (2008). Coding of auditory-stimulus identity in the auditory non-spatial processing stream. *Journal of Neurophysiology, 99*, 87–95.

Rutkowski, R. G., Wallace, M. N., Shackleton, T. M., & Palmer, A. R. (2000). Organisation of binaural interactions in the primary and dorsocaudal fields of the guinea pig auditory cortex. *Hearing Research, 145*, 177–189.

Ruusuvirta, T., Penttonen, M., & Korhonen, T. (1998). Auditory cortical event-related potentials to pitch deviances in rats. *Neuroscience Letters, 248*, 45–48.

Saberi, K., Dostal, L., Sadralodabai, T., Bull, V., & Perrott, D. R. (1991). Free-field release from masking. *Journal of the Acoustical Society of America, 90*, 1355–1370.

Saberi, K., & Perrott, D. R. (1999). Cognitive restoration of reversed speech. *Nature, 398*, 760.

Saberi, K., Takahashi, Y., Farahbod, H., & Konishi, M. (1999). Neural bases of an auditory illusion and its elimination in owls. *Nature Neuroscience, 2*, 656–659.

Sanes, D., & Rubel, E. (1988). The ontogeny of inhibition and excitation in the gerbil lateral superior olive. *Journal of Neuroscience, 8*, 682–700.

Schneider, P., Scherg, M., Dosch, H. G., Specht, H. J., Gutschalk, A., & Rupp, A. (2002). Morphology of Heschl's gyrus reflects enhanced activation in the auditory cortex of musicians. *Nature Neuroscience, 5*, 688–694.

Schneider, P., Sluming, V., Roberts, N., Scherg, M., Goebel, R., Specht, H. J., et al. (2005). Structural and functional asymmetry of lateral Heschl's gyrus reflects pitch perception preference. *Nature Neuroscience, 8*, 1241–1247.

Schnupp, J. W. (2008). Auditory neuroscience: Sound segregation in the brainstem? *Current Biology, 18*, R705–706.

Schnupp, J. W., Booth, J., & King, A. J. (2003). Modeling individual differences in ferret external ear transfer functions. *Journal of the Acoustical Society of America, 113*, 2021–2030.

Schnupp, J. W., & Carr, C. E. (2009). On hearing with more than one ear: lessons from evolution. *Nature Neuroscience, 12*, 692–697.

Schnupp, J. W., Hall, T. M., Kokelaar, R. F., & Ahmed, B. (2006). Plasticity of temporal pattern codes for vocalization stimuli in primary auditory cortex. *Journal of Neuroscience, 26*, 4785–4795.

Schnupp, J. W. H., King, A. J., Walker, K. M. M., & Bizley, J. K. (2010). The representation of the pitch of vowel sounds in ferret auditory cortex. In E. A. Lopez-Poveda, A. R. Palmer, & R. Meddis (Eds.), *Advances in auditory physiology, psychophysics and models* (pp. 407–416). New York: Springer.

Schnupp, J. W., Mrsic-Flogel, T. D., & King, A. J. (2001). Linear processing of spatial cues in primary auditory cortex. *Nature, 414*, 200–204.

Schonwiesner, M., & Zatorre, R. J. (2008). Depth electrode recordings show double dissociation between pitch processing in lateral Heschl's gyrus and sound onset processing in medial Heschl's gyrus. *Experimental Brain Research, 187*, 97–105.

Schorr, E. A., Fox, N. A., van Wassenhove, V., & Knudsen, E. I. (2005). Auditory-visual fusion in speech perception in children with cochlear implants. *Proceedings of the National Academy of Sciences of the United States of America, 102*, 18748–18750.

Schreiner, C. E., & Langner, G. (1988). Periodicity coding in the inferior colliculus of the cat. II. Topographical organization. *Journal of Neurophysiology*, *60*, 1823–1840.

Schulze, H., Hess, A., Ohl, F. W., & Scheich, H. (2002). Superposition of horseshoe-like periodicity and linear tonotopic maps in auditory cortex of the Mongolian gerbil. *European Journal of Neuroscience*, *15*, 1077–1084.

Schwarz, D. W., & Tomlinson, R. W. (1990). Spectral response patterns of auditory cortex neurons to harmonic complex tones in alert monkey (*Macaca mulatta*). *Journal of Neurophysiology*, *64*, 282–298.

Scott, S. K., Blank, C. C., Rosen, S., & Wise, R. J. (2000). Identification of a pathway for intelligible speech in the left temporal lobe. *Brain*, *123*, 2400–2406.

Scott, S. K., & Wise, R. J. (2004). The functional neuroanatomy of prelexical processing in speech perception. *Cognition*, *92*, 13–45.

Seidl, A., & Grothe, B. (2005). Development of sound localization mechanisms in the Mongolian gerbil is shaped by early acoustic experience. *Journal of Neurophysiology*, *94*, 1028–1036.

Shackleton, T. M., & Carlyon, R. P. (1994). The role of resolved and unresolved harmonics in pitch perception and frequency modulation discrimination. *Journal of the Acoustical Society of America*, *95*, 3529–3540.

Shackleton, T. M., Liu, L. F., & Palmer, A. R. (2009). Responses to diotic, dichotic, and alternating phase harmonic stimuli in the inferior colliculus of guinea pigs. *Journal of the Association for Research in Otolaryngology*, *10*, 76–90.

Shahidullah, S., & Hepper, P. (1994). Frequency discrimination by the fetus. *Early Human Development*, *36*, 13–26.

Shamma, S., & Klein, D. (2000). The case of the missing pitch templates: How harmonic templates emerge in the early auditory system. *Journal of the Acoustical Society of America*, *107*, 2631–2644.

Shannon, R. V. (1983). Multichannel electrical stimulation of the auditory nerve in man. I. Basic psychophysics. *Hearing Research*, *11*, 157–189.

Shannon, R. V., Zeng, F. G., Kamath, V., Wygonski, J., & Ekelid, M. (1995). Speech recognition with primarily temporal cues. *Science*, *270*, 303–304.

Sharma, A., & Dorman, M. (2006). Central auditory development in children with cochlear implants: Clinical implications. *Advances in Oto-Rhino-Laryngology*, *64*, 66–88.

Shelton, B. R., & Searle, C. L. (1980). The influence of vision on the absolute identification of sound-source position. *Perception & Psychophysics*, *28*, 589–596.

Shepherd, R., & Hardie, N. (2000). Deafness-induced changes in the auditory pathway: Implications for cochlear implants. *Audiology and Neurotology*, *6*, 305–318.

Sinex, D. G., Li, H. (2007). Responses of inferior colliculus neurons to double harmonic tones. *Journal of Neurophysiology, 98,* 3171–3184.

Skottun, B. C., Shackleton, T. M., Arnott, R. H., & Palmer, A. R. (2001). The ability of inferior colliculus neurons to signal differences in interaural delay. *Proceedings of the National Academy of Sciences of the United States of America, 98,* 14050–14054.

Slattery, W. H., III, & Middlebrooks, J. C. (1994). Monaural sound localization: Acute versus chronic unilateral impairment. *Hearing Research, 75,* 38–46.

Smith, S., Gerhardt, K., Griffiths, S., Huang, X., & Abrams, R. M. (2003). Intelligibility of sentences recorded from the uterus of a pregnant ewe and from the fetal inner ear. *Audiology & Neuro-Otology, 8,* 347–353.

Solis, M., & Doupe, A. (1999). Contributions of tutor and bird's own song experience to neural selectivity in the songbird anterior forebrain. *Journal of Neuroscience, 19,* 4559–4584.

Spitzer, M. W., & Semple, M. N. (1998). Transformation of binaural response properties in the ascending auditory pathway: Influence of time-varying interaural phase disparity. *Journal of Neurophysiology, 80,* 3062–3076.

Stecker, G. C., Harrington, I. A., & Middlebrooks, J. C. (2005). Location coding by opponent neural populations in the auditory cortex. *PLoS Biology, 3,* e78.

Stecker, G. C., & Middlebrooks, J. C. (2003). Distributed coding of sound locations in the auditory cortex. *Biological Cybernetics, 89,* 341–349.

Stein, B. E., Huneycutt, W. S., & Meredith, M. A. (1988). Neurons and behavior: The same rules of multisensory integration apply. *Brain Research, 448,* 355–358.

Stein, B. E., Meredith, M. A., & Wallace, M. T. (1993). The visually responsive neuron and beyond: Multisensory integration in cat and monkey. *Progress in Brain Research, 95,* 79–90.

Steinschneider, M., Fishman, Y. I., & Arezzo, J. C. (2003). Representation of the voice onset time (VOT) speech parameter in population responses within primary auditory cortex of the awake monkey. *Journal of the Acoustical Society of America, 114,* 307–321.

Stevens, S. S. (1972). Perceived level of noise by mark VII and decibels (E). *Journal of the Acoustical Society of America, 51,* 575–601.

Sucher, C. M., & McDermott, H. J. (2007). Pitch ranking of complex tones by normally hearing subjects and cochlear implant users. *Hearing Research, 230,* 80–87.

Suga, N., & Ma, X. (2003). Multiparametric corticofugal modulation and plasticity in the auditory system. *Nature Reviews Neuroscience, 4,* 783–794.

Szymanski, F. D., Garcia-Lazaro, J. A., & Schnupp, J. W. (2009). Current source density profiles of stimulus-specific adaptation in rat auditory cortex. *Journal of Neurophysiology, 102,* 1483–1490.

Tomlinson, R. W., & Schwarz, D. W. (1988). Perception of the missing fundamental in nonhuman primates. *Journal of the Acoustical Society of America, 84*, 560–565.

Tong, Y. C., Blamey, P. J., Dowell, R. C., & Clark, G. M. (1983). Psychophysical studies evaluating the feasibility of a speech processing strategy for a multiple-channel cochlear implant. *Journal of the Acoustical Society of America, 74*, 73–80.

Tramo, M. J., Cariani, P. A., Delgutte, B., & Braida, L. D. (2001). Neurobiological foundations for the theory of harmony in western tonal music. *Annals of the New York Academy of Sciences, 930*, 92–116.

Trehub, S. (2003). The developmental origins of musicality. *Nature Neuroscience, 6*, 669–673.

Ulanovsky, N., Las, L., & Nelken, I. (2003). Processing of low-probability sounds by cortical neurons. *Nature Neuroscience, 6*, 391–398.

Unoki, M., Irino, T., Glasberg, B., Moore, B. C., & Patterson, R. D. (2006). Comparison of the roex and gammachirp filters as representations of the auditory filter. *Journal of the Acoustical Society of America, 120*, 1474–1492.

van Hoesel, R., & Tyler, R. (2003). Speech perception, localization, and lateralization with bilateral cochlear implants. *Journal of the Acoustical Society of America, 113*, 1617.

Van Noorden, L. P. A. S. (1975). *Temporal coherence in the perception of tone sequences*. Eindhoven: The Netherlands Technical University.

Van Wanrooij, M. M., & Van Opstal, A. J. (2004). Contribution of head shadow and pinna cues to chronic monaural sound localization. *Journal of Neuroscience, 24*, 4163–4171.

Van Wanrooij, M. M., & Van Opstal, A. J. (2007). Sound localization under perturbed binaural hearing. *Journal of Neurophysiology, 97*, 715–726.

van Wassenhove, V., & Nagarajan, S. (2007). Auditory cortical plasticity in learning to discriminate modulation rate. *Journal of Neuroscience, 27*, 2663–2672.

Vandali, A. E., Sucher, C., Tsang, D. J., McKay, C. M., Chew, J. W. D., & McDermott, H. J. (2005). Pitch ranking ability of cochlear implant recipients: A comparison of sound-processing strategies. *Journal of the Acoustical Society of America, 117*, 3126–3138.

Vongpaisal, T., & Pichora-Fuller, M. K. (2007). Effect of age on F0 difference limen and concurrent vowel identification. *Journal of Speech, Language, and Hearing Research, 50*, 1139–1156.

Wada, J., & Rasmussen, T. (1960). Intracarotid injection of sodium amytal for the lateralization of cerebral speech dominance. *Journal of Neurosurgery, 17*, 266–282.

Walker, K. M., Schnupp, J. W., Hart-Schnupp, S. M., King, A. J., & Bizley, J. K. (2009). Pitch discrimination by ferrets for simple and complex sounds. *Journal of the Acoustical Society of America, 126*, 1321–1335.

Wallach, H., Newman, E. B., & Rosenzweig, M. R. (1949). A precedence effect in sound localization. *Journal of Psychology, 62*, 315–336.

Wang, X., & Kadia, S. C. (2001). Differential representation of species-specific primate vocalizations in the auditory cortices of marmoset and cat. *Journal of Neurophysiology, 86*, 2616–2620.

Wang, X., Merzenich, M. M., Beitel, R., & Schreiner, C. E. (1995). Representation of a species-specific vocalization in the primary auditory cortex of the common marmoset: Temporal and spectral characteristics. *Journal of Neurophysiology, 74*, 2685–2706.

Weinberger, N. (2004). Specific long-term memory traces in primary auditory cortex. *Nature Reviews Neuroscience, 5*, 279–290.

Wenzel, E., Arruda, M., Kistler, D., & Wightman, F. (1993). Localization using nonindividualized head-related transfer functions. *Journal of the Acoustical Society of America, 94*, 111–123.

Werner-Reiss, U., Kelly, K. A., Trause , A. S., Underhill, A. M., & Groh, J. M. (2003). Eye position affects activity in primary auditory cortex of primates. *Current Biology, 13*, 554–563.

Wightman, F. L., & Kistler, D. J. (1989). Headphone simulation of free-field listening. II: Psychophysical validation. *Journal of the Acoustical Society of America, 85*, 868–878.

Wightman, F. L., & Kistler, D. J. (1992). The dominant role of low-frequency interaural time differences in sound localization. *Journal of the Acoustical Society of America, 91*, 1648–1661.

Wightman, F. L., & Kistler, D. J. (1997). Monaural sound localization revisited. *Journal of the Acoustical Society of America, 101*, 1050–1063.

Wilson, B. S. (2004). Engineering design of cochlear implants. In F.-G. Zeng, A. N. Popper, & R. R. Fay (Eds.), *Cochlear implants: Auditory prostheses and electric hearing* (pp. 14–52). New York: Springer.

Wilson, B. S., & Dorman, M. F. (2009). The design of cochlear implants. In J. K. Niparko (Ed.), *Cochlear implants: Principles & practices* (2nd ed., pp. 95–135). Philadelphia: Lippincott Williams & Wilkins.

Winkler, I., Denham, S. L., & Nelken, I. (2009a). Modeling the auditory scene: Predictive regularity representations and perceptual objects. *Trends in Cognitive Sciences, 13*, 532–540.

Winkler, I., Háden, G., Ladinig, O., Sziller, I., & Honing, H. (2009b). Newborn infants detect the beat in music. *Proceedings of the National Academy of Sciences of the United States of America, 106*, 2468–2471.

Winkler, I., Teder-Sälejärvi, W. A., Horváth, J., Näätänen, R., & Sussman, E. (2003). Human auditory cortex tracks task-irrelevant sound sources. *Neuroreport, 14*, 2053–2056.

Winter, I. M., & Palmer, A. R. (1995). Level dependence of cochlear nucleus onset unit responses and facilitation by second tones or broadband noise. *Journal of Neurophysiology, 73*, 141–159.

Winter, I. M., Wiegrebe, L., & Patterson, R. D. (2001). The temporal representation of the delay of iterated rippled noise in the ventral cochlear nucleus of the guinea-pig. *Journal of Physiology, 537*, 553–566.

Wood, S., & Lutman, M. (2004). Relative benefits of linear analogue and advanced digital hearing aids. *International Journal of Audiology, 43*, 144–155.

Woods, T. M., Lopez, S. E., Long, J. H., Rahman, J. E., & Recanzone, G. H. (2006). Effects of stimulus azimuth and intensity on the single-neuron activity in the auditory cortex of the alert macaque monkey. *Journal of Neurophysiology, 96*, 3323–3337.

Wright, B. A., & Zhang, Y. (2009). A review of the generalization of auditory learning. *Philosophical Transactions of the Royal Society B. Biological Sciences, 364*, 301–311.

Wunderlich, J., & Cone-Wesson, B. (2006). Maturation of CAEP in infants and children: A review. *Hearing Research, 212*, 212–223.

Yin, T. C., & Chan, J. C. (1990). Interaural time sensitivity in medial superior olive of cat. *Journal of Neurophysiology, 64*, 465–488.

Young, E. D., & Sachs, M. B. (1979). Representation of steady-state vowels in the temporal aspects of the discharge patterns of populations of auditory-nerve fibers. *Journal of the Acoustical Society of America, 66*, 1381–1403.

Zatorre, R. J., & Penhune, V. B. (2001). Spatial localization after excision of human auditory cortex. *Journal of Neuroscience, 21*, 6321–6328.

Zella, J. C., Brugge, J. F., & Schnupp, J. W. (2001). Passive eye displacement alters auditory spatial receptive fields of cat superior colliculus neurons. *Nature Neuroscience, 4*, 1167–1169.

Zhang, L., Bao, S., & Merzenich, M. (2001). Persistent and specific influences of early acoustic environments on primary auditory cortex. *Nature Neuroscience, 4*, 1123–1130.

Zilany, M. S. A., & Bruce, I. C. (2006). Modeling auditory-nerve responses for high sound pressure levels in the normal and impaired auditory periphery. *Journal of the Acoustical Society of America, 120*, 1446–1466.

Zwislocki, J., & Feldman, R. S. (1956). Just noticeable dichotic phase difference. *Journal of the Acoustical Society of America, 28*, 152–153.

Index